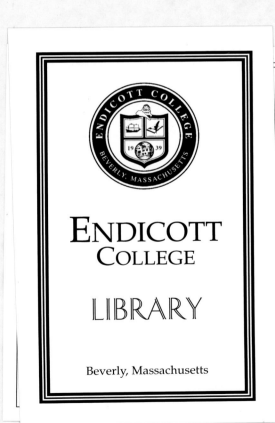

AIDS

PREVENTION THROUGH EDUCATION:
A WORLD VIEW

AIDS

Prevention Through Education:
A World View

Edited by

Jaime Sepulveda M.D. Dr. Sc.
Vice-Minister of Health, Mexico

Harvey Fineberg, M.D. Ph.D.
Dean, Harvard School of Public Health

Jonathan Mann, M.D. M.P..H.
Professor, Harvard School of Public Health

New York   Oxford
OXFORD UNIVERSITY PRESS
1992

Oxford University Press

Oxford New York Toronto
Delhi Bombay Calcutta Madras Karachi
Kuala Lumpur Singapore Hong Kong Tokyo
Nairobi Dar es Salaam Cape Town
Melbourne Auckland

and associated companies in

Berlin Ibadan

Published by Oxford University Press, Inc.,
200 Madison Avenue, New York, New York 10016

Oxford is registered a trademark of Oxford University Press

ISBN 0-19-506882-3

Printing (last digit) : 987654321

CONTRIBUTORS

Jeanne Blake
Medical reporter for WBZ-TV

Maryan Pye
AIDS Programme for the Health
Authority in the U.K.

David J. Hunter
Harvard School of Public Health

Claire M. Cassidy
At the University of Maryland
–College Park

Mark L. Rosenberg
Division of Injury, Epidemiology
and Control at the Center for
Environmental Health and Injury
Control

Mukesh Kapila
Senior Health & Population Adviser
Overseas Development
Administration, U.K.

Marcie L. Cynamon
Division of Health Interview
Statistics, at the National Center
for Health Statistics

Jaime Sepulveda
Under Secretary of Health, Mexico

Milton Gossett
Harvard School of Public Health

G. Stephen Bowen
Bureau of Health
Resources Development

Michael L. E. Ramah
Porter/Novelli

Jose Antonio Izazola
Fogarty fellow in the doctoral
program at the Harvard School
of Public Health

Lincoln C. Chen
Harvard School of Public Health

Gil Schwartz
Group W Television of
Westinghouse Broadcasting .
Company, Inc

Lloyd J. Kolbe
Centers for Disease Control

Mary Debus
International Division for
Porter/Novelli

Federick Kroger
U.S. Centers for Disease Control

Mervyn F. Silverman
National spokesperson for the
American Foundation for AIDS
Research

William DeJong
Center for Health Communication
at Harvard School of Public Health

Peter Lamptey
AIDSTECH Project ar Family Health
International

William A. Smith
Social Development Programs
at the Academy for Educational
Development

Harvey V. Fineberg
Harvard School of Public Health

Jonathan M. Mann
Harvard School of Public Health

Dennis D. Tolsma
Public Health Practice at the
Centers for Disease Control

Laurie Garret
Medical reporter for Newsday

Thomas W. Netter
Harvard University

Jeremy S. Warshaw
Saatchi & Saatchi Advertising

Thomas Goodgame
Harvard Institute for
Social Research

June E. Osborn
School of Public Health at
the University of Michigan

Sharon Weir
Research associate with the
AIDSTECH program at Family
Health International

Steven L. Gortmaker
Harvard Institute for
Social Research

Richard G. Parker
Institute of Social Medicine at the
State University of Rio de Janeiro

Jay A. Winsten
Harvard School of Public Health

ACKNOWLEDGMENTS

The original idea of writing this book developed after the First Symposium on AIDS Education and Communication, sponsored by the World Health Organization and held in Ixtapa, Mexico at the end of 1988. The editors and many of the co-authors of the book were present at the Symposium. All the material included here, however, is new and updated as much as possible.

In any collective effort, it becomes difficult to give appropriate credit to every participant. More people contributed to this book than can be acknowledged in justice.

Kelly Scoggings acted as an assistant editor for the early drafts of the book; Bethania Allen took over the responsibility until the manuscript was finished. Both of them did it with skill and grace.

Several contributors of this book sent their chapters in a computer diskette. Other chapters had to be retyped. The process of transferring files and making the computer environments compatible is to be credited to the assistant editors. At Harvard, Roberta S. Hirshson and Bernita Anderson were responsible for proof-reading and copy-editing at various stages of the process.

Edith Velasco played an important role throughout the making of the book; she typed parts of the manuscript and was also responsible for the computerized formatting of this product. Blanca Rico provided useful ideas and moral support. Carlos del Rio helped reviewed and updated some of the chapters on national experiences. Rodolfo Casillas and Hector Gomez produced the camera-ready copy of the book with outstanding dedication. Mario Bronfman supervised the overall printing process with exquisite obsessiveness. William Krutzfeldt provided expert editorial advice.

Our special gratitude goes to Mr. Jeffrey House, our publisher, for the patience, trust and encouragement.

Jaime Sepulveda
Harvey Fineberg
Jonathan Mann

CONTENTS

Prevention Through Information and Education: Experience from Mexico 127
Jaime Sepulveda

Targeted AIDS Intervention Programs in Africa 145
Peter Lamptey, Sharon Weir

The Role of Behavioral Sciences and Health Education in HIV Prevention: Experience at the U.S. Centers for Disease Control 175
*Mark L. Rosenberg, Dennis D. Tolsma, Lloyd J. Kolbe,
Fred Kroger, Marcie L. Cynamon, G. Stephen Bowen*

The European Response to AIDS 199
Mukesh Kapila, Maryan J. Pye

IV. STRATEGIES FOR COMMUNICATION AND THE MEDIA

Preface 237
Harvey Fineberg

The Media and AIDS: A Global Perspective 241
Thomas W. Netter

The Strategic Use of the Broadcast Media for AIDS Prevention: Current Limits and Future Directions 255
William Dejong, Jay A. Winsten

I. OVERVIEW

Introduction

Jaime Sepulveda
Harvey Fineberg
Jonathan Mann

Ten years after AIDS was first recognized, the often repeated dictum that education is the most effective weapon to prevent infection remains valid. This is true because AIDS will not disappear, just as the majority of infectious diseases have not disappeared, even those for which effective methods of treatment and prevention already exist. Therefore, education is not a transitory strategy; if and when effective drugs and vaccines are developed, education will still play a major role in contending with the epidemic. Too much emphasis, human and financial resources, and hope have been directed toward the development of drugs and vaccines, without realizing that even with these resources, AIDS will continue to exist, especially in underprivileged populations.

For most unaffected people, AIDS has lost the interest it originally elicited. Individuals in many societies perceive AIDS as a problem of others, of deviates. The media show signs of fatigue. For most government officials the difficulties, expenses and controversy related to AIDS make it attractive to turn their minds to other problems. This widespread indifference is explained in part by the lack of spectacular results in therapeutics and immunoprevention, and the failure to achieve tangible results from massmedia campaigns against AIDS.

AIDS prevention requires a collective effort, both from society as a whole and from individuals. The safety of blood and blood products should be a societal and, more specifically, a governmental responsibility, because individuals must be protected from modes of transmission that are beyond their individual means of control. It is also a societal duty to ensure adequate information for all and to provide access to preventive devices. At the same time, individuals have an obligation to adopt responsible behaviors to protect themselves and others. Here we have a paradox: AIDS must be conceived as a global, societal problem, but its control also depends on active individual participation.

Enough has been learned about AIDS prevention through education during the last decade to merit reflection on both the failures and successes of this short, tragic but also intense and vital period. The original education models based on fear have been replaced with more optimistic and even humorous campaigns. Health promotion has moved to center stage in the global fight against AIDS.

This book is based on a simple premise: AIDS is completely preventable with adequate information and the adoption of appropriate measures. It is by now a *cliché* to say education is the only weapon we have to fight AIDS, but no text has attempted to systematize the diverse body of knowledge on the subject. This book is an effort to collect and organize a wealth of global experience from many experts and to consolidate new information. Of course, this is not an "AIDS education cook book." Instead, the book offers the reader a range of views and perspectives from experts in the varied disciplines that make up the very broad field of AIDS education.

Qualitative and quantitative behavioral research are more than complementary. The first allows us to gain deeper understanding of human behavior and its determinants, while the latter permits us to assess that behavior and its consequences. To be effective, as the chapters in the section on methods indicate, AIDS programs should combine both quantitative and qualitative research methods.

In contrast to biomedicine, where most of the resources are concentrated and most modern medical breakthroughs have occurred, innovations in health promotion are open to all societies, regardless of their economic status. From this premise comes this book's emphasis on a global perspective on AIDS education and prevention. Global learning —the process of communities and countries learning from each other— must accelerate. There are many AIDS-prevention community efforts worldwide, of which we have included only a few. If innovations can be more quickly shared and disseminated, we will do a better job of fighting AIDS everywhere.

Information is a necessary but not sufficient condition for behavioral change; we must not only inform, but persuade. This is essential for behavior modification to be adopted and sustained. The chapters on the media and communication conclude that news broadcasting, print media and social marketing are effective first steps toward behavior change by lessening fear through repeated reassurance and by wearing away attitudes of denial. Also, by promoting compassionate attitudes toward people with AIDS this type of campaign can affect positively how the public deals with the politics of AIDS.

The fight against AIDS will be a long one. Unfortunately, humans are better prepared biologically and psychologically to confront acute crises than chronic ailments. Therefore, we must make a special effort not to succumb to resignation or complacency. AIDS poses challenges for science and societies, placing stress on weaknesses in such areas as human rights and international access to health care. We must rise to these challenges and strengthen these weaknesses. We must overcome the behavioral, biological and economic obstacles to prevention.

Health Promotion Against AIDS: A Typology

Jonathan M. Mann

Against HIV/AIDS, health promotion can not be modest. Confronted with the challenges of the global pandemic and strengthened by decades of thought and action, health promotion occupies the central role in the global AIDS strategy. This chapter seeks to place experience with HIV/AIDS health promotion into a global and historical perspective and to develop a typology of national HIV/AIDS health promotion programs.

HIV/AIDS AND HEALTH PROMOTION

While the capacity to identify historical trends in recent events is limited, the history of global AIDS appears thus far to be divisible into three periods, of silence, initial discovery and global mobilization; the shape, meaning and appropriate title for the current period can not yet be discerned.

The period of silence started during the mid-1970s, as the human immunodeficiency virus (HIV) began to spread in epidemic form around the world. As the events of HIV infection and transmission are silent, and the clinical manifestations of infection do not become apparent for months, and usually years or even decades later, the world remained ignorant of the new epidemic. From the mid–1970s until 1981, when the disease AIDS was first recognized, HIV spread, silently and unnoticed, to five continents; at least 100 000 people became infected.

The recognition of AIDS in the United States in 1981 ended the period of

21

silence and inaugurated the period of initial discovery (1981–1985). During this time, the causative virus (HIV) was discovered, its modes of transmission were identified and tests were developed to detect HIV infection. Rapidly, studies using this information and technology produced three vital facts about the pandemic. First, at this stage of the epidemic at least, many more people in any population are HIV-infected than have AIDS (i.e., AIDS is the "tip of the iceberg" of HIV infection). Second, the time between HIV infection and development of disease is measured in months, usually in years, and perhaps in decades. Third, studies during the mid-1980s showed that HIV infection was truly pandemic, affecting, although not uniformly, all regions of the world.

However, this period involved much more than biomedical discovery; substantial research was also directed at the individual and social dimensions of HIV-related risk and behavior. In the social sciences (as in the biomedical sciences) HIV/AIDS-related questions and concerns focused attention on the limits of our knowledge about human behavior (or virology and immunology). Around the world, those seeking to learn about HIV/AIDS-related behaviors by building upon knowledge of sexuality and self-injecting drug behavior, found that little reliable or useful information was available on these subjects. In addition, the social dimensions of HIV/-AIDS became a major challenge, as social scientists witnessed the emergence of discrimination, stigmatization and other forms of HIV–related prejudice, hysteria, and individual or collective and contemporary forms of witch-hunting.

The third phase in the history of global AIDS started in early 1985, at the First International AIDS Conference in Atlanta (U.S.). Information presented at that meeting convincingly demonstrated the global nature of HIV/AIDS; immediately following the meeting the World Health Organization convened a group of experts which recommended a global approach to the problem. The World Health Organization (WHO) is the specialized agency of the United Nations with responsibility to direct and coordinate international health work. The Global AIDS Strategy of the WHO is the first truly global strategy against a communicable (or any other) disease. While large-scale programs against diseases (i.e., smallpox eradication) have occurred in the past, they have only really involved certain areas of the world.

One of the early challenges was to define and conceptualize the HIV/AIDS problem, for this would determine the shape of the response to the pandemic. Health promotion was then explicitly recognized as the central element in the global strategy with all its associated dimensions of support, and repressive and discriminatory approaches were rejected.

The Global AIDS Strategy has three objectives:

* to prevent HIV transmission;
* to reduce (control) the personal and social impact of HIV/AIDS;
* and to unify national and international efforts against the disease.

This Global AIDS Strategy, which provides guidance to national and international programs linked in common purpose, was developed by the WHO in 1986 and approved by the World Health Assembly in May 1987. Then, an unprecedented development occurred, for in October 1987, the General Assembly of the United Nations held an extraordinary session to discuss AIDS. This was the first time that a disease was debated by this highest international political forum. The historic resolution which emerged declared AIDS to be a global problem warranting great energy and commitment, and called upon the vast network of United Nations agencies and organizations to join together in a global effort under the leadership of the WHO and in conformity with the Global AIDS Strategy.

The WHO created the Global Program on AIDS as its instrument to develop, help implement and evaluate the Global AIDS Strategy. From four professional staff in February 1987, the Global Program on AIDS had grown, by mid-1989, to become the WHO's largest single program, with over 250 staff in Geneva, regional offices of the WHO and in country posts.

By mid-1989, the Global Program on AIDS was collaborating actively with over 155 countries, through a well-defined and systematic process. First, upon receiving a country request, the Global Program on AIDS organizes a technical visit to help assess the general epidemiological and organizational situation. Then, urgent support (financial and technical) is provided to nascent national AIDS committees and programs. The Global Program on AIDS develops a conceptual framework for national AIDS program development, and supports short-term (usually 6-18 month) and medium–term (three to five year) planning. Resources for short and medium–term plan implementation are obtained from development assistance agencies through a process coordinated by the national AIDS program with support from the Global Program on AIDS.

The result of this work has been a truly global mobilization in support of HIV/AIDS prevention and control. Many countries who were reluctant to admit the presence of HIV/AIDS developed open and active programs; guidance and resources were provided to accelerate program implementation; and the spirit of global solidarity grew stronger.

However, HIV infection and associated disease also progressed rapidly during this period. By 1989, an estimated five to ten million people had become HIV infected worldwide. From 1980-85, an estimated 70 000 people developed AIDS; from 1986–88, an additional 300 000 people were estimated to have developed AIDS. By mid-1989, the global cumulative total of people with AIDS exceeded 500 000.

Therefore, from 1986–89, during the period of global mobilization, the face of the world's confrontations with HIV/AIDS changed dramatically and irrevocably. The challenges for the early 1990s are in many ways derived from the successes and the failures in the approach to global AIDS prevention and control which was adopted during the mid–to–late 1980s.

HEALTH PROMOTION IN THE GLOBAL AIDS STRATEGY

In late January 1988, there was another unprecedented event—a global summit of ministers of health on AIDS prevention and control. Jointly organized by the United Kingdom and the WHO, the summit was attended by more ministers of health than had ever assembled, for any purpose, at any time. The ministers spoke openly about their national programs, obstacles faced and difficulties yet to be overcome. Then, the London Declaration was issued, which is a milestone in awareness of the importance and the dimensions of health promotion. The Declaration stated: "the single most important component of national AIDS programs is information and education… individuals, governments, the media and other sectors all have major roles to play in preventing the spread of HIV infection."

From the beginning, the Global AIDS Strategy focused on information and education as the critical elements in national strategy development. The Global Program on AIDS Health Promotion unit developed guidelines and related materials. Working with new national AIDS programs worldwide, the Global Program on AIDS provided training and technical support for information, education and communication programs, and promoted international exchange of information and experience.

In general, national HIV/AIDS health promotion strategies and activities have been based on experience in health promotion work of the past decades, tailored to some of the specific features of HIV/AIDS. Yet as in many other areas, the HIV/AIDS challenge has clarified weaknesses, imbalances and inequities in past health promotion efforts. Therefore, HIV/AIDS health promotion is not simply a challenge of how to apply what is already known. Facing HIV/AIDS, health promotion itself must learn, grow and evolve.

One powerful source of inspiration is international exchange of experience. In AIDS prevention and control, these exchanges (symbolized by the International Information and Education Conferences in Ixtapa, Mexico in 1988 and in Yaounde, Cameroon in 1989) are particularly important. An image from pharmacology (provided by a Danish colleague) may be useful to explain how vital such exchanges can be. In searching for new pharma-cologic agents, efforts are made to find "rare plants" which, thriving in their particular ecologic niche, can make an unexpected yet invaluable contribution to the whole world. To find such plants, the search must be thorough, alert and imaginative.

In AIDS health promotion, local experiences, reflecting creative adapta-tion to a specific context and environment, can be a source of insight and inspiration. For it is clear that in HIV/AIDS education, the boundaries of creativity are not limited by economics, and no society has a monopoly on intelligence, imagination or the strength to bear the burden. The Global Program on AIDS serves as a forum for such a search for "rare plants" in health promotion, through exchange of information and experience unim-peded by geographical, social or political borders.

Research is a second source of inspiration for health promotion. The central problem of "risk behavior" is immediately relevant to HIV/AIDS prevention and control. This concern includes how to reach risk behavior populations and understanding how risk behaviors are initiated, main-tained and modified. Research can also help clarify social dimensions of risk perception and behavior, including constraining and facilitating factors and the nature of HIV–related prejudice.

A third way to enhance progress is to strengthen the assessment capabil-ity of health promotion. In many aspects of public health, evaluation is more frequently discussed than effectively practiced. Progress in HIV/AIDS health promotion is critically dependant upon the intensive technical support and training required to strengthen assessment capacity.

GLOBAL HIV/AIDS HEALTH PROMOTION

By mid-1989, nearly every country in the world had a national AIDS commit-tee and a national AIDS program. A tremendous reservoir of experience now exists to illustrate how similar or related HIV/AIDS health promotion chal-lenges have been addressed in different epidemiological, social, economic and political settings.

From among the many dimensions of health promotion programs, twel-ve particularly important elements can be identified, which can be incorpo-rated into a typology of national HIV/AIDS health promotion programs. Within each element, a gradient can be described, extending from ini-tial/less–developed to advanced/well–developed approaches and activities.

The elements and gradients are outlined first, followed by outlines of three general types of national HIV/AIDS health promotion programs. The typology proposed in this chapter is provisional. While descriptively useful, the individual elements, gradients and typology itself need to be assessed. The relationship between elements, gradients, typology and documented HIV/AIDS health promotion program effectiveness must remain the touchstone of validity for any such effort at categorization.

KEY ELEMENTS AND ASSOCIATED GRADIENTS

Information content

Central to all programs is a need to explain how HIV is transmitted. This information can be linked either with recommendations about personal protection against HIV or to appeals for tolerance and non-discrimination. Also important is guidance on how to obtain further information. Advanced programs link transmission information with both protection and non–discrimination and provide specific guidance on obtaining further information.

Message and materials development

All programs develop messages which are carried through specific materials. The process of message/material development in advanced programs involves extensive and repeated consultation with target audiences and includes field testing.

Perception of HIV/AIDS

There are two major issues regarding how HIV/AIDS is conceptualized: whether the disease is presented as "our" problem or "their" problem; and whether HIV infection is accorded a pejorative moral dimension. Advanced programs express a global perspective and stress solidarity, and while a moral dimension may be present, it is not pejorative, particularly regarding already infected persons (e.g., no talk of "innocent victims").

Audiences

Definition of audience is essential. Advanced programs may continue to address the general public but focus mainly on segment audiences. In addition, advanced programs try to access not only the "easy to reach" target groups such as school children and health workers, but also the "hard to reach," such as prostitutes and their clients, self–injecting drug users, and out–of–school youth.

Channels

Major channel choices include mass media, "little media" (posters, brochures, flyers), and face–to–face approaches. While an advanced program will generally mix all three, it emphasizes approaches in which discussion and dialogue are possible.

Attitudes towards sexuality

Programs vary widely regarding the explicitness of sexual content and the extent to which moral judgments accompany this information. An important specific issue is the attitude toward condoms and the extent to which they are promoted. More advanced programs adjust the level of explicitness in consultation with target audiences and avoid a prejudicial moral dimension. In such programs, the implicit and explicit attitude toward condoms is positive and while targeted, the condom promotion effort also reaches the general public.

Institutional networks

While HIV/AIDS is first a health issue, its social, cultural, economic, legal, ethical and political dimensions and impact are now widely appreciated. More advanced national HIV/AIDS health promotion programs form links with and generate institutional networks which reflect this broad social impact, including community–based and non–governmental organizations.

Linkage with health and social services

There are two vital dimensions to this linkage. First, information about HIV/AIDS should be provided along with information about specific services which can help the individual to prevent or modify HIV–related risk behaviors (e.g., condom availability, confidential HIV test sites, access to needle–exchange programs). More advanced HIV/AIDS health promotion programs are carefully tailored to establish explicit linkage with already available services and/or with services developed specifically in association with the health promotion program. The second dimension of linkage involves integration of HIV/AIDS health promotion within existing health and social services. Advanced programs will have established close ties with such programs, particularly in maternal and child health, family planning, and sexually transmitted disease control contexts.

Political and social leadership

While HIV/AIDS health promotion programs all require some level of social and political acceptance, the extent and manner of involvement of political and social leaders varies widely. More advanced programs have explicit and highly visible linkages with selected political and/or social leaders.

Assessment capability

HIV/AIDS health promotion programs can only improve if they are monitored for program efficiency and evaluated for effectiveness (or impact).

More advanced programs are aware of this dimension and are developing and strengthening their assessment capability.

Institutional base

At one level, the institutional relationship between HIV/AIDS health promotion and the national AIDS committee and program involves issues of staff, budget, policy and strategy formulation. More advanced programs have adequate staff of sufficient grade and professionalism, a well–identified budget, and close linkage with the overall national AIDS program and policy process. In addition, advanced programs are decentralized from headquarters and capital cities to district and community levels. Decentralization involves delegation of both responsibility and authority (including financial resources).

Strategic capability

HIV/AIDS health promotion must be integrated within broad strategies for preventing HIV infection, reducing its personal and social impact, and unifying national and international efforts. More advanced programs have a substantial capability for strategic thinking and action as part of a well-functioning national AIDS program.

TYPOLOGY OF HIV/AIDS HEALTH PROMOTION PROGRAMS

National HIV/AIDS health promotion programs can be divided into three groups, based on these 12 elements and the gradients within each.

Information type programs are least developed and focus on information. Empowering type programs are moderately developed and include efforts to enhance self–empowerment as well as providing information. Finally, community advocacy type programs not only deliver information and address self–empowerment, they also strengthen community advocacy.

Broadly considered, these three program types correspond to different levels in conceptualizing health promotion itself. The more limited view–point (information type) defines its task as provision of information. Such programs often disseminate this information from a central source, using mass media channels and time–limited campaigns in an effort to reach many people. The information provided is often imbued with consensus attitudes regarding risk behaviors. As HIV/AIDS is considered a health problem, information emanates from health institution sources or is quoted by others from such sources. Little attention may be given to health and social service linkages. Information type programs are often observed during the first year or so of national AIDS program activity, with subsequent evolution toward Types II and III. However, information type programs may persist beyond the initial period if the entire national AIDS program operates in an ambivalent or frankly hostile social and political environment.

The next stage in thinking about health promotion reflects awareness of the need to examine closely the motivating factors and constraints operating on the individuals whose past, present and future behavior is at issue. The "individual locus of control" perspective leads to concern that information be well–targeted. Information is therefore designed with input from target audiences and includes explicit attention to health and social services needed to support, immediately and over time, specific behaviors and behavior change. In empowering type programs, HIV/AIDS is generally described as a global problem which concerns everyone; awareness of the social dimension is reinforced by clear messages about non–discrimination. Empowering type programs use a broader mix of media, with increasing emphasis on person–to–person approaches. The attitude toward sexuality is neutral or positive and can be quite explicit depending upon the target audience; the approach to condom promotion is also targeted. Recognizing that people are influenced and reached by many channels and institutions, the program seeks integration in the national health system and forms alliances with other sectors of government and with other agencies and groups. Realizing that people are best reached in and through their communities, the national HIV/AIDS health promotion program seeks to decentralize. Overall, the empowering type program is integrated within, and supported by, the national AIDS program, the health sector and the broader community. In sum, the emphasis of the empowering type program is on motivation and support for informed individual behavior change.

The third stage of health promotion recognizes the broad policy and social dimensions of health promotion. Information provided by community advocacy type programs, developed with the target audiences, emphasizes solidarity and the need to protect the rights and dignity of HIV–infected persons. The community advocacy type program is decentralized, so that information is provided from within many different institutions and organizations.

The community advocacy type program distinguishes itself particularly in the areas of linkage with health and social services, its relationship with social and political leadership and its strategic capability. Community advocacy type programs include elements of Types I and II, but go beyond these to consider the cultural, economic and political impediments to promotion of health. For community advocacy type programs, information about HIV/AIDS is only useful when it takes both individual and social realities into account. Therefore, such issues as women's capability in a given social system to refuse intercourse without a condom, or the availability of truly confidential diagnostic or support services, or the realities of condom distribution, availability and cost, are seen as central concerns.

From this viewpoint, the "right to information" means also that informed decisions about HIV/AIDS can not be separated from freedom to act and access to requisite social support. In sum, the community advocacy type program sees strategic action and community advocacy as inseparably linked with other dimensions of HIV/AIDS health promotion.

When this typology is applied to current national HIV/AIDS health promotion programs, many countries are seen to remain in information type programs. Indeed, it appears particularly difficult to advance beyond information type programs in countries with low HIV prevalence and few AIDS cases. However, most countries have empowering type programs, with varying levels of progress along the gradients towards more advanced program development.

FUTURE CHALLENGES

Looking toward the future, several issues may be usefully considered. First, how can the WHO and other organizations best support national HIV/AIDS programs to move out of information type into empowering type and then towards community advocacy type?

What are the linkages between overall national AIDS program development and its health promotion component? A deeper understanding of factors which enhance or limit national HIV/AIDS health promotion program development would be useful, to help accelerate program evolution. While preliminary, there are several roles for a typology of national HIV/AIDS health promotion programs. A typology can help identify programs at similar levels, in order to enhance the specificity and relevance of information and experience exchange. Such comparative efforts may identify particular barriers and facilitating factors in program development for which research and evaluation efforts can be targeted.

This first effort at creating a broad typology will hopefully stimulate further discussion, so that the best criteria can be selected and most relevant indicators identified, thereby strengthening the process of national and global assessment of HIV/AIDS health promotion efforts.

This chapter must end, as it started, with a historical perspective. The WHO projects that the decade of the 1990s will be more complex and challenging than the 1980s, in terms of numbers of HIV–infected persons, persons developing HIV–related diseases, and associated social, economic and political stresses.

The pressures, the expectations and the opportunities for HIV/AIDS health promotion during the next decade are likely to be even greater than in the past few years. Biomedical research will provide improved tools for diagnosis, treatment and even prevention. Yet, as with other diseases today and in the past, it is also clear that these technologies, by themselves, will not be sufficient to prevent and control HIV/AIDS.

As we review the decade passing and the decade to come, we can identify several reasons why the world was fortunate that the HIV pandemic occurred now, rather than 50 years ago. One reason is the strength of modern science, which was able to identify the causative agent, develop powerful diagnostic tests and make rapid progress in developing therapeutic agents and preparing for vaccines. A second reason is global communications, which allow useful information (as well as viruses) to move rapidly, to the benefit (or danger) of all. A third reason is the existence of the United Nations system and of international development assistance; if they did not already exist, both would have had to be created to deal with HIV/AIDS. Fourth, today there is evidence of a new globalism, an international solidarity toward issues facing all, such as the degradation of the global environment and HIV/AIDS.

There is yet another major factor which distinguishes our world and which gives us confidence as we face HIV/AIDS. This is the development of health promotion itself, its philosophy and practice, and its integration in strategies for "Health for AIDS. The conceptual framework of health promotion is essential to our work today and to our vision of the future. In this regard, we pay tribute to the thinkers and doers of health promotion for, as always, we can see far, "for we stand on the shoulders of giants." In the face of AIDS, we must deepen and broaden the philosophy and the practice of health promotion, for it will lead us to the very frontiers of our knowledge of others, and of ourselves.

II. METHODS FOR BEHAVIORAL RESEARCH

Preface

Jonathan Mann

The global HIV/AIDS epidemic represents an enormous, and in some ways unprecedented challenge to health professionals.

The magnitude of the task makes it essential for people at all levels of the health and social system to have a common understanding of the approach to be taken. Good intentions are not enough; as Michael Ramah and Claire Cassidy point out, information campaigns have potential for harm as well as good.

Therefore, before examining national experiences, or considering the role of the media or the broader context within which AIDS information and education programs will be developed and implemented, it is important to consider some methodological issues. The three excellent chapters in this section describe key concepts and tools which must be understood by decision–makers and other health officials, as well as by the practitioners of AIDS education themselves.

The first chapter in this section, by Steven Gortmaker and Jose Antonio Izazola, provides a framework for quantitative analysis of behavior. The emphasis is on the proper role of quantitative analysis and its limitations. As in other parts of this book, the reader is encouraged to seek elsewhere for detailed methodology.

In the second chapter, by William Smith and Mary Debus, the problem of describing behavior is approached from a related yet quite different perspective. Qualitative research is quite appealing, especially at first glance, as it appears to offer a simpler and quicker path to acquisition of key information

35

to guide AIDS education programs. The apparent simplicity of qualitative research is deceptive; the authors explain why and argue persuasively for methodological rigor as a safeguard against excessively biased results.

The reader will note that quantitative and qualitative research are not proposed as discrete alternatives; their appropriate use, as always, depends on an understanding of the strengths and limitations inherent in each approach.

The third chapter in this section, by Michael Ramah and Claire Cassidy, takes the reader directly into the world of social marketing. For those unfamiliar with its concepts and language, this chapter deserves the closest attention; readers already aware of social marketing will find the material on the specific application of social marketing to AIDS education lively and provocative.

It is hoped that these chapters will familiarize the reader with concepts and language in quantitative and qualitative analysis and social marketing. Then, after reading the remainder of the book, the reader is advised to re–read this section, to gain further insight into the application of these concepts and methods. For ultimately, this book seeks to motivate and guide *action* in AIDS education; the next step is up to the reader.

The Role of Quantitative Behavioral Research in AIDS Prevention

Steven L. Gortmaker
Jose Antonio Izazola

Quantitative behavioral research plays a central role for scientists as they work to describe, monitor, understand and evaluate the AIDS epidemic. There is the need to describe human behaviors which are known risk factors for the spread of HIV–1, to monitor change in these behaviors (or to document a lack of change), to understand what causes behavioral change, to test hypotheses concerning the effects of behaviors upon the spread of HIV–1, and to evaluate the effects of behavioral interventions. Quantitative methods are utilized to measure and evaluate not only behaviors related to the spread of HIV–1, but also attitudes and knowledge which may be important determinants of behavioral change.

In this chapter we review the impact that quantitative behavioral research has had upon our understanding of the HIV–1 epidemic and discuss the limitations of this research caused by poor measurement, weak research designs and biased sampling plans.

We point out the insights into prevention made possible by quantitative modeling of behavior, discuss the importance of employing clear theories of behavioral change and of carrying out process evaluations, and outline critical issues which arise as we attempt to tie quantitative behavioral research to health policy.

THE IMPORTANCE OF QUANTITATIVE BEHAVIORAL RESEARCH IN AIDS PREVENTION

The global nature of AIDS has highlighted quantitative estimates of the spread of the epidemic which appear almost daily in the international press. Estimates are published concerning numbers of cases and prevalence rates of AIDS in local, risk–group specific and national populations. Researchers have similarly estimated the seroprevalence of HIV–1 in multiple local and population–based samples. Studies from throughout the world now appear which estimate the prevalence of risky sexual behaviors and IV drug use, describe changes in these behaviors over time, and which document the lack of preventive behaviors, e.g. the infrequent use of condoms. Knowledge (and ignorance) concerning AIDS and HIV–1 are regularly described, and attitudes about the disease and the virus are regularly sampled in opinion polls throughout the world.

Without a doubt our knowledge concerning the epidemic and our ability to plan scientifically for strategies to prevent further spread of HIV–1 have benefitted enormously from quantitative estimates of knowledge, attitudes and behaviors. While there are some very important limits placed on the quality of these estimates—which we will describe in detail below—the fact remains that it has been our ability to quantify these aspects of the AIDS epidemic which has furthered our understanding of both the enormity of the epidemic and the tremendously difficult task ahead of working to prevent further spread through behavioral interventions.

The advantages of quantitative measures are quite clear: for example, quantitative estimates can clearly document the relative frequency and distribution of behaviors, attitudes and knowledge in different risk groups and populations. Change in behaviors over time can be assessed. Quantitative measurement also makes possible the replication of results, a key to validation of scientific inference. Models which utilize quantitative measures can provide useful projections of future trends, can lead to estimates of the relative effects of social and behavioral influences upon the course of the epidemic, and permit calculations of the relative efficacy and cost–effectiveness of intervention strategies. Wide dissemination of preventive programs aimed at behavioral change may be unlikely in the absence of solid quantitative experimental data concerning intervention effectiveness.

THE LIMITATIONS OF QUANTITATIVE BEHAVIORAL MEASURES

A major limitation to the usefulness of behavioral measures is poor measurement quality. We can describe the quality of measures by referring to both their reliability and their validity. We will discuss these concepts in substantial detail, at the same time illustrating their application by refering to the measurement of selected areas of importance in AIDS research. We will discuss the measurement of whether a person is infected with the HIV–1 virus, and contrast the quality of these biological measures with indicators of risky sexual behaviors, use of drugs, use of condoms, and knowledge and attitudes about AIDS. We have chosen to contrast the quality of behavioral measures with measures of viral infection because of the familiarity many professionals have with the quality of tests for HIV–1 antibodies and virus.

A lack of reliability in a measure refers to random measurement error, and concerns the extent to which measurements are repeatable. A reliable measurement is one which will be stable over a variety of conditions in which essentially the same results should be obtained; i.e. when there has been no true change in the measure. Reliability can be expressed quantitatively via a reliability coefficient (ranging from 0.0 to 1.0) which estimates the amount of true score variance (and conversely, the amount of error variance) in a measure.[1] A highly unreliable measure is thus mostly "noise" and will be characterized by a reliability coefficient between 0.0 and 0.5.

To illustrate how this concept works in practice, we can examine the reliability of measures of the presence of antibodies to HIV–1 virus such as the ELISA and the Western Blot. Studies of these measures indicate very high repeatability, and reliability coefficients are thus probably .99 or higher. It is important to note, however, that a measure can be highly reliable but not necessarily perfectly predictive of the construct or variable of interest (the intended construct or variable in this case could be infection with the HIV–1 virus). Thus, while the ELISA may be highly reliable, it is not a perfect indicator of infection with HIV–1, because some individuals may be infected but not exhibit antibodies.

Measures of knowledge, attitudes and behavior can be assessed with varying levels of reliability. In AIDS–related research, this assessment has not often been made. One published report indicates that the reliability of multi–item scales which measure knowledge and attitudes concerning AIDS ranged from .52 to .68.[2] This level of reliability is considered moderate. It should be possible, however, to increase the reliability of these scales by increasing the number of items which are used to make up the scales (e.g. increase the number of items from five to ten).[3]

Few estimates of the reliability of measures of risky sexual behaviors have been reported; one recent study indicates moderate levels of reliabil-

[1] J. Nunnally, *Psychometric Theory*. (New York: McGraw-Hill, 1978.)

[2] J.G. Joseph, S.B. Montgomery, C.A. Emmons, R.C. Kessler, D.G. Ostrow, C.B. Wortman, K. O'Brien, M. Eller, S. Eshleman, "Magnitude and Determinants of Behavioral Risk Reduction: Longitudinal Analysis of Cohort at Risk for AIDS," *Psychology and Health* 1 (1987): 73–96.

[3] *Op. cit.* J. Nunnally, 1978.

ity for measures of these behaviors,[4] meaning a substantial portion of the variance in these measures is noise. The reliability of drug use behavior measures, in contrast, has been studied for quite some time, and quite good reliability has been documented for self–reported measures.[5] Unreliability in these measures is caused by a variety of factors including the limitations of short–term memory, subjects not wanting to report behavior perceived as deviant, and the difficulty of characterizing complex behaviors in terms of simple responses.

The validity of a measure refers to whether that measure is useful scientifically. There are three major aspects to validity:

- Predictive validity;
- Construct validity; and
- Content validity.[6]

It is important to emphasize that both validity and reliability are not all–or–none properties: these are characteristics which have broad ranges, and measures with imperfect reliability and limited validity can still serve important purposes, both in population research and in applied clinical settings.

Predictive validity concerns whether a measure is predictive of some important criterion. For example, we can refer to the predictive validity of the ELISA test as a measure of infection with the HIV–1 virus. Or, we can ask whether a particular sexual behavior may be predictive of infection with HIV–1. Another example of predictive validity is the extent to which a person's knowledge (or lack of knowledge) may predict whether that person decides to start using condoms.

The predictive validity of a measure can be characterized quantitatively via a number of approaches: sensitivity and specificity are terms used by epidemiologists to indicate how well a dichotomous measure accurately predicts a dichotomous outcome.[7] Predictive validity can also be characterized by other statistical terms such as positive predictive values, odds ratios, correlations and regression coefficients.

[4] S.P. Saltzman, A.M. Stoddard, J. McCusker, M.W. Moon, K.H. Mayer, "Reliability of self–reported sexual behavior risk factors for HIV infection in homosexual men," *Public Health Reports* 102 (6) (November–December 1987): 692–697.

[5] R. Smart, "Recent studies of the validity and reliability of self–reported drug use, 1970–1974," *Canadian Journal of Criminology and Corrections* 17(4):326–33.

[6] *Op. cit.* J. Nunnally.

[7] J.L. Fleiss, *Statistical Methods for Rates and Proportions* (New York: John Wiley and Sons, 1981).

Table 3-1. *Predictive value of HIV-l infection ELISA detection test, according to the prevalence in fictitious populations of 100 000 each.*

True prevalence in population	Truly infected	Detected as positive	PPV[a]	NPV[b]
20.00%	20 000	19 660	99.2%	99.6%
0.07%	70	69	25.6%	99.9%

Sensitivity – 98.3%; The probability of tested positive given truly infected.
Specificity – 99.8%; The probability of tested negative given truly not infected.
[a] PPV - Positive Predictive Value; the probability that given a positive test being really infected.
[b] NPV - Negative Predictive Value; The probability that given a negative test being really not infected.
Source: Adapted from P.D. Cleary, M.J. Barry, K.H. Mayer, A.M. Brandt, L. Gostin, H.V. Fineberg, "Compulsory premarital screening for the Human Immunodeficiency Virus," *Journal of the American Medical Association* 258(13) (1987): 1757-62.

For example, we know that the predictive validity of an ELISA test for seropositivity followed by confirmation with a Western Blot is in general excellent, with very high sensitivity and specificity.[8] Thus, for most behavioral research, the measurement quality associated with seropositivity is quite high, and we do not need to be too concerned about measurement errors in the seroprevalence variable when estimating associations between risky behaviors and seropositivity.

However, there are some serious limitations to use of the ELISA and Western Blot tests when examining populations with a low seroprevalence of HIV–1. In examining the policy of mandatory HIV–1 screening in low prevalence populations, for example, one study points out that in such populations the low positive predictive value (i.e. the probability that given a positive test one is really infected) negate the usefulness of mandatory screening. Table 3-1 provides a hypothetical illustration of this result, which indicates that in a low seroprevalence population, 74% of the seropositives identified by the ELISA will not in fact be infected.[9] As a general rule, then, the predictive validity of these tests is higher (more accurate) in populations with a higher seroprevalence.

[8] P.D. Cleary, M.J. Barry, K.H. Mayer, A.M. Brandt, L. Gostin, H.V. Fineberg, "Compulsory premarital screening for the Human Immunodeficiency Virus," *Journal of the American Medical Association* 258(13) (1987):1757–62.
[9] *Ibid.*

In contrast to the generally excellent predictive validity of measures of seropositivity, the predictive validity of knowledge and attitudes concerning HIV–1 and the predictive validity of risky behaviors can be very limited. For example, longitudinal data concerning 637 participants in the Multicenter AIDS Cohort Study in Chicago indicated very little relationship between measures of knowledge of AIDS, perceived risk of AIDS, perceived efficacy of behavioral change and measures of actual behavioral change in risky sexual practices.[10] It is a fact that attitudes are simply not very often strongly predictive of behavior. There are many factors which influence human behavior, and attitudes are only part of the picture—sometimes a relatively small part.[11]

At the same time, approaches to behavioral change should not necessarily be dismissed because of relatively low predictive validity. Small effects upon behavioral change can accumulate just like money in the bank can accumulate at low interest rates[12] and even low levels of predictive validity can be important, particularly if the associated costs are low and effects accumulate over time.

Construct validity concerns whether a measure is really measuring what is intended. This can include ascertaining whether the measure includes all relevant components, whether these components measure the same underlying construct, and whether within experiments and studies of individual differences the measure performs as predicted by highly accepted theoretical hypotheses.[13]

The use of tests of seropositivity to infer infection with HIV–1 offers an excellent example of the issues surrounding construct validity. If our goal is to measure infection with HIV–1, seropositivity is not ideal, and is only an approximate indicator of infection; antigen measures would be more accurate. Following infection, some individuals do not demonstrate seropositivity to HIV–1 for six months. Thus while seropositivity may be a perfectly adequate measure for many behavioral studies (because it is highly correlated with infection), it is clear that we are not measuring precisely what we really want to measure, and hence we have some construct invalidity. This construct invalidity will then imply lowered predictive validity.

For some behavioral studies it could furthermore be argued that the real construct of interest is infectivity. Recent research appears to indicate that

10 C.A. Emmons, J.G. Joseph, R.C. Kessler, C.B. Wortman, S.B. Montgomery and D.G. Ostrow, "Psychosocial predictors of reported behavior change in homosexual men for risk of AIDS," *Health Education Quarterly* 13(4) (1986): 331–345.

11 M.H. Becker and J.G. Joseph "AIDS and behavioral change to reduce risk: a review," *American Journal of Public Health* 78(4), (1988): 394–410.

12 Gilbert, Light and Mosteller, "How well do social innovations work?," in *Statistics: A Guide to the Unknown*, eds. Tanur *et al.* (San Francisco: Holden–Day, 1978), pp. 125–138.

13 *Op. cit.* J. Nunnally.

infectivity is greatest immediately following infection, then declines (perhaps among some individuals to a noninfectious state) and increases again as symptoms of AIDS appear and as the disease progresses.[14] It is quite clear that tests like the ELISA and Western Blot are limited indicators of infectivity.

When measuring sexual behaviors and condom use, even seemingly minor variations in question wording and methods of data gathering can result in different measures and hence differential construct validity. Data from KAP surveys in six cities in Mexico in 1988 illustrate these issues. In these surveys of the general population, homosexual/bisexual males and prostitutes, one question asked about the number of sexual partners in the previous month. While respondents from the general population, and gay and bisexual men understood the question, female prostitutes seemed to equate this question with the number of "steady" partners, since their answer to the question was an average of four partners for the last month. For the prostitutes, the questions concerning the average number of days that they worked every week and the average "clients" per day resulted in a reported 48 client partners in a month (Table 3-2). In some situations, then, different questions need to be asked of different risk groups to measure the same underlying construct: number of sexual partners.

Obviously the meaning of questions concerning use of a condom during the last month and use during last intercourse will depend upon the frequency of intercourse: a prostitute with 200 clients in the last month is very likely to have used a condom at least once, even if her rate of use is low during an average encounter (Table 3-2). This fact also illustrates how construct validity can vary across populations.

Our illustration also points to the continuing need for basic research into how people behave sexually and how they verbally describe their sexual behavior; this is one of the basic functions of qualitative research.

Finally, measures need to contain a representative sample of content from a specified domain; this is content validity. This aspect of validity is particularly relevant for measures of knowledge and attitudes: multiple questions are needed to adequately sample all the relevant areas of knowledge. For example, one would not want to assess the mathematical knowledge of college students with a single multiple–choice question. Similarly, the assessment of AIDS knowledge requires more than a single question.

MEASUREMENT QUALITY AND SCIENTIFIC INFERENCE

It is clear that some of the variables we utilize in research concerning AIDS

[14] D. Baltimore and M.B. Feinberg, "HIV revealed: toward a natural history of the infection," *New England Journal of Medicine* 321 (1989):1673–75.

Table 3-2. *Measure of partners and condom use among samples of the general population, prostitutes and homosexual/bisexual men in six Mexican cities, 1988.*

	General Population		Female Prostitutes	Gay and Bi-Sexual Men
	Men (N=350)	Women (300)	(700)	(715)
Average No. of sexual partner (last 4 months) (client partners)	1.0	0.7	216	4.0
Recognized a condom visually	88%	66%	94%	97%
Have ever used a condom	49%	34%	73%	60%
Use a condom at least once in last 4 month (last month)	19%	7%	57%	43%
Average No. of condoms used in last month	2.7	2.8	18.9	4.1
Used a condom in last intercourse	9%	3%	37%	30%
Willing to use a condom in next intercourse	50%	28%	85%	82%

prevention are measured with high reliability and validity, while others are lacking in one or more of these attributes. Limited reliability and validity of measures can significantly affect the inferences we can draw from scientific studies.

Perhaps the most serious effect of low reliability of measures is that relationships will be attenuated (e.g. a true correlation of 0.50 could be attenuated to 0.20 by an unreliable measure).[15] Predictive validity will decrease as measurement error in the predictor variable increases. One serious consequence of this type of measurement error is that researchers can conceivably report no association between a risk factor and disease, even though in fact one exists. If researchers are looking to test the "riskiness" of a particular sexual behavior (e.g. receptive anal sex), but individuals unreliably report this behavior (for many reasons, including stigma, forgetting, etc.), the chances of finding a relationship between the behavior and a measure of infection will be lowered as the reliability of the measure decreases.

Because we can quantify reliability, we know the levels of reliability at which this attenuation becomes an important concern: if the reliability of a measure is below .80 (and certainly below .70), this attenuation can significantly reduce the estimated relationship.[16] For example, because risky sexual behaviors are probably unreliably measured, we can assume that the reported associations between these behaviors and seroprevalence is probably attenuated. Similarly, we know that unreliability in the dependent measure can also weaken relationships.[17] In the present example, however, the reliability of the serological tests is well above .90 and thus the effects of unreliability in this measure should be minimal.

The effects of other aspects of poor measurement will also limit the inferences which can be drawn from studies. Poor construct validity may mean that measures are in fact tapping the wrong domain of behavior, as we saw above in the questions concerning sexual activity of prostitutes. In assuring construct validity, qualitative research is essential: sexual behaviors are still not well understood, and our ability to understand risky sexual behaviors and their modification are still severely limited by this lack of knowledge. There are enormous cultural and ethnic variations in sexual behaviors, in the language used to describe and speak of these behaviors, and very little of this has been systematically studied.

In spite of these imitations, we need to be very careful not to discard study results simply because of imperfect measures. As we have already noted, small effects can accumulate over time into large effects, and these small effects can sometimes be masked by poor measurement. Thus, even weak indications that a behavioral change program can be effective in reducing the risk of seroconversion can provide important clues to reduce the impact of the AIDS epidemic.

Even in the face of measurement problems we can at times come to clear policy implications. This is the situation with data concerning condom use

---

15 *Op. cit.* J. Nunnally.
16 *Ibid.*
17 *Ibid.*

among populations during risky practices such as receptive anal sex. A survey of homosexual and bisexual males in six cities in Mexico indicates that only about 30% used a condom during their last sexual encounter.[18] Low rates of condom use were also obtained from a survey of over 2000 individuals tested for HIV-1 at the one government run testing and counseling center in Mexico City.[19]

Based upon numerous prior studies of the reliability and validity of questions concerning condom use (particularly in fertility studies), we know that there are significant limitations to these quantitative measures—both gaps in reliability and validity. In addition to the problem of unreliable reporting of behavior, there is the issue of condom breakage, as well as other aspects of contraceptive failure.[20] However, it is important to recognize that even though these measures may be imperfect, we can still derive policy–relevant results by estimating the inaccuracies and by placing limits on our estimates. For example, we can assume that some individuals will overreport condom use in order to give a "socially desirable" response. Conversely, we can argue that underreporting of condom use occurs because of faulty recall (short–term memory). We may therefore assume that true estimates of use could be lower or higher than this 30%, perhaps ranging from 10% to 50%.

However, as has been pointed out by one study, changes in condom use of this order of magnitude (i.e. from 30% to 50% use) may not effect much of a long–term change in the risk of infection, although higher use rates of condoms should slow the course of the epidemic.[21] Certainly those individuals who always use condoms will be more protected, but to have a substantial impact on the course of the epidemic, much higher rates of condom use are required than those seen in these Mexican surveys.[22] Thus, in this example, poor measurement quality will not really affect a main policy implication: that rates of condom use in these populations from Mexico are too low, and need to be increased dramatically if the epidemic is to be halted via this preventive behavior.

---

[18] J.A. Izazola Licea, J.L. Valdespino Gomez, S.L. Gortmaker, J. Townsend, J. Becker, M. Palacios Martinez, N.E. Mueller, J. Sepulveda Amor, "HIV-1 seropositivity and behavioral and sociological risks among homosexual and bisexual males in six Mexican Cities," *Journal of Adquired Immunodeficiency Syndroms*, 4 (1991): 612-22.

[19] M. Hernandez, P. Uribe, S. Gortmaksa C. Avila, L. E. De Caso, M. Hernandez, P. Tovar, P. Garcia, S. Gortmaker, J. Sepulveda. "Sexual Behavior and Status for Human Immunodeficiency/virus type1 among homosexual and bisexual males in Mexico City," *American Journal of Epidemiology*, 135 (992): 883-94.

[20] J. Trussell and K. Kost, "Contraceptive failure in the United States: A critical review of the literature," *Studies in Family Planning* 18(5) (Sept./October 1987): 237–83.

[21] H.V. Fineberg, "Education to prevent AIDS: prospects and obstacles," *Science* 239(4840), (February 5, 1988): 592–6.

[22] *Ibid.*

A Mexican Case Study: Quantitative Measures of Bisexuality and Insertive and Receptive Behaviors

Some other problems with construct and predictive validity can be illustrated with recent data from Mexico: one topic of interest concerns both the definition and measurement of bisexuality. The second topic concerns the fact that measures of sexual practices may be confounded with the risk posed by different partner pools. For example, individuals practicing only insertive or only receptive anal sex may be interacting with partner pools that exhibit very different seroprevalences of HIV–1, and thus we may erroneously infer that these sexual behaviors are the only important risks, when in fact the associated serological status of the partner pool may be the more important causal factor.

Defining and Measuring Bisexuality

Sexual behavior is of great importance to the AIDS epidemic, yet scientific studies of these behaviors are quite limited. Sexual practices refer to whom sexual activity is done with, and sexual techniques refer to what is done among the subjects of sexual activity. Value judgments about sexual activity must be avoided, and the analysis and description of it must be carried out as objectively as possible. Many problems arise when trying to define practices, and even some commonly used terms are not clearly defined. For example, many studies report distinctions between bisexual and homosexual men, but this term is often used indiscriminately. Homosexuality/bisexuality/heterosexuality is a complex continuum variable, where preferences, conscious or unconscious, may or may not be reflected in sexual practices. What most often matters in the study of HIV/AIDS are the practices and the techniques and not the preferences. Thus, the variable of interest is often the sexual practice.

In different surveys among Mexican men with homosexual practices, heterosexual practices were present in varying degrees. For example, in a survey of 715 homosexual and bisexual men in six Mexican cities in May 1988, men were asked to define themselves according to whom they usually have sex with on a five point scale (from only with men to only with women). 39% reported they had sex with persons of both genders. When asked in a separate question about ever having sex with a female, 52% answered in the affirmative. In another question, 27% reported having sex with a female in the past year. Thus, heterosexual practices were reported more or less frequently than the reported "identity" depending upon the time frame used in recall.

Another issue in measuring "identity" is that some males playing the anal insertive role may not identify themselves as homosexuals.[23] Which method one uses to define bisexuality will depend on what is being looked for: measures of ever heterosexually active, recently heterosexually active, or self identification. Sometimes the number of sexual partners per each gender in a recent period is the most appropriate measure.

Measuring Insertive and Receptive Behavior

When measuring sexual techniques which can be seen as risk factors for acquiring HIV, caution must be used in interpreting associations of reported behaviors with HIV–1 seropositive status. For example, the major sexual risk for acquiring HIV–1 in gay and bisexual men has been reported as having unprotected anal receptive intercourse.[24] This increased risk has been explained on a physio–pathological and anatomical basis. However, it could also be the case that distinctive sociological networks of partners—partner pools—are associated with these behaviors, and that estimates of the risk of HIV–1 seroconversion associated with receptive anal intercourse are confounded with the risks posed by the serological status of these networks.

In Mexico it has been noted that there is significant stigma attached to an individual engaging in receptive anal intercourse:[25] Although the motivations of males participating in homosexual encounters are unquestionably diverse and complex, the fact remains that in Mexico cultural pressure is brought to bear on effeminate males to play the passive insertee role in sexual intercourse, and a kind of *de facto* cultural approval is given (that is, no particular stigma is attached to) masculine males who want to play the active inserter role in sexual intercourse.[26]

Therefore, it is very likely that there are distinctive pools of partners for those individuals practicing only insertive or only receptive anal sex in Mexico.

In order to differentiate these partner pools, in our studies in Mexico we have constructed a measure of insertive and receptive behavior (IRB) for anal intercourse according to reported practices in the previous four months: six categories are delineated: those with no or almost no activity, exclusively anal receptive, mainly receptive, both receptive and insertive half of the time or more ("mixed" behavior), mainly insertive and exclu-

---

[23] J.M. Carrier, "Participants in Urban Mexican Male Homosexual Encounters," *Archives of Sexual Behavior* 1(4) (1971):279–291; and J.M. Carrier, "Cultural Factors Affecting Urban Mexican Male Homosexual Behavior," *Archives of Sexual Behavior* 5(2) (1976):103–24.

[24] L.A. Kingsley, R. Kaslow, C.R. Rinaldo Jr. K. Detre, N. Odaka, M. Van Raden, R. Detels, B.F. Polk, J. Chmiel, S.F. Kelsey, D. Ostrow, B. Visscher, "Risk Factors for Seroconversion to Human Immunodeficiency Virus Among Male Homosexuals," *Lancet* (February 14, 1987): 345–348.

[25] *Op. cit.* J.M. Carrier, 1971; and *op. cit.* J.M. Carrier, 1976.

[26] *Ibid.*

sively insertive. The greatest prevalence of HIV–1 infection was associated with mixed behavior.[27] Conversely, low seroprevalences were found among those practicing either exclusively insertive or exclusively receptive anal sex. Two explanations can be given for these findings: one is that "mixed" behavior could more efficiently transmit the virus from partner to partner, and hence the mixed partner pool could have a greater reservoir of infection. A second explanation is that individuals practicing only receptive behavior could be having sex with individuals with lower seroprevalence rates of HIV–1, including those practicing only insertive behavior, and those who identify themselves as heterosexual.[28]

In describing and measuring sexual behaviors, other factors beyond those already discussed need to be taken into account. Often individuals do not practice a single pattern of sexual techniques; combinations of techniques are common. For oral–genital and anal intercourse, two roles may be played, isolated or mixed: insertive and receptive, protected or unprotected (through condom use) and with or without ejaculation (through *coitus interruptus*). It can be imagined that the possibilities also vary from partner to partner. The risks associated with all these varieties of practice have not been clearly delineated.

LIMITATIONS POSED BY WEAK RESEARCH DESIGNS

While poor quantitative measurement can impair our scientific understanding of behavioral issues concerning AIDS, the most serious threat probably comes from the lack of strong research designs which permit clear causal inferences to be drawn. Problems with these designs include nonprobability samples, non–experimental research, lack of random assignment to treatment, and a lack of attention to issues of efficacy, effectiveness, and efficiency.

THE DIFFICULTY OF CONSTRUCTING RANDOM SAMPLES

A major issue with respect to studies of risk groups such as prostitutes, homosexuals, bisexuals, intravenous drug users and their sexual partners is the difficulty of assembling population–based sampling frames from which to draw true probability samples—ideally simple random samples. Often samples are based upon frames constructed upon geographic locales where risk groups gather: bars, discos, parks, hotels, shooting galleries, etc. The

[27] *Op. cit.* J.A. Izazola Licea *et al.* Manuscript under review.
[28] *Ibid.*

biases in estimates produced because of these sampling frames are often unknown.[29]

NON-EXPERIMENTAL RESEARCH AND EVALUATION DESIGNS

Non-experimental designs for research are those in which the investigator does not explicitly manipulate the treatment or variable under investigation.[30] For example, this could be a behavior, an educational intervention, or a new preventive behavior program. Unfortunately, almost all of the knowledge we have to date concerning the HIV epidemic comes from research which is non-experimental in nature (see table of reported studies in Becker and Joseph, 1988).

With non-experimental designs it becomes very difficult to make clear causal inferences concerning the effectiveness of intervention programs. For example, it has been reported that the behavioral changes seen in some gay and bisexual populations may be "the most rapid and profound response to a health threat which has ever been documented."[31] However, because of the (unavoidably) non-experimental nature of this research, it is unclear just what causal factor changed behavior. Was the change caused by people knowing via the media that there was a severe health threat, and these individuals then acting accordingly? If this were the case, then perhaps we have some evidence that increases in knowledge in the population leads to behavior change. A counter hypothesis, however, might suggest that dramatic changes in the behavior of gay and bisexual males in certain locales could have been more profoundly influenced by the very substantial seroprevalence in the local population, and the many AIDS cases which had already appeared. No one would want to suggest that an effective intervention for behavior change would be to wait for a population seroprevalence rate to increase to 30%.

Besides the lack of experimental data, few studies of behavioral interventions randomly assign participants to treatment conditions. This lack of control also significantly impairs our ability to evaluate the effectiveness of behavioral change programs to reduce the spread of HIV–1. While substantial knowledge can result from poorly controlled experimental or even non-experimental studies (witness the very substantial knowledge we have concerning economic science: a discipline based almost entirely upon non-experimental or quasi–experimental studies), the fact remains that many of

[29] S. Sudman, *Applied Sampling* (New York: Academic Press, 1976).

[30] T.D. Cook and D.T. Campbell, *Quasi–Experimentation: Design and Analysis Issues for Field Settings* (Boston, M. A.: Houghton Mifflin Company, 1979).

[31] *Op. cit.* M. H. Becker and J.G. Joseph.

the effects observed in behavioral interventions are often relatively small, and weak designs make it more difficult to detect small effects.[32] Weak experimental designs as well as poor quality measurement can thus make it difficult to substantiate the effectiveness of social and behavioral intervention programs.

EFFECTIVENESS AND EFFICIENCY

Another advantage to quantitative behavioral studies is that estimates of cost effectiveness can be calculated.[33] This issue is extremely important for the evaluation of behavioral interventions which can be personnel intensive and which can demonstrate relatively low levels of effectiveness. Some behavioral change interventions may be quite feasible and effective but very expensive.

A related issue concerns the targeting of intervention groups. It sometimes may be more cost–effective to offer help to individuals who seek it versus spending substantial resources in outreach programs if difficult–to–reach subjects also fail to comply with interventions. If the risk is great enough, however, extensive outreach may be called for because of the relative isolation of high-risk groups.

PREVENTION IMPLICATIONS OF QUANTITATIVE MODELS

In spite of the limitations posed by poor measurement, non–random samples and weak research designs, quantitative behavioral models can provide important insights into the causal processes underlying the AIDS epidemic. One such model has been constructed by making a series of assumptions regarding the risk of infection with HIV–1 from a single unprotected anal sexual exposure, and the level of effectiveness of protection afforded by condom use. This model of the cumulative probability of infection affords us an indication of the relative impact of three determinants of the risk of infection:

- the prevalence of HIV–1 among the available partner pool,
- the frequency of condom use, and
- the number of sexual partners.[34]

---

[32] Op. cit. Gilbert, Light and Mostelle.

[33] M.C. Weinstein, J.D. Graham, J.E. Siegel, H.V. Fineberg, "Cost-effectiveness analysis of AIDS prevention programs: concepts, complications, and illustrations," in *AIDS: Sexual Behavior and Intravenous Drug Use*, eds. C.F. Turner, H.G. Miller and L.E. Moses (Washington D.C.: National Academy Press, 1989).

[34] Op. cit. H.V. Fineberg.

Table 3-3. *Cumulative probability of HIV-1 infection from 1000 sexual exposures.[1]*

Prevalence of HIV–1 among potential partners	Frequency of Condom Use		
	Never	Half the time	Always
	One partner		
0.01	0.01	0.01	0.006
0.50	0.50	0.50	0.32
	Five partners		
0.01	0.04	0.03	0.009
0.50	0.94	0.87	0.38
	Fifty partners		
0.01	0.09	0.05	0.01
0.50	0.99	0.93	0.39

[1] Assumptions include: 1) risk of infection from a single unprotected exposure = .01; 2) reduction in risk per exposure through use of condoms = .89; 3.) prevalence of HIV-1 among potential partners is constant and selection of partners is random with respect to their probability of infection.
SOURCE: adapted from H.V. Fineberg, "Education to prevent AIDS: Prospects and obstacles," *Science* 239 (4840) (February 5, 1988): 592-6.

Some predictions of this simple model are tabulated in Table 3-3. They indicate the extreme behaviors that are needed to reduce the risk of infection by a single individual (particularly when the HIV–1 prevalence in the partner pool is 50%—remember that it only takes one exposure for the possibility of transmission). This model also indicates that condom use can reduce risk, but that if HIV–1 is prevalent in the partner pool the risk may still be substantial (because of the imperfect effectiveness of condoms.) While these changes in individual risk can be quite small, the impact of such change on slowing the course of the epidemic could be more substantial.[35]

While this mathematical model is extremely limited, and depends upon the validity of the underlying assumptions, the model's implications are suggestive and point out important areas for research. Recent studies of our own in Mexico using mutivariate logistic regression models indicate the limited predictive value of condom use and numbers of sexual partners, and the substantial predictive value of the infection rate among local partner pools.[36] Other models indicate greater effectiveness of condom use among subpopulations, e.g. among adolescents.[37]

[35] *Ibid*.
[36] *Op. cit.* J.A. Izazola Licea *et al*. Manuscript under review.
[37] *Op. cit.* M.C. Weinstein *et al*.

If the predictions of this model are at all accurate, there are important implications for AIDS campaigns. A common recommendation of education and behavioral change campaigns is to limit the number of sexual partners as a means of reducing the risk of HIV–1 infection. The effect upon risk of seroconversion of reducing the number of partners from 50 to five, although the change sounds dramatic, can actually be relatively small, as indicated in Table 3-3. The key behavioral issue for individuals is not just to reduce their partners, but to reduce their contacts with infectious partners. Unfortunately, data concerning infectivity are not often known to either the researcher or the individual, and often only crude sociological or behavioral indicators are available.

LIMITATIONS OF INTERVENTIONS AND THE IMPORTANCE OF PROCESS EVALUATION

While limited measurement and weak research designs hinder the development of programs to slow the HIV epidemic, a lack of powerful intervention strategies is at the root of the difficulties. While it is quite clear that risky behaviors have dramatically changed in some populations, and some information programs have been effective in increasing knowledge, no powerful, low-cost interventions have been documented. Part of the problem is the complexity of the human behavior change required and the biological roots of these behaviors, as well as the extreme behavioral changes needed to substantially slow the epidemic.[38]

In the search for more effective intervention programs, it is important not to focus all effort upon mere outcome prediction. Behavioral change is a complex process, and attention to measurement of the process of change can reap dividends in terms of improved understanding and improved program effectiveness. Process evaluations can provide more sensitive measures of program achievements which can lead to an understanding of how behavioral change occurred.

Evaluation of behavioral change programs can take place at three levels: in terms of process, in terms of impact and in terms of outcome. In process evaluation the object of interest is professional practice; quality aspects may be monitored through various means such as audit, peer review, accreditation, certification and government or administrative surveillance of contracts or grants. Standards of acceptability can be established by means of consensus among health education specialists.

Impact evaluation of a program refers to the immediate results of the program, in specific behaviors and/or in their predisposing, enabling and

---

[38] *Op cit*. H.V. Fineberg, 1988.

reinforcing factors: for example, knowledge and attitudes related to contributory behaviors to the health problem, or the practice itself of this behavior, such as the availability and accessibility of condoms or sterile syringes.

The final objective of behavioral intervention programs is to decrease the incidence of a health problem and thus acquire a social benefit. In the case of HIV/AIDS, an important goal is to decrease new infections, but also to decrease the socio–psychological impact for those already infected, to slow the progress of AIDS in an infected individual and alleviate the social impact of AIDS cases and deaths.

LINKING RESEARCH AND POLICY

While quantitative research can provide important insights and results in reportable data, these results do not often easily translate into effective programs or policies. For example, KAP surveys can indicate deficient knowledge in the population, but this identification is only a first step in building an effective education program. One useful framework to employ in planning health education and behavior change programs is the PRECEDE model.[39] This model has seven phases:

- Phase 1: Assessment of quality of life concerns.
- Phase 2: Identification of those specific health problems that appear to be contributing to the social problems noted in phase 1.
- Phase 3: Identification of the specific health–related behaviors that appear to be linked to the health problem chosen as deserving of most attention in phase 2.
- Phase 4: Identify three classes of factors that have potential for affecting health behavior: predisposing, enabling and reinforcing factors.
- Phase 5: Selection of the specific factors to be focused on in an educational intervention;
- Phase 6: Development and implementation of the program.
- Phase 7: Evaluation.

This algorithm is based on two basic propositions: that health and health behavior are caused by multiple factors, and that health education efforts to affect behavior must be multidimensional.[40] The beginning step is an epidemiological and social diagnosis of health and non–health factors

---

[39] L.W. Green, M.W. Kreuuter, S.G. Deeds, K.B. Partridge, *Health Education Planning: A Diagnostic Approach* (Mountain View California: Mayfield Publishing Company, 1980).
[40] *Ibid.*

affecting quality of life, and proceeds backward through behavioral, educational and administrative diagnoses to identify the desired content and delivery of a program. Epidemiological methods and information are the basis for the first, second and part of the third phases described above; social and behavioral theory and concepts are used for phases three through six, and the evaluation utilizes quantitative and qualitative methods. Quantitative research, in the case of HIV/AIDS, may be used to identify specific behavioral factors that contribute to the disease, e.g. particular sexual behaviors, partner pools, intravenous drug use, etc.

Each individual or social behavior is influenced by a set of factors that are labeled as predisposing if they provide the motivation for the behavior, enabling if they allow the motivation to be realized, and reinforcing if they provide the incentives, rewards or punishments that maintain or stop continuation of the behavior (see Table 3-4).

Factors and behaviors can be classified by their importance for the disease and by their degree of changeability. Estimates of changeability are arrived at via evaluation of previous programs. Changeability and importance of the behaviors can also be determined through the theory of diffusion of innovations, where behavior change is analyzed over time, and the stages by which behavior is adopted. The stages individuals pass through are "awareness," "interest," "trial," "decision" and "adoption," and the individuals may be innovators, early adopters, early majority or late majority. Behavioral influences may be individual, institutional or social: for instance, availability of condoms is a social or institutional characteristic that contributes to the frequency of unprotected sexual intercourse as an enabling factor.

CONCLUDING THOUGHTS

Quantitative behavioral measures and models have substantively improved our understanding of the magnitude and course of the HIV-1 epidemic, and have led to the identification of risk factors for infection. Problems with the validity and reliability of behavioral measures—particularly behavioral measures of sexual activity—often impose severe limits on our ability to interpret study results. We thus need to be careful in interpreting risk factor estimates: measurement error can lead to an attenuation of associations, and this means we could unknowingly be discounting the impor-tance of some risks.

Poor construct validity may mean that we are not measuring the aspects of sexual behavior of greatest importance: new qualitative and quantitative research is needed to further our understanding of the limits of currently available measurement approaches.

Table 3-4. *Selected predisposing, enabling and reinforcing factors related to unprotected sexual intercourse that contributes to HIV transmission.*

Importance	Changeability	Factors	Behavior	
		Predisposing		
Medium	High	Lack of knowledge of paths of HIV infection	U N	
High	High	Lack of knowledge of condom use as a preventive measure	P R	
High	High	Belief that condoms fail	O	I
High	Medium	Unwillingness to use condoms	T	N
Medium	Low	Religious beliefs	E	T
Medium-High	Low	Demographic variables	C	E
		Enabling	T	R
High	High	Availability and accessibility of condoms	E D	C O
High	High	Skills in proper condom use		U
Medium	Medium	Cost of condoms	S	R
		Reinforcing	E	S
High	Medium	Partner reaction and fear of it	X U	E
High	Medium	Bad previous experiences with condoms	A L	
Medium	Low	Media emission of "not-proven news"		
Medium	Medium	Alcohol and drug use		

Better sampling methods and stronger intervention and evaluation designs need to be developed and implemented. Low cost and effective interventions must be a high priority for future behavioral studies.

This research has been supported by an ICAR grant (PO1 AI26487) from NIAID, National Institute of Health. The Ministry of Health, Mexico, The Population Council under contract C187.32A, and the Fogarty International Center, National Institutes of Health, Program of International Training Grants in Epidemiology Related to AIDS, grant D43TW00004 supported the time of Dr. Izazola.

The Role of Qualitative Research in AIDS Prevention

William A. Smith
Mary Debus

The AIDS epidemic dramatizes what we do not yet know about human sexuality, exposing the limitations of our behavioral research technology and challenging us to develop new ways to learn about some of humanity's most private and taboo behaviors. To help people protect themselves from HIV infection we must offer alternative practices which are acceptable to those at risk. We must present information in ways which not only inform but persuade. We must find the means to overcome fear, prejudice and denial among groups of people who feel victimized and ostracized by society as a whole. This task requires not only good epidemiology and excellent survey research; it demands that we find new ways to collect data and understand the relationship of knowledge and attitudes to the behaviors which place people at risk of HIV infection.

This chapter provides an overview of qualitative research—a group of techniques which were developed to gain deeper insight into human behavior—and makes the case that integrating qualitative research with quantitative techniques in an AIDS education program will significantly enhance our understanding of how to promote AIDS prevention.

For the purpose of this chapter, qualitative research will be defined as the use of in–depth interviewing and observational techniques on small samples of target groups to investigate the attitudes, beliefs and social contexts associated with human behavior. Qualitative approaches have evolved from several disparate fields of inquiry. Anthropology has contri-

57

buted techniques such as in–depth interviews, participant observation and ethnographies, which were traditionally used to understand communities and the context of social interaction. Social marketing has added techniques such as focus group interviews, its own version of in–depth interviews, and tracking studies for the monitoring of advertising impact. Behavioral psychology has contributed observation studies, while other social sciences have developed case study and documentary techniques which are part of the evolving qualitative methodology.

In the last ten years, education and communication specialists have adopted many of these techniques to complement quantitative research. These qualitative approaches provide insight into complex beliefs and behaviors and can help to increase our understanding of the antecedent and consequence factors which influence behavior and behavior change. Because qualitative techniques use small samples of people, researchers often have the luxury of flexibility and depth of inquiry. However, care must be taken when attempting to generalize conclusions from these data. Qualitative researchers can expand beyond the frameworks required of quantitative techniques but they must also be respectful of the limitations of subjectivity. Qualitative data is "attractive... a source of well–grounded, rich descriptions and explanations of processes occurring in local contexts... [which] preserve chronological flow, assess local causality, and derive fruitful explanations."[1]

Qualitative techniques can be useful to understand the context and language of behavior in a community, using ethnographies to observe and interact within a neighborhood setting. For example, how are young boys "initiated" into sexual behavior and what language is used when they try out these new skills? Qualitative techniques can be used to generate hypotheses about a problem. For example, why do adolescents feel particularly invulnerable to the risks of HIV infection? Data from qualitative research can aid the development of a questionnaire for a large–scale study of adolescent behavior to generate concepts and strategy for a communication program directed at adolescents. Once the strategy is developed, "concept testing" can help to try out a specific approach with a targeted segment of adolescents. Messages and materials are then produced in draft form. Once again, qualitative techniques can be utilized to pretest those messages and materials to ensure that they are appropriate for a specific segment of adolescents and that they have the intended impact. Finally, qualitative research can be used to monitor or track the development of a program over time, using rapid assessment techniques to check for flaws or identify changing audience response.

[1] Miles and Huberman (1984).

This chapter will describe the practical usefulness of qualitative research in an AIDS prevention education program. Examples from two case studies will be given showing how two kinds of qualitative research can be used to learn about specific behaviors in a particular target group. The program areas in which qualitative research techniques can be usefully employed within an AIDS prevention program will be discussed. It will describe several qualitative techniques and lay out a set of criteria against which the authors believe qualitative research should be measured. It will not attempt to duplicate other excellent manuals on how to conduct qualitative research. The reader who wishes a greater understanding of how to collect and analyze qualitative data should refer to the bibliography at the end of this chapter for a list of recommended texts on qualitative methods.

This chapter is a plea for the integration of qualitative and quantitative studies. The combination of techniques will enable us to develop more accurate and sensitive understanding of HIV–related behavior. This chapter aims to demonstrate how and why qualitative research can complement the already extensive agenda of quantitative studies on AIDS prevention and education programs.

WHAT IS QUALITATIVE RESEARCH?

Qualitative research is holistic. It is also inductive, context–based and narrative. It uses small samples studied in great depth. It is holistic because it provides information and insight into a wide variety of aspects of a situation. This allows the research to assemble a more complete picture of an event. For example, many women who practice prostitution are also mothers. Their self–image as women, professionals, and mothers often differs from that which society as a whole has developed to describe their behavior. To understand to what lengths these women might go to protect themselves and their clients from HIV infection, we must understand them as people with many facets to their lives. Qualitative research also helps to determine not only what happened (e.g. that a condom was not used in the last sexual encounter) but also what led up to the event and what followed it (e.g. she tried to find one but couldn't; she wanted to use the condom but the partner refused; she wanted to use it but felt embarrassed to mention it).

Qualitative research is inductive. It does not begin with all the variables clearly defined. It imposes fewer concrete expectations on the study situation than survey research and therefore increases the chance of finding unanticipated outcomes. Often a topic guide is prepared by the qualitative researcher but the order of questions is not fixed and the discussion follows unexpected leads that arise during the interview. During in–depth interviews with adolescent men regarding dating practices, the subject of condoms came up unexpectedly. These men revealed during probing questioning that what truly bothered them about using condoms was neither discomfort, the lack of sensation, nor the inconvenience, but rather the fear that they would not be able to perform adequately. Direct questioning about condom attitudes had not revealed this insight.

Qualitative research is also context–based. It uses observations and in–depth interviews under conditions that are as natural as possible. If the goal is to understand why female sex workers use condoms and the alternatives are to interview these women at STD clinics or in their places of work, the qualitative researcher would almost always choose the place of work. The assumption is that people feel more at ease and in control in their own environments and are therefore more likely to be comfortable talking about sensitive subjects.

Qualitative analysis is also narrative rather than numerical. Data are not summarized as "percentage of respondents who," but rather as themes which recur, insights which emerge, ideas which may explain why someone feels at risk or why he or she may deny personal risk. For example, rather than report that "80 percent of women responded that men don't like condoms," the text of a qualitative report might be phrased, "Women in the groups often mentioned that they feel powerless if the man doesn't want to use a condom."

Like quantitative research, the interpretation of qualitative data requires an experienced analyst. The majority of qualitative analysis is done by hand immediately after the interview. There are many examples of summary forms which are particularly useful for the initial steps of data analysis.[2] The need for immediate analysis is primarily to capture the feeling of participants' responses. Rapid data analysis also makes results available to help guide future research. One significant difference between qualitative and quantitative research is that with the former, the goal is not "significance" but an emerging and consistent pattern. Once this goal has been reached in a particular subject area (behavior or belief), the researcher has the luxury of omitting it from future topic guides. Using qualitative techniques is similar to learning a language or filling in a jigsaw puzzle. Once researchers understand the syntax and how new pieces of information fit together with others they have heard, they can reasonably assume that a part of the "puzzle" is solved.

Finally, qualitative research typically uses small samples. Observation studies, for example, while not particularly inductive, are qualitative because they try to observe small samples of behavior under naturalistic

[2] Miles and Huberman (1984).

conditions. The small sample size permits investigators to conduct research under conditions which allow for analysis of complete detail, unrestricted by the constraints of having to replicate the research event (question or observation) hundreds of times. Ethnographies are conducted in communities by anthropologists who observe small samples of people in great detail. They combine in–depth interviewing and participant observation skills, and make use of the local context and language. Ethnographies are particularly helpful to understand the antecedents and consequences of behavior because they often span a longer period of time than quantitative research techniques.

In sum, qualitative research is open–ended and unbounded by predetermined variables. It is contextual. It is summarized by narrative rather than numerical statements. Large sample sizes are not required. For the most part, it is characterized by in–depth interviews and observation studies.

The next section of this chapter will describe these two methods and give examples of how in–depth interviews and observation studies are used to elicit information which could be useful for an AIDS prevention education program.

TWO QUALITATIVE RESEARCH TECHNIQUES: IN–DEPTH INTERVIEWS AND OBSERVATION

Interviews

Interviews include both in–depth individual interviews and group interview techniques, ranging from conversational formats, to counseling encounters, to projective techniques. The reader may be more familiar with interviewing in conversational or counseling formats. Popular projective techniques include role playing of key interactions and association techniques, in which an individual is asked to relate one word to another, or to complete a sentence. Cartoon completion and storytelling allow participants to discuss and interpret experiences. Thematic aperception tests ask participants to create stories based on the presentation of selected pictures. The roles, sentences, cartoons or pictures used in projective and association techniques are carefully chosen to elicit information in an open–ended but structured sequence.

In an interview, the selection of questions, the sequences in which they are presented, the setting in which they are asked, and the skill with which a mediator can probe and follow up an answer without leading to a conditioned response, are fundamental to qualitative success. An interview often lasts up to one and one half hours and may or may not cover all the topics listed on the topic guide. A researcher may go back to the same respondent several times over the course of a few days to complete or follow up on the discussion for clarification.

Group interviewing has become particularly popular through the focus group format. The focus group evolved from group therapy practices. It has been used for many years in marketing and is being used in ethnographic studies (the study of communities) as well. Although methods and applications of focus groups vary widely, basic principles and quality standards can be described.

There is general agreement that focus groups work best with eight to twelve individuals who represent a narrow, homogeneous segment of the population to be studied (for example, gay men with multiple partners or sexually active females, grouped into users and nonusers of condoms). Recruitment is an important factor in good focus group research. As in any study, participants must be "well qualified" and actually represent the study group under investigation. Poorly selected respondents can produce misleading results. A trained interviewer uses a topic guide to explore individual and group feelings and experiences. It is imperative that the moderator be unbiased, skillful in group facilitation, and familiar with the subject matter and research objectives. Focus groups are most useful when a wide range of information is needed, when group discussion may facilitate thinking or help reduce personal inhibitions, and when speedy data collection is desirable.

Observation

Observation studies constitute a second category of qualitative research. They help to describe the setting of a particular event, the event itself, the people who participate in the event, and the timing, frequency and sequence of events which both precede and follow the specific event being studied. Observation studies can employ a range of techniques. These are often broken down into two categories: participant observation, in which the observer also participates in the activity; and covert observation in which the observer is hidden behind a one–way mirror or other device which screens his or her presence from the group. Much debate has raged over the relative merits of each technique.[3]

Observational studies also vary in terms of their purposes. Some are designed to enumerate the details of an event in order to examine how that behavior is carried out and reinforced. Other observation studies have more in common with an ethnographic approach, in which the setting or "culture" of the event is of principal importance. All of these approaches can be

---

[3] For further discussion on this issue see J.P. Spradley, *Participant Observation* (New York: Reinholt and Winston, 1980); and M.Q. Patton, *Qualitative Evaluation Methods* (Beverly Hills, CA: Sage Publications, 1980).

useful in the study of HIV–related behavior (although some require considerable ingenuity in their undertaking).

There are many uses for observation techniques in an HIV–related study, such as observing pick–up techniques in bars to determine how safe–sex behavior might be introduced; observing physician/patient interactions[4] to improve the quality and amount of counseling provided; and conducting longitudinal observations of HIV–infected people in their communities to see how they are cared for or ostracized, to study community care and possible transmission.

Two Case Studies

Each technique, whether individual or group, observation or interview, has its own standards of rigor and quality. Each must be understood as a separate qualitative method useful for specific purposes and applicable to specific settings. This section will present two case studies. The first is a hypothetical example of how in–depth interviews can be used to understand why a woman at high risk of infection might choose not to use a condom to protect herself. The second example is a real life study conducted in the Dominican Republic which demonstrates the use of observation techniques in a simulated exercise to understand condom use among female sex workers at high risk of HIV infection.

Case Study #1:
Maria's Story, A Hypothetical Example

Our heroine is named Maria. She is 18 years old and lives in a large Latin American city. Maria is unmarried, but she is the mother of a two–year–old daughter named Consuelo. Maria is also a prostitute, a professional sex worker.

Maria knows the basic facts about AIDS; she knows condoms can provide protection. She has a ready supply of condoms on her dressing table. And she has heard radio broadcasts which report that many women like herself, in her own community, are already infected with the AIDS virus. Yet she has decided for some reason not to use that knowledge to protect herself. Clearly there is some critical gap between Maria's knowledge and her practices.

Our present understanding of AIDS and its impact on people who practice high–risk behaviors suggests that three factors may help to explain Maria's decision. First, even though Maria knows about AIDS, she herself may not feel susceptible to infection; she may not feel at personal risk. In study after study we continue to find people who know about AIDS and who are prac-

4 Roter (1984).

ticing high–risk behaviors, who say things like, "AIDS No, not me—it won't happen to me. Who knows if AIDS is real anyway?" A second hypothesis to explain Maria's behavior is that she doesn't feel AIDS is as serious as other problems in her life. The loss of her livelihood, the inability to support her daughter, and her self–esteem as a working woman may take priority in Maria's life even over the threat of death. Death seems remote and distant to Maria; it is not sufficiently concrete to seem to be a real threat.

A third explanation centers on Maria's feelings toward condoms. Maria may feel at risk—she may even take AIDS seriously—but if she does not like or trust condoms, she may fail to use them to protect herself.

A personal sense of susceptibility, the perceived seriousness of the consequences, and the attractiveness or practicality of a proposed solution such as condoms—these are three of many possible explanations for Maria's behavior. Each explanation, however, leads us towards a quite different educational intervention. The first view should make us ask ourselves if, as educators, we should personalize the risks of a behavior. The second would challenge us to dramatize the deadly consequences of the behavior. The third would suggest we improve the image of condoms or the product itself.

In order to decide what specific educational intervention would be effective for a woman like Maria, we might invite her to participate in a qualitative in–depth interview. In such an interview, Maria would first be asked to complete the sentence: "When I think about AIDS, the thing I worry about most is..."

Maria's first answer would be followed by a series of spontaneous probing questions, such as: "Why do you feel that way?" "Tell me more about that." "Can you think of other reactions you have had in the past?" Second, using a projective technique, Maria would be shown photos showing two sets of couples. While she was looking at the pictures, she would be asked: "Which of these couples do you think will use a condom tonight?" This would be followed by probing questions such as: "Why do you think so, Maria?" "Tell me more about the couple on the right." "What about the other couple?"

Viewing these pictures, Maria might have responded that the couple on the left would use condoms. She might have explained that the couple on the right "look like lovers... like steady partners...they have been together for several months." She might have remarked several times during the interview that "lovers don't need condoms."

Next, a laddering technique would be used, in which a series of questions would move Maria backward in time from a key event. This "laddering" approach helps to reveal how Maria perceives the event and its relationship to other important facets of her life. The interview would continue with the following questions: "Maria, what would happen if you got AIDS?" Maria's first answer might be: "I might die." Follow–up questions would include: "What would happen right before you die? What would happen to your friends? To your family? To your daughter?"

The technique of laddering is particularly useful in establishing links between factors not immediately obvious to the interviewers or program directors. In the interview, Maria might have mentioned her daughter over and over again. "My daughter, she's the only thing that's really mine... What would happen to Consuelo if I got AIDS?"

These techniques and others would reveal that Maria feared AIDS, but that she worried more about her daughter than herself. She seemed to trust condoms, but didn't think they were necessary with a steady partner. In fact, the study would reveal that the reason Maria selectively used condoms with some men and not with others is that she had told herself that her "steady" partners wouldn't be infected with AIDS, and therefore if she continued to see a man for several months she would "know" he was safe.

This in–depth interview and others like it would give program planners insight into behavior among other women like Maria which could then be developed into concepts to test on a larger scale and ultimately lead to an educational program.

Case Study #2:
Condom Proficiency among Women who Practice High Risk Behavior in the Dominican Republic

The National AIDS Control Program in the Dominican Republic had been aggressively distributing condoms to female prostitutes throughout the island for several years. Educational materials were principally focused on motivational appeals—why condoms are necessary. Usage levels had risen but not as rapidly as program directors expected or wanted and anecdotal data suggested that women believed condoms broke very easily and very frequently. The program directors suspected that condom proficiency, that is, the dexterity with which a person placed and removed a condom, might be influencing the perception or the reality of condom breakage. They hypothesized: if a woman or her partner is unfamiliar with how to put on and take off a condom, she or he might be more prone to break the condom and therefore more reluctant to use one in the future. The problem became: How could such behavior as condom use be studied?

Aside from "participant observation" methods which seemed impracti-cal for such a private behavior as condom use, three options remained: self–reports, covert observation or simulation. Self–reports of behavior were eliminated for their predictable lack of validity. Covert observational studies, using a one–way mirror to observe sexual encounters, were considered unethical and unacceptable to program directors. A group of simulation studies, in which a plastic model of a penis would act as a surrogate, was a potential solution. Women could be asked to demonstrate how they would put on and take off the condom using the surrogate model. A detailed observation guide was created, including 23 specific skills to observe and code.

Three distinct groups of women were identified and included in the study: sex workers in brothels; salaried sex workers located at bars, hotel cafeterias and restaurants; and sex workers working on their own or as street walkers. The study was conducted in work–place environments. The women who participated were asked to carry out a demonstration consisting of placing a condom on an artificial penis, to determine whether or not the correct procedure was followed. The researchers were trained through activities which also tested the observation guide and developed quick coding procedures.

The coding consisted of a set of behavioral options, such as:

- Women had long finger nails?   Yes   No
- Women unrolled condom before
  placing on model?   Yes   No
- Women covered (? %) of the
  model with condom?   25%   50%   75%   100%

The interviewers were taught to check appropriate blanks while observing each participant. This part of the process proved quite simple, but required several practice sessions.

The biggest difficulty was imparting the interpersonal skills to researchers to help them set participants at ease during the interview and observation. Some participants were amused when the model was shown, others didn't like touching the condoms, others were casual and facile with the exercise. But all the female respondents found the exercise unusual, and needed to be supported in one way or another as they went through the steps.

The results of this simulation exercise showed that most of the women placed the condom incorrectly in several ways. This included unrolling the condom and re–rolling it completely with their fingertips before placing it on the model, much like they would a stocking. Seven percent of the condoms broke during this unrolling process. This was the most important finding of the research and led to a totally unanticipated but vital educational effort on condom usage, including the creation of a simple visual instruction stressing that a condom should not be unrolled before placing it on the penis.

OTHER APPLICATIONS OF QUALITATIVE RESEARCH FOR EDUCATION AND COMMUNICATION FOR AIDS PREVENTION

The AIDS educator has thousands of possible messages, approaches, and channels. But which is best for a given population? We have seen that qualitative techniques can help to examine a behavioral problem within its social context. But qualitative research also provides a means for concept testing, and for pretesting specific messages and materials. While detailed discussion of these areas is beyond the scope of this text, a brief overview will illuminate the usefulness of concept testing and pretesting for the AIDS educator.

Concept Testing

Concept testing is "a market research technique used to evaluate a concept's potential and to discover ways of improving it. A concept test involves exposing an idea to consumers and getting their reaction to it... [their] emotions, reactions and opinions."[5]

Concept testing can be used to test ideas, tactics and strategies, such as whether or not to promote the concept that "steady" sex partners need to practice safe sex, and how condoms should be promoted as a protective device for this target group. The following are examples of questions concept testing can be used to help answer:

- Are adolescents more motivated by "fun" appeals or by peer identification?
- Which of the different roles (mother, casual partner, steady partner) could women play to increase their effectiveness as AIDS educators?
- What is the optimum price of condoms for the low income user?

Concept testing can also be used to discuss an embarrassing topic that requires sensitivity and rapport. For example, how can married bisexual men be urged to consider the risk posed to their spouses? It is useful to understand how a particular action or behavior fits into a whole pattern. For example, what is the range of unsafe sexual experience of newly recruited sex workers?

Concept testing is useful when creating a questionnaire for a large sample survey. It can help to identify the vocabulary, concepts, and even some of the multiple choice answers in quantitative studies. For example, it is important to know what words will most clearly distinguish between condom use in receptive versus insertive sexual partners among a specific group of bisexual men. Qualitative studies can explore this vocabulary in simpler ways than surveys can. Finally, these techniques can be useful to

[5] D. Schwartz, *Concept Testing* (New York: American Management Association, 1987).

understand the results of a survey. For example, consider the finding that intravenous drug users commonly share needles despite high levels of knowledge that this is extremely risky behavior. Focus groups or in–depth interviews may illuminate why these people ignore their own knowledge.

Pretesting

Pretesting, on the other hand, is a systematic process of testing target audience reactions to specific messages, vocabulary, visuals, sequences and materials before they are produced in final form. Pretesting allows programmers to determine if materials are clear, persuasive, attractive, and seen as relevant among a particular audience.

The sequence and presentation of materials or messages for testing in focus groups or individual interviews is critical. Several formats are available to program designers. Comparative tests, in which several alternative formats are shown at once, help to identify those images which stand out from the others. The order in which different treatments are presented must be varied from individual to individual, so the sequence of presentation does not influence results. The visual quality of the material being pretested need not be as high as that of the final product —draft art work is adequate for this purpose— but the quality must be high enough to communicate the central ideas clearly and effectively.

In Trinidad and Tobago, a condom brochure was tested in a series of in–depth interviews and focus groups. The results of the pretesting exercise contributed to significant changes in the condom brochure. Comments on the first version, showing a picture of a condom and the words "STOP AIDS," included:

- The picture of the condom on the front and back did not look like a condom.
- The wording "STOP AIDS" was inappropriate because participants thought it was impossible to "stop" AIDS. The recommendation was made for a more positive approach, such as "PROTECT YOURSELF."
- Since most participants were unfamiliar with condoms, they thought that specific suggestions on how to use them would be helpful.

Changes were made and a second version was produced after the pretesting exercise that reflects these important perceptions.

THE LIMITATIONS OF QUALITATIVE RESEARCH

Interpretations of qualitative research data are subject to important limitations. The first and most obvious concern is researcher bias. The predisposition of a researcher toward a given area of study can affect his or her conduct of the study and the subsequent interpretation of the narrative results. This is particularly true with subject matter as sensitive and personal as sexual practice. Qualitative research often brings the interviewer into close contact with the study situation. A person researching sexual practices may find the practice of some behaviors unexpectedly distasteful when first encountered. A competent qualitative researcher does not display approval or disapproval of respondents. He or she may use judgment to interpret the findings but should not impose personal value judgments about the behavior upon the data. For AIDS programs in particular, it may be important for the researchers to explore their feelings about sexuality, about same–gender sex, and about prostitution before conducting research. Where possible, using transcriptions (tapes) or videos will allow individual interpretation to be subject to the analysis of other researchers. If researchers are working in teams, switching interview transcriptions so that interviewers are not analyzing their own results can improve objectivity as well. In the case of HIV–related research, people who are affected by the disease are also excellent resources as interviewers or moderators if properly trained.

The second major danger inherent in qualitative research is the temptation to treat results as if they were quantitative in nature. Qualitative results cannot be "counted" or projected to a larger population. Rather, they must be seen as experiences indicative of feelings or beliefs that surround particular behaviors.

Poorly structured or sequenced questions, poorly trained or selected interviewers, and superficial or precocious analysis can also undermine the reliability of qualitative information. Participants in focus groups, for example, must be selected to reflect precisely the type of person proposed for an intervention. Interviewers must be experienced at helping respondents feel relaxed, at using group dynamics, at asking open–ended questions without biasing answers, and at posing questions that follow the respondents' own thought processes.

The researcher's presence in a home, bar or street may also influence the way the respondents perform, presenting an unrepresentative behavioral sample to the observer. While this is also a possible pitfall with quantitative research, the intensity, closeness, and context–based character of qualitative research make it particularly susceptible to this problem.

Understanding the limitations of qualitative research is of critical importance so that precautions are taken to minimize their effects and results are not used to generalize to much larger population samples.

MEASURING RIGOR AND QUALITY

Effective qualitative research has its own standards of quality and rigor. Not every casual conversation is an "in–depth interview," not every group meeting is a "focus group," and not every neighborhood visit is an "ethnographic study." A number of quality checks can help ensure that qualitative research methods are carried out rigorously. The following questions are useful check points for assuring that the information collected will be valuable. Program planners are encouraged to consider the following factors when reviewing any qualitative data.

Rival Hypotheses
In their analysis do the researchers consider rival hypotheses? Is the analysis too neat, too clean? Is there evidence the researchers considered other explanations?

Exceptional Case
Are the negative or exceptional cases considered? Almost all research will turn up outlying cases—cases which do not "fit." Are these cases mentioned, or discarded in the analysis?

Triangulation
Is there triangulation of data? Is other information used to support the basic analysis? Are several observers' comments included to help control for individual bias?

Common Sense
Is there evidence that the researchers have seen beyond superficial answers? Do many comments seem to represent rationalizations or socially desirable responses that do not "ring true"?

Transcriptions
Were transcripts, tapes or other records kept of the research, or did the researcher appear to rely solely on memory and first impression?

Quotes
Is actual data included—for example, quotes from participants as well as paraphrased remarks—which permit the planner to get a direct feel for the data?

Design Checks
Are there design checks to help determine if the observed situation is typical or abnormal? Is it possible to determine if the time period or the people observed are special in some way which is likely to bias the results?

Methodological Description
Do the researchers describe their methodology fully? Do they give enough detail for reviewers to assess where bias might have occurred?

Peer Review
Is peer review a part of the analysis process—have other experienced researchers been able to review raw data and make comments?

Experience
Were the researchers experienced in qualitative techniques? Did they have track records of useful qualitative research behind them?

This list demonstrates that there are many ways to check the rigor of qualitative research. As with quantitative methods, there is a need to establish the quality of a given analysis. These checks are particularly important for qualitative data, because many health professionals are unfamiliar with these methods and approaches. Only by maintaining consistently high standards can we ensure that qualitative research avoids both superficiality and bias, and remains persuasive and useful to decision–makers.

MIXING QUALITATIVE AND QUANTITATIVE RESEARCH TECHNIQUES

The previous sections have referred to studies in which qualitative and quantitative techniques have been used in a complementary fashion. Qualitative research can be used before a survey to develop hypotheses, test concepts and identify precise vocabulary. It can be used after a survey to illuminate seemingly contradictory results.

Qualitative research is attractive because it uses smaller numbers of respondents and it can be done more quickly than many large–scale surveys. To some, qualitative research seems like a quick and practical alternative to replace survey research. However, it must not be given this role. Qualitative research—even when executed brilliantly—is not sufficient in itself to guide most of our programs. It is limited by subjectivity and bounded by a lack of generalizability.

Indeed, no single research technique is capable of giving us the depth of insight required to address AIDS effectively. The challenge we face is to build a research agenda broad enough to cover all the critical areas, but narrow enough to be practical and affordable. Six priorities stand out as critical to program development in most AIDS prevention programs today:

- the epidemiology of AIDS;
- the nature of high–risk behavior;
- the prevailing public image of AIDS;

- the services and products available and acceptable for fighting AIDS;
- the kinds and power of different communication channels to reach and persuade specific audiences;
- and the specific obstacles and constraints (political, economic and technical) likely to be encountered.

Some of this information is amenable to qualitative studies. Some of it is more appropriately studied through quantitative methods. Within each type of research there is an issue of depth. How much do we have to know in order to know enough? In many cases we will have to build field programs on inadequate data. We will have to move ahead quickly and learn from mistakes.

The following matrix (see table 4–1) outlines distinctions between qualitative and quantitative research. It is included to assist AIDS educators, program planners and researchers to develop new avenues and investigative approaches for combining qualitative and quantitative research in the study of communities and HIV–related behaviors.

Table 4–1. *Distinctions between qualitative and quantitative research.*

Qualitative	Quantitative
Provides depth of understanding	Measures level of occurrence
Asks "why?"	Asks "How many?", "How often?"
Studies motivations	Studies actions
Is subjective	Is objective
Enables discovery	Provides proof
Is exploratory	Is definitive
Allows insights into behavior, trends, etc.	Measures level of actions, trends, etc.
Interprets	Describes

Summary

The most effective AIDS programs today combine qualitative and quantitative research methods. They use focus groups and ethnographies to develop hypotheses which survey research then validates for large–scale populations. The critical role for qualitative research in AIDS prevention is to deepen our understanding of the beliefs and practices previously assigned to Knowledge and Practice (KAP) surveys. Qualitative research provides insights into beliefs which affect behavior and helps bridge the gap between knowledge and practice. It provides information about how people feel about themselves, about their relationship to AIDS, and about the proposed alternatives for AIDS prevention. Qualitative research is no quick fix, but it can be a vital partner in the search for ways to help people protect themselves from HIV infection and AIDS.

The authors wish to express their appreciation to Dr. Deborah Helitzer–Allen for her contribution to the form and content of this chapter.

REFERENCES

Agar, M. (1980). *The professional stranger*. Academic Press, New York.

Agar, M. (1986). *Speaking of ethnography*. Sage Publications, Beverly Hills, CA.

Bogdan, R.C. and Viklen, S.K. (1982). *Qualitative Research for Education: An introduction to Theory and Methods*. Allyn and Bacon, Boston.

Cook, T.D. and Reinhardt, C.S. (1979). *Qualitative and Quantitative Methods in Evaluation Research*. Sage Publications, Beverly Hills, CA.

Fetterman, D.M. (1989). *Ethnography. Step by Step.* Sage Publications, Beverly Hills, CA.

Goetz, J.P. and Le Compte, M.D. (1984). *Ethnography and Qualitative Design in Educational Research*. Academic Press, New York.

Patton, M.Q. (1980). *Qualitative Evaluation Methods*. Sage Publications, Beverly Hills, CA.

Pelto, P.J. and Pelto, G.H. (1978). *Anthropological Research: The Structure of Inquiry*. Cambridge University Press, Cambridge.

Schwartz, D. (1987). *Concept Testing*. American Management Association, New York.

Spradley, J.P. (1980). *Participant Observation*. Reinholt and Winston, New York.

Social Marketing and Prevention of AIDS

Michael Ramah
Claire M. Cassidy

Communications approaches are central to the control of HIV infection because we have neither vaccine nor curative treatments and because transmission occurs primarily through the practice of specific behaviors. Social marketing provides a perspective, a set of techniques and a process which can be successfully applied to helping people choose HIV–protective alternative behaviors.

AIDS and Social Marketing

HIV is transmitted by behaviors involving sexual intercourse, by blood during transfusions, as a result of accidental needle sticks or by the sharing of needles, or from the mother to her fetus or newborn.

These few emotionally neutral lines hide a wealth of issues that complicate the HIV–prevention marketing mission. This mission, baldly stated, is to reduce the transmission of the virus by encouraging people and organizations to stop practicing behaviors that can transmit HIV and to start practicing other safer behaviors.

This mission might be easier to address were we dealing with a simpler choice like choosing between two commercial products. Of course, we are not, and HIV disease is perhaps uniquely frightening. It is a disease that activates some of people's deepest fears and prejudices, and its control requires people to think and speak about subjects that have been tradition-

75

ally private or taboo. This point is worth analyzing briefly in the light of the early history of the social response to AIDS.

The first official recognition of a new disease appeared in a report published by the Centers for Disease Control on June 5, 1981. This report described a puzzling finding—the formerly rare *Pneumocystis carinii* pneumonia was becoming much more common. All the reported cases were in gay men, and at the time no connection was made with the so–called "junkie pneumonia" that had been killing drug addicts. Within a short time, AIDS had been socially characterized as a "gay" disease, and as a "venereal" disease, labels that are culturally interpreted as pejoratives. This helped fuel an outflow of prejudice including public expressions of homophobia, and governmental slowness to respond to the new disease by publicizing its dangerous potential or by funding research on it.

One result of this situation was that grass–roots, community–based organizations were the first to respond to the AIDS threat, seeking ways to inform their constituents of the danger and of how to avoid infection. These organizations often developed knowledge and skills that continue to be valuable in current communications efforts.

Other early efforts actually set up roadblocks to effective communications that are demanding continuing mop–up activities to modify public images. For example, mid–1980s efforts to tell the U.S. public that AIDS was not limited to homosexual communities took as their "hook" the idea that "AIDS is everybody's problem." But because most Americans were not HIV positive and did not know anyone who was, this message activated a good deal of disbelief and denial, what social marketers call the "NOT ME" syndrome. In short, people stopped paying attention to AIDS information messages, feeling it was just one more bit of advertising overload in their lives. A more accurate message—one which was later promulgated—is that "Anybody who practices certain behaviors may be at risk, but everybody is not." This phrasing puts the emphasis on the behavior, which is what the marketing message aims to change, rather than on the person or the society.

It is risk behaviors that must be targeted, not risk groups. The reasons are several. For example, if a person does not define himself as belonging to a "risk group" he or she may simply ignore useful AIDS prevention information. Bisexual men are recognized as important transmission agents of HIV into the heterosexual population, often beginning with their wives. Research has shown that bisexual men typically do not define themselves as "homosexual." Thus they may not respond to messages aimed at homosexuals. They may think something like "The guy I sleep with, not me," a logic analogous to claiming that women have all the responsibility for birth control. Bisexual men may not view themselves as homosexuals because they see homosexuality as a lifestyle choice (rather than as a behavior), whereas they have chosen to be married men with families, who occasionally visit male partners. AIDS information that focuses on the desired behavior—protected anal intercourse or a safer substitute—is potentially more effective because it maybe "heard by" both self–defined homosexual men and bisexual men, as well as by heterosexual partners who practice anal sex.

A second reason to avoid targeting "risk groups" is because this has the untoward effect of activating prejudice, with all its socially destructive outflow. In the case of AIDS, because transmission is via behaviors that are emotionally laden, there is a very great potential for "blaming the victim."

A third reason relates to the process of the communications endeavor itself. Specifically, it is often impossible to access "groups" because they simple do not exist. That is, in many cases, there are no sanctioned environments—no clubs, health clinics, neighborhoods or other settings—where many who practice risky behaviors may be found grouped together. Instead, communications efforts must reach out to individuals who practice specific behaviors.

Semantics will always be centrally important to effective AIDS communication. Two recent efforts to alter the AIDS image are the result of improved understanding of the syndrome. The first effort involves encouraging people to see AIDS as the end of a lengthy process that begins with infection with the HIV virus. In epidemiological contexts, this idea is sometimes illustrated using an "iceberg" analogy, showing AIDS as its visible tip, and non–symptomatic infection and AIDS Related Complex (ARC) as "submerged" aspects of the whole syndrome. Such imagery is intended to re–focus attention and defuse anxiety by emphasizing "infection" and "long development," with their implicit promises of hope for medical intervention. The second effort consists in redefining HIV/AIDS as a "lifestyle" rather than as a venereal disease. Using the lifestyle concept puts AIDS in the same perceptual arena with other health issues such as heart disease, cancer, diarrheal disease of infancy and alcoholism. The new label both emphasizes that control is possible, and suggests that social marketing will be a powerful control tool. Indeed, social marketing lessons learned from intervention in these diseases do have direct applicability to the control of HIV infection.

Because HIV infection, and AIDS, produce fear in people, and because one's addictive habits, sexuality and death are difficult to talk about, social marketing for AIDS prevention presents possibly unique challenges. People must be enabled to think and speak frankly about private acts. They must learn new skills, such as how to negotiate condom use with a partner. They must also find ways to redefine the meaning of existing behaviors—for example, by learning to find non–penetrative sexual activities, often culturally categorized as "foreplay," as satisfying as the penetrative behaviors they replace. All these lessons and skills can be imparted using the methodology of social marketing. However, due to the sensitive nature of the subject, most campaigns will have only one chance to communicate such information successfully. Therefore, AIDS prevention strategies need to be unusually professional and thorough both in research and in communication, covering every base so as not to alienate or miscommunicate. Beyond these caveats, social marketing efforts for AIDS prevention are not very different from social marketing for other behavior changes.

OVERVIEW OF SOCIAL MARKETING STRATEGIES

Social marketing is defined as "the design, implementation and control of programs designed to ultimately influence individual behavior in ways that the marketer believes are in the individual's or society's interests." Social marketing is a science that has grown, in the last 30 years, out of precursors in advertising and communications. More complex than its parent disciplines, a complete social marketing strategy consists of a planned process involving:

- data gathering (market research);
- efforts to ensure the goodwill of all groups directly or indirectly involved (public relations);
- the design and dissemination of effective behavior change messages (communications and advertising);
- the provision of support modalities to encourage continuation of new behaviors (maintenance); and
- continuous monitoring of effectiveness (evaluation).

The major steps in this sequential process are summarized in figure 5–1. In the remainder of this section, we examine these activities in relation to social marketing for AIDS prevention.

WHY SOCIAL MARKETING?

A social behavior is an intangible "product" which, experience has shown, can be "sold" using techniques that are similar to those applied to selling tangible products like soap and soup.

A most important characteristic of social marketing is that it is, first and foremost, consumer–centered. This means that while the marketing organization —the local library, the Audubon Society, Family of the Future— has a defined mission involving social change, it recognizes that it cannot accom-

FIGURE 5–1. *Social Marketing Wheel*

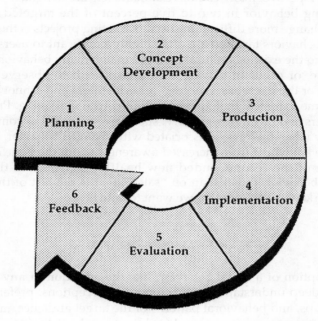

plish its aims without knowing a great deal about its consumers, and without responding to their knowledge, attitudes and practices.

A second important attitude that social marketers bring to their work is the commandment: Do No Harm. Particularly in the case of AIDS control, insufficient or inaccurate data collection, or the misapplication of behavior modification techniques, can set up resistance in target populations that is both difficult and costly to erase. Because the AIDS issue is delicate, it is immensely important that social marketers use their talents judiciously from the outset.

If social marketers are to ask the right questions and design effective messages, they must keep in touch with the target population. For AIDS specialists this means that they need to visit and work with people with AIDS, and must try to keep open lines of communication with communities that tend to experience high rates of HIV seroconversion. Each such community is unique, as are the issues of people with AIDS in different countries; keeping contact will help the social marketer respond more accurately to local situations and concerns.

For many health projects, the hope is that a majority of the target population—even 80–90%—can be convinced that the proposed change is in their best interests, and can be assisted in changing their behavior. To put this goal in perspective, many commercial marketers are delighted with changed purchasing behavior in two to five percent of the targeted population. Making change more difficult in social marketing projects is the fact that the kinds of behaviors targeted are often highly significant to users, and tightly bound into the existing cultural matrix. Finally, many behavior changes are intangible, or occur in private, and are difficult to observe or measure directly. For these reasons, "success" at social marketing cannot be measured by the same yardstick that applies to commercial marketing. Prize–winning AIDS posters and brochures, and T.V. spots, are successful as communications tools only when their use is associated with changed behavior. Such change can range anywhere from increased awareness about the issue addressed to adoption of the recommended new health practice. It is this focus on changed behavior, rather than on "sales," that is the last of the distinctive social marketing attitudes that we want to note here.

MARKET RESEARCH

"The adoption of a social behavior, like the adoption of any product, re-quires a deep understanding of the needs, perceptions, preferences, refer-ence groups, and behavioral patterns of the target audience, and the tailor-ing of messages, media, costs and facilities to make changing easy."

To be effective, practitioners must aim behavioral change messages correctly. That is, messages must be expressed in language, and using symbols, images, and concepts that speak as directly as possible to the real concerns of the target audience. This is the burden of the statement that social marketing is consumer–centered. To achieve this end, however, so-cial marketers must first know as much as possible about the potential consumers of their behavioral product.

Market research is designed to gather information about the existing knowl-edge, attitudes and practices —the "KAP"— of potential consumers. (Some social marketers prefer to speak of the "KAB," that is, knowledge, attitudes and behaviors.) During the KAP process, marketers also learn about sources of resis-tance among consumers, and about better and worse options for channeling the behavioral change messages. The actual techniques that market researchers use to gather information on KAP will not be discussed here.

However, one aspect of the method is unusually important and deserves mention. Many of the persons presently in greatest danger of AIDS —bisexual men, sex workers, intravenous drug users— are isolated or live in socially peripheral communities. As such, they are difficult to reach by standard research (and communications) techniques, and often require personal contact approaches. Market researchers must find ways to approach such individuals, and must also use good public relations to maintain their lines of access Some approach techniques used include meeting target audiences on their own territory (e.g. in bars or drug shooting galleries, on the street), and using the vocabulary or clothing symbolism of the people they want to meet. An important behavior, non–quantifiable, but essential to an interviewer, is also that of appearing approachable, that is, harmless but not helpless. Lines of access can be jeopardized if actions in the central community, such as media attacks, threaten the peripheral community. Market researchers prefer to predict such events and head them off (using public relations techniques), because it is often difficult to repair lines of access.

Useful Results of Market Research

General market research has revealed that the consumer decision process is complex. Market research for AIDS prevention has revealed that popular images of many of the target audiences for AIDS education are well off the mark. Finally, specific projects reveal the particular attitudes and needs that constitute the "windows of opportunity" for effective AIDS communication.

Consumer decisions are complex. Many decisions that involve behavioral change, from the decision to eat more whole grains to the decision to will half of one's future to a conservation organization, are highly involving and require the consumer to balance many issues against one another. The Fishbein Model (Figure 5–2) summarizes this process from the point of view of the consumer and underlines the importance of doing careful market research.

Note, first, that behavioral intention does not guarantee behavioral outcome: a woman may wish and intend to talk her partner into wearing a condom but she may not succeed in convincing him. She may lack the necessary negotiation skills, or she may have forgotten to buy one, broken the only one she had, or gone to a store that was all out. Even if she is skilled at negotiation and prepared with a condom, he may flatly refuse her request. Each of these may be an unexpected situational inhibitor; actual social marketing campaigns try to reduce the probability of such inhibitors. Situational promoters are also possible, such as a partner who surprises the woman by providing a condom.

Second, even reaching the level of behavioral intention is highly complex. The consumer's decision to try the new behavioral product can be viewed as the sum of that consumer's knowledge, attitudes and practices (KAP) of the behavior, combined with her previous experience with the issue, the kinds of messages she gets from others in her circle, and the risk she thinks is associated with trying, or not trying, the new behavior.

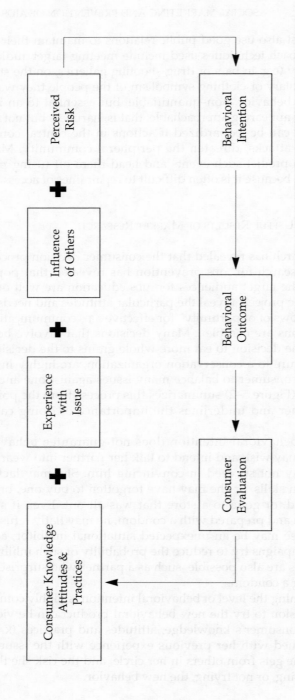

FIGURE 5-2. *Fishbein Consumer Decision Model**

*Modified from Kotler and Andreasen 1987:86.

WASHINGTYPE, INC., 1001 30th Street, N.W. #380, Washintom, D.C. 20007, (202) 298-7171 FAX 963-TYPE

The sum of this equation yields the consumer's choice set: cumulative data from many consumers yields a choice set that characterizes that group or locale. The social marketer's task is to learn about and then use the contents of the choice set to design effective intervention.

Accurate KAP research is the cornerstone upon which good communications strategies are build. Current levels of information can be modified by education, but this must be done using language and concepts that "make sense" to the target audience. These concepts, often not easily discussed by users because they are so tied to perceptions of reality as to seem simply "normal" and "natural," provide the windows of opportunity for tailoring culturally sensitive, hence effective, behavior change messages. Consider the problem of reaching adolescents. Social marketing projects often target adolescents because it is thought that youths have less deeply ingrained habits, and may adopt new behaviors more easily. However, messages that may sway adults—such as those emphasizing longer life—strike many teens as irrelevant. On the other hand, teens enormously value certain trappings of adulthood, and the fear of loss of these can motivate safer behavior. One U.S. social marketing project put this finding to good use: An effective print ad countering drunk driving showed two teens, certainly old enough to drive themselves, and looking highly embarrassed, being driven by their mother. The text said: "If the thought of death doesn't scare you, think of losing your driver's license!"

An AIDS prevention social marketing project in Tijuana, Mexico, targeted female sex workers for increased condom use. The first need was to determine the KAP of the sex workers to AIDS and condom use. Among other things, research showed that the women were not motivated by the idea "I want to live." They felt that the everyday need to put supper on the table was far more important than the possibility of dying of AIDS five years down the road. On the other hand, the research also revealed that many of the women had children, and were deeply concerned for their welfare. Because they were responsible parents, they responded to the query "If something happens to you, what will happen to your child?" Accepting this finding, communications experts designed a small comic book, distributed inside a two–condom pack, which features "Barbara" explaining to her sex worker friend one reason why she uses condoms: "Quiero cuidar a mi hijo, por eso no expongo mi salud" (I want to protect my child, so I take no chances with my health).

A couple of counter examples emphasize the dangers of doing inadequate market research leading to inaccurately aimed behavior change messages. Consider the social issue of convincing people to stop smoking. For years, organizations dedicated to decreasing the number of smokers in the U.S. assumed that the reason people did not quit was because they did not realize that smoking was dangerous to their health. Finally, the National Cancer Institute did a retrospective review of existing consumer studies and found that the "product" they were trying to sell was already sold. People did know that smoking was bad for them; however, they did not know how to quit. In fact, many had tried sincerely to quit, had failed repeatedly, and had finally come to ignore anti–smoking messages which seemed to them simply to be asking them to "fail again." Once social marketers understood this situation, they were able to develop new strategies that combined warnings about smoking aimed at potential smokers (i.e. teens), with messages that indicated where one might go for help in really quitting. This example has particular applicability to AIDS social marketing. Continuing to bombard people who already fear AIDS with its danger is counter–productive if they do not know how to avoid the disease. They can be immobilized by their fear, their sense of being ignorant, and their sense of guilt, and come to behave as if thinking, "Why bother? I'm damned anyway." Communications strategies that give information that people need (need being established on the basis of market research) are most effective.

Parallel with the smoking example is the frequent assumption that a major reason why people do not use condoms is because they do not know about them. However, studies suggest that often people do know about condoms and are even willing to use them, but do not know how to use them correctly. A training project in Trinidad and Tobago noted that all participants had seen a condom before and nearly nine out of ten had used them. However, many made mistakes in putting on or removing the condom that decreased their utility in preventing the transmission of disease. A two–phased training intervention significantly raised individual "condom skill scores" and group skill levels.

In the spring of 1989, a proposed AIDS prevention headline concept intended for Caribbean audiences began: "Stop AIDS." When tested in focus groups, however, this headline was scrapped in favor of another: "Protect yourself." "Researchers made the change in response to comments by members of the focus group among whom they tested their headline concepts. These respondents had emphasized two things. First, they found the phrase "Stop AIDS!" misleading. To some, it implied that a cure was in sight—yet they knew it was not. To others, it suggested that humans were overstepping the boundaries of their capacities, for "only God could stop AIDS." Second, participants kept returning to the issue of protection, and agreed that it was a priority. Analyzing this event one step further, we suggest that people were more motivated with the close–up and accessible concept of personal and familial safety—"Protect yourself!"—than with what must have appeared as a cosmic abstraction, "Stop AIDS!"

The end of the consumer decision (Fishbein) model emphasizes that people will judge the new behavior or product that they have tried. Only if they judge it worthy of further trials and adoption can it be integrated into their lives as a lifestyle change. The aim of social marketing for AIDS prevention is, in fact, to promote lifestyle change—that needle users will always use sterile needles, and that persons in a relationship with an HIV—infected or potentially infected partner will always practice safer sex. These are ambitious goals, and success at achieving such thorough–going results is, not unexpectedly, mixed. However, it is often encouraging. A condom education project in Kenya found that before the project began, condom use among prostitutes was at only eight percent; five months into the program 85% reported using condoms. A survey in Uganda found that after an AIDS education project aimed at the general public, 95% of those surveyed knew about AIDS, and 86% could name at least two protective measures. Unfortunately, no pre–project survey had been conducted. Much more detailed information exists for urban centers in Europe and America; all suggest that a significant proportion of target populations, met by well–aimed AIDS communication projects, can and will change their behavior in directions favoring AIDS prevention. Some will remain resistant; we will return to this issue below.

Market research reveals sources of resistance to behavior change. As noted, effective communications strategies must respond knowledgeably to popular anxieties about the behavior change "product." Especially with AIDS, assumptions abound.

A major source of resistance in AIDS education arises from the existing plenitude of public misinformation, sometimes the result of "scare" stores in the media, also a result of pejorative labeling of the syndrome. Because of its association with sex and with intravenous drug use, AIDS also tends to activate social conservatism. It is common for AIDS to be discussed as a "moral" issue; religious arguments sometimes blind consumers to the true threat of AIDS. Additionally, in some locales, existing laws—such as those prohibiting "unnatural" sex acts—may further complicate the communications effort. Fortunately, communicators often find astute ways to work around such limitations.

Another source of resistance arises from having false—often stereotypical—images of target communities. For example, outsiders to a community easily see that community as homogeneous. Extensive ethnographic and market research has shown, in contrast, that adolescent, homosexual, intravenous drug user and sex worker communities are heterogeneous, and commonly organize themselves as along the same lines of social valuing that are found in mainline communities. To take just two examples: Sex workers often distinguish class lines among themselves such that those who work for higher fees and out of the same room every time have more status than those who work out of bars and hotels; at the bottom are those who work on the street. This pattern, found widely, has also been documented recently in the Dominican Republic. Again, homosexual communities are often complexly patterned. Homosexual men in Mexico also distinguish among "committed homosexuals" (of whom some are passives, some actives and some called *internacionales*, take both sides), "independent operators" (swingers, and others), and "exploiters," who are violent, and may entrap, blackmail, or steal from other homosexual men. Wherever detailed data are available similar evidence of heterogeneity emerges.

As a final comment on the danger of stereotyping, consider how different an AIDS communication strategy built upon a common popular image of sex workers, rather than on the image of these workers that emerged from market research, would have been. A KAP survey noted that at the outset, health and media personnel viewed female sex workers in a stereotypical manner: the sex worker community was perceived as homogeneous, women were thought to sell sex for clothes, money and drugs, and were perceived as "fast women." It was also assumed that the women could leave prostitution if they wanted to. Results of the KAP survey revealed a significantly different picture: the sex workers tended to be young women who had migrated to the city, and who worked through economic necessity with little sense that they could escape a job many did not enjoy. Many were married, and felt trapped into their jobs by the demands of providing food, clothing and shelter for their children.

THE IMPORTANCE OF GOOD PUBLIC RELATIONS

Research and communications are infinitely more effective if they occur in a supportive environment. The environment of AIDS social marketing, because of the syndrome's transmission pattern, severity and endemicity, is the entire world; additionally, the HIV syndrome is such as to easily inflame public opinion. In this setting, it is extremely important that AIDS social marketing projects include attention to public relations from the outset.

Public relations is really a matter of getting people on one's own side, so they see one's own point of view. As such, it is simply a subset of good communications.

A useful perspective is to realize that AIDS communication projects cannot remain localized. Therefore they must be acceptable to persons who are not part of the target audience. One way marketers try to ensure that projects do not backfire is to bring the leaders of a society in on the issue and the planning from the outset. A recent project in the Philippines provides an excellent example. Before any public communication was begun, a national program focused on educating opinion–leaders and media personnel. A series of workshops was held, by invitation only. The first set was for the media. This workshop emphasized the power of a free press, showed the dangers of journalistic misinformation in increasing people's fear of AIDS and provided accurate information about AIDS. It emphasized the role and the responsibility of the press in informing the public about AIDS, and it indicated that the government had determined upon a humane policy. In support of the workshop, a "media hotline" was set up to provide scientific AIDS updates upon request. A second series of workshops was held to provide similar education to and elicit cooperation from opinion–shapers in industry, education, health administration, advertising and others whose jobs involved influencing public opinion from the top down. Social marketers judged the workshop approach highly effective. The frequency of media "scare" stories about AIDS fell markedly and the "hot–line" was used to prepare numerous accurate stories, while opinion–shapers used their weight to promote more positive public attention to AIDS.

A second way to help ensure the success of communications projects is to run two in parallel. One is aimed at educating the general public, arousing appropriate concern and providing information about the disease while encouraging compassion for people with AIDS. The second, more complex parallel project, is aimed at specified target audiences, and may contain material that might have offended the public had it not also been the focus of an information campaign.

It is also often effective public relations to get private industry involved in the research or education effort. For example, some companies may be glad to share KAP data with AIDS social marketers if they perceive some benefit to themselves, such as the right to publicize their public service activities.

Another important issue concerns language. We have already noted the importance of presenting the HIV syndrome accurately, and with labels that are not pejorative and do not stereotype. The social marketer must try to "speak the language" of both the target and non–target audiences. Thus, social marketers should be familiar with the jargon and concerns of the professionals they work with as well as with the vernacular of target audiences. Marketers must also be alert to how this vernacular strikes the public, including key decision makers: Readers can probably recall instances in which comics or brochures using "street language" have offended public officials and others and aroused resistance that might have been avoided had the need for direct communication with target audiences been made clear to opinion–leaders from the outset.

COMMUNICATIONS STRATEGIES

Intervention ideally moves consumers from unawareness of need or opportunity to adoption of a new behavior (Figure 5–3). The adoption model, in contrast to the consumer decision Fishbein model, above, takes the perspective of the communicator. Thus, KAP data is used to divide a population into sub–groups who are "unaware," "aware" and so forth, and different communications strategies are set up to address these subpopulations, always with the ultimate goal of encouraging adoption of the new behavior.

Technically, communicators segment and target audiences. In any large population, there is a range of attitude and readiness to change. A single message will reach only a part of the potential audience. A message which appeals too far down the readiness continuum will similarly fall short of effectiveness. Therefore, different messages are constructed for different segments of the audience, and a particular audience is given several messages in sequence to lead them gradually from mere "awareness" through to trial of the new behavior.

KAP data allows researchers to segment populations according to geographic, demographic and psychographic variables. The latter include markers of social class and of lifestyle preference. In addition, in some cases, there are core concepts that reach across such lines, linking people at a fundamental cultural level. For example, KAP researchers have repeatedly found that sex workers are motivated to use condoms out of concern for the future of their children. Concern for children runs deep in most societies and may prove to be an effective motivator of safer sex in groups that usually do not come into contact with each other, from rural villagers to middle class suburbanites to inner city sex workers. Segmentation helps communicators determine how many messages, and of what type, are needed to reach target audiences.

A target audience is one that has been selected out of the whole population, to receive social marketing messages. Typically, for any social change, there are true or primary target populations (i.e. people who practice behaviors that enhance their likelihood of infection with HIV), as well as secondary audiences such as health–related institutions and the public. While the latter are in less direct danger of HIV infection, their opinions count, for they often have the power to short–circuit or destroy communications campaigns aimed at primary target populations. Equally, they have the power to support and magnify the beneficial effect of target messages. Institutional targets are additionally important because most social marketing campaigns are of limited duration. If the benefits of behavior change are to be maintained, institutions—health ministries, schools, hospitals,

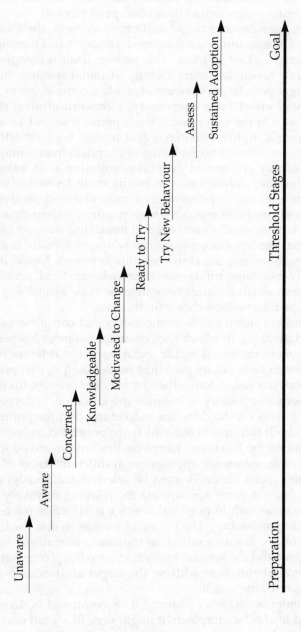

Figure 5.3. Behavior Change Continuum Model*

Unaware → Aware → Concerned → Knowledgeable → Motivated to Change → Ready to Try → Try New Behaviour → Assess → Sustained Adoption → Goal

Preparation

Threshold Stages

*Simplified from "Health Behavior Change Continuum, A Framework for Measurement"
by Mary Debus, Porter/Novelli Internal Memo 2/21/89.
A version of the "Buyer Readiness" model.

medical schools—must integrate the concern and the solutions promoted by the social marketing program into their concept of mission.

Communicators segment and target audiences to break their task into manageable parts. Once an audience is defined, concepts and messages can be constructed, tested and set in place. This process itself is complex. "For example," comments researcher Mary Debus, "if initial research indicates that a high risk target population is aware of AIDS but complacent or unconcerned that AIDS will affect them personally, a concern arousal strategy might be warranted. On the other hand, this approach would be entirely off the mark among a highly sensitized and fearful (concerned) target population. Panic management might be the appropriate intervention strategy in this case, highly concerned general population with substantial incorrect knowledge may warrant a mass media myth reduction strategy, whereas gay men who are appropriately concerned and motivated to change but who find condoms repulsive may require condom desensitization counseling. A mass media campaign glamorizing the condom may help overcome social barriers among teenagers whose motivation is daunted by fear of disapproval or stigma. However, this approach would be inappropriate for highly motivated rural sex workers who are 'sold' on condoms but simply find them unaffordable. Promoting the wide availability of free condoms may be the intervention choice (in this case)."

It is often helpful to conceive of communicators and consumers as being in an exchange relationship in which the consumer balances his perceived costs against the benefit promised by the social marketer. (Market research allows the specialist to flesh out an exchange model such as that presented as Figure 5–4.) Social marketers know they must either account for or minimize the consumer's costs so as to balance the equation in favor of the consumer's benefit. This can be done for individuals and for populations. Specific issues are built into messages, which are presented in sequence to move consumers along the behavior change continuum toward adoption.

Different types of messages are appropriate at different stages of awareness, and communications channels must be selected judiciously. A mass medium like television is most appropriate for relaying relatively simple informational messages, while personal contact is effective for teaching specific skills and for counseling. The timing of messages, and the intensity of message promotion, are also issues in the communications strategy. Whenever the budget and the societal infrastructure permit, communicators prefer to use several channels to address the target audiences, a process known as an "integrated approach.

Consider the sentence: "Use a condom." This command is deceptively simple. If it should lead off a campaign, it might very likely fail to convince many to change their behavior, because this idea really falls near the end of

FIGURE 5–4. *Exchange Model**

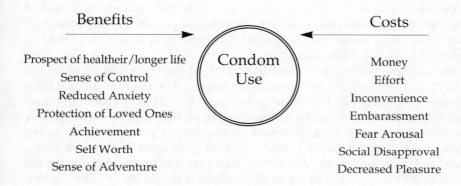

Benefits   Condom Use   Costs

Benefits	Costs
Prospect of healtheir/longer life	Money
Sense of Control	Effort
Reduced Anxiety	Inconvenience
Protection of Loved Ones	Embarassment
Achievement	Fear Arousal
Self Worth	Social Disapproval
Sense of Adventure	Decreased Pleasure

*Source" Modified from "Concept of Exchange" model by Mary Debus, for AIDSCOM.

WASHINGTYPE. INC., 1001 30th Street, N.W. #380, Washintom, D.C.
20007, (202) 298-7171 FAX 963-TYPE

the behavior change continuum (step seven in Figure 5–3). Most people need to be led up to this point through a series of iterations before they can act on the message. Part of the problem lies in the fact that condoms "have a bad reputation." They are used by people "not like me," or if people are willing to consider using them, they have perceived disadvantages. More than that, condoms begin behind in the race for public acceptance because the modified behavior is only subtly different from the familiar behavior. "Yes/No" (e.g. "Sex/No Sex") messages are easier for people to comprehend and choose; asking for "more protected sex" is easily perceived as asking for "less immediate sex." It also sets up a need for negotiation between partners that is more complex and demands more skill than giving a simple Yes/No answer.

Condom use is still struggling to overcome image roadblocks in the United States. For example, early efforts to encourage condom use to protect people from AIDS fell into a social context in which the disease was perceived as a gay disease, and condoms were perceived as useful only for those who practiced anal intercourse. In this setting, if you tell me that I must use a condom, you also suggest that I practice anal intercourse. Well, who says I do? And if I do, why should I tell you? And I'm a woman anyway, so why do I need anal sex? For the communicator, such attitudes constitute a people hurdle: Communicators must make it possible (for example) for people to understand that it is O.K. to practice any type of penetrative sex, that different practices imply little about one's sexual orientation, but that in an era of AIDS unprotected penetrative sex is dangerous. Once those points are made and accepted, people can more readily accept the solution: "Use a condom!"

Social marketers have worked hard to limit the costs and magnify the benefits that consumer's associate with condoms. For example, people have been helped to change the value weightings they attach to condoms from negative to positive. Sometimes, the tangible product has been changed. A condom company in the U.S. aimed a campaign at young sexually active women. They developed a "new" condom, packaged in a stylish purse pack, and contained in an "applicator" that prevents users from putting the condom on incorrectly. The top of the condom is ringed by an adhesive that prevents its coming off prematurely. Finally, this condom comes in several colors and textures.

Alternately, the condom may be presented in a light that makes it seem desirable either because it is erotic, or because it is a way to be concerned and loving; this approach is described in more detail in the case history which ends this chapter. Other communication approaches have helped people accept condoms by noting neglected positive consequences of using them. For example, one can counter the objection that condoms reduce sensitivity by noting the increased pleasure to be derived from a prolonged sexual encounter.

Of course, much of condom communications work focuses on altering people's beliefs about alternatives —specifically, that unprotected sex is dangerous to one's health. However, for some, there is another alternative— a woman may fear that if she insists on a condom, she will anger her partner and put herself in physical or economic danger. The "Empower" project in Thailand addressed this issue by providing female sex workers not only with AIDS information, but also with assertiveness and negotiation training so that they would be better able to convince their partner to accept a condom. These women also received language training—many of their customers are foreign—and counseling to help them find other remunerative work.

MAINTENANCE OF COMMUNICATIONS EFFECTIVENESS

Marketing strategies do not consist entirely of communications messages. Very often they also include two types of support activities: offerings that make adoption of the new behavior easier for target populations, and offerings that help institutionalize the new behavior.

Target populations need more than information to choose a new behavior. Often, people need to know where to learn how to practice or solve problems connected with the new behavior. People also need to be able to find the equipment that will help them use the new behavior. Many people want to feel that others are also adopters. Thus, smoking cessation campaigns tell people where to go for retraining and provide special courses, while AIDS campaigns make sure that condoms of the right kind are available where target audiences will look for them, distribute sterile needles or bottles of bleach to intravenous drug users, provide assertiveness training to sex workers so they can negotiate condom use with their customers, provide counselling and "buddies" to people with AIDS so they can live most fully, or establish "hotlines" so that journalists can easily get hold of the most accurate new information on AIDS. Practically speaking, most social marketing projects include adoption support activities.

Less obvious than the provision of such support activities is the need to ensure that once the social marketing campaign is complete, adoption of the new behavior continues to be encouraged, and adoption continues to occur. The latter happens most effectively when institutions that are appropriately linked to the new behavior actually choose to encourage it themselves. Institutional changes are most lasting when they are widely accepted as modifications of mission and formalized in writing. Institutionalization of the AIDS prevention effort occurs, for example, when a Ministry of Health establishes a new office of, say "health communications," funds it appropriately, and monitors it to make sure that it continues to encourage AIDS–protective behaviors. Similarly, institutionalization of a new behavior occurs when a governing body enacts laws that mandate communications and support for the new behavior and when school systems require schools to teach about AIDS prevention, provide courses and training to teachers, respond constructively to parental anxieties or resistance, and ensure that the students are receiving the information. Finally, institutionalization may be said to be occurring when opinion–leaders take the topic in stride, are informed, and inform others as a matter of course.

EVALUATION AND FEEDBACK

Evaluation, also called monitoring, is ideally an ongoing process that tells marketers how well they are doing.

It is used to determine if messages are having the intended effect, or if they need modification as to content, channel, or pacing. It is used to identify gaps in market research. It is used to measure the level and rate of acceptance and institutionalization of the new behavior.

Effectiveness at encouraging safer sex or drug use behaviors is difficult to measure directly, since these behaviors occur in private. However, effectiveness of AIDS social marketing projects has been judged based on such markers as falling rates of sexually transmitted disease, rising condom sales, and raised frequencies of self–reported condom use. A study in New York City established that messages warning intravenous drug users about the dangers of sharing needles were being heard because demand for sterile needles was so high that a black market arose in used needles, repackaged to appear new and sterile.

Ongoing evaluation can warn marketers that a message is misfiring or that its impact is waning. In any marketing process, impact is higher earlier than later, with the same marketing mix, because those who are susceptible to the message move quickly toward adoption. This leaves behind those who do not respond as rapidly or effectively. The fact that buyers do not respond identically underlines why a good marketing strategy involves a phased and integrated approach.

Evaluation studies have also shown that fears expressed initially that set up resistance to AIDS prevention campaigns may actually have little basis in fact. For example, a common objection to distributing sterile needles to people who use intravenous drugs has been that a while such distribution may decrease the likelihood of AIDS, it might also increase the rate at which people took up intravenous drug use. Part of the problem stems from the fact that observers tended to think of drug users as driven by their habit, and unable to control themselves even enough to understand the purpose of sterile needles. Work in Amsterdam, in Baltimore, in Philadelphia and elsewhere shows that addicts can change their behavior. Needle distribution programs are typically linked to drug treatment programs, thus providing a pathway by which drug users can find their way to help. Alfred Allen, director of a "needle exchange" program in Washington State, comments, "We're establishing ongoing contact with drug addicts, and we're there when they're ready to accept a referral to drug treatment." Because it has been documented that "no addict starts using drugs just because clean needles are available," cities that have been reluctant to distribute clean needles are beginning to.

CASE HISTORY:
A PILOT AIDS SOCIAL MARKETING PROJECT IN MEXICO

While many AIDS prevention communication campaigns are currently underway, relatively few are complete enough to allow analysis of the level of behavioral change that occurred concomitant with the campaign. The following pilot project was designed as a demonstration project and is complete.

The Setting

The pilot project was carried out among sexually active gay men in the city of Guadalajara, Mexico, from November 1987 to August 1988. During this period, the Mexican Government's National AIDS Education Campaign was in full swing, providing informational messages in several media including television, radio and print, and also including periods of free condom distribution. CONASIDA (Consejo nacional para la prevencion y control del SIDA—National Council for the prevention and control of AIDS), with the support of the Population Council (United Nations), completed KAP surveys in six Mexican cities, one of which was Guadalajara, in November 1987 and May 1988. CONASIDA in collaboration with AIDSCOM (USAID), used data from the November 1987 KAP to develop a communications campaign in July 1988 evaluated with a mini–KAP survey in August 1988.

Sexually active gay men in Guadalajara were targeted for a social marketing project for several reasons. First, in Mexico, AIDS continues to be more common among homosexual men than among other population subgroups. In 1987, the rate was approximately 20 AIDS cases among men for each case in women, with most of the affected men being homo–or bisexual. Second, Mexican (like many peoples) resist holistic interventions—people prefer messages directed specifically toward the group with which they identify. Thus, while gay men are not segregated in Mexico as they tend to be in some other countries, they nevertheless live outside the population mainstream in terms of culture, ethos and sexual behavior, and therefore may often ignore communications aimed at the general public. Finally, gay men in Guadalajara are well organized, congregating in certain bars, discos and parks, and preferring particular health clinics, which makes them relatively identifiable and accessible to research and communications.

KAP Results

The lengthy KAP survey completed by CONASIDA indicated that gay men in Guadalajara were relatively well educated and both aware of the AIDS threat and knowledgeable about modes of transmission and means of self–protection. Nevertheless, actual use of condoms was quite low. Only 55% stated that they had ever used a condom, and of those, only 33% did so all of the time, for a total "all the time" usage of just 18%. Another 27% claimed they used condoms "most of the time."

Accordingly, the goal of the pilot intervention became that of increasing the prevalence and frequency of condom use. The method selected to achieve this goal was that of intensive and targeted distribution of condoms along with educational support materials.

Strategy for Meeting the Objective

These independent creative teams were assembled and given the same brief—they were to develop artistic concepts and supportive materials that would encourage condom use. To increase the probability that these materials would successfully communicate with the target audience, the designs were to reflect information about attitudes and concerns garnered from the November 1987 KAP survey.

Each team presented its recommended concept materials for approval and refinement. However, in accordance with the social marketing goal of being consumer–centered, the final selection was made by members of the target audience. The research team rented a suite in a local hotel. They then contacted gay men in gay bars, in health clinics, during lectures about AIDS, and in parks, inviting them to attend a focus group discussion about AIDS prevention.

During the focus group, the several artists' concepts were presented and the men were invited to comment upon them. In time, a clear consensus emerged; however, it was one that the researchers had not expected. Researchers had predicted that only one would be preferred; in fact, opinion among the men was split almost evenly. The younger men desired a multi–partner erotic lifestyle, and liked a straightforward command to "Use a condom!" Older men, on the other hand, idealized a single–partner lifestyle and responded to a logic that emphasized responsibility: "Prevenir el SIDA es responsabilidad de ambos. Por eso usamos condom." (Both of us are responsible for preventing AIDS. That's why we use condoms.)

This preference split actually represented an attitudinal split in the homosexual community (later confirmed in the post–intervention mini–KAP) that had not emerged during the KAP survey. On this basis, two of the posters were developed so as to respond to the concerns of both subcommunities. Condoms were packaged for both lifestyle groups in a paper "wallet" containing two condoms and an eight–page mini–comic in which "Un Chico Diferente" (A Different Kind of Guy) explains about AIDS and why he uses condoms. Ten thousand of each poster and 20000 wallet packs (40000 condoms) were prepared and distributed over a two–week period in July 1988. At the same time, a multi–channel AIDS prevention campaign attempted to reach all members of the gay community via messages on T.V. and radio, articles in magazines and the newspaper, and information in free brochures that were handed out in parks, bars, health clinics and elsewhere.

Success at Meeting the Objective

The effectiveness of the project was measured in August 1988 via a "mini–KAP" survey. As with the focus group work, researchers met gay men in bars, discos, the park and in other settings where they congregated, and invited them to answer an oral questionnaire about AIDS.

A total of 260 men were interviewed. Thirty–seven percent were ages 15–20, 38% 21–25, 15% 26–30 and 10% over 30. Those encountered in the park tended to be under twenty. About two–thirds stated that they had sexual relations strictly with the same sex and an additional 20% mainly with the same sex. Almost 40% claimed they had had sex with people they did not know well, and an additional 30% reported having had sex with foreigners in the last five years. At least 20% had had a sexually transmitted disease, and 46% reported that they had been tested for the AIDS virus. One–fourth of respondents said that they had not had sexual relations in the last four months. Of those who had had relations, half stated that they had had only one partner, 38% had had two to five partners, and 14% had had six or more. Those with numerous partners tended to be over thirty.

As predicted by the health continuum model (above) respondents were at different levels of awareness and concern about AIDS. Thus, asked how much the information provided by the CONASIDA campaign (as opposed to other sources) had influenced their sexual behavior in the previous month, 54% said very much, 18% somewhat, 12% a little, and 13% not at all, while four percent remained completely unaware of the campaign. Those who were more aware and better able to receive its message were men who used condoms, men ages 21–25, and men who knew someone with AIDS. Those least aware or least accepting included men over 26, men who were more sexually active, men who were not aware of the time lag between infection and symptoms, and men who did not believe the disease was fatal.

Approximately two–thirds of the men had what was judged as accurate general knowledge of AIDS transmission, prevention and symptoms, but 25% continued to believe that AIDS could be passed on by casual contact or by insects. Older men and those contacted in discos/bars or who had attended an AIDS prevention lecture had better knowledge. Youths under 20 were most likely to believe that there was a medical way to prevent or cure AIDS.

Awareness of Condoms

Over half of the respondents stated that they practiced oral–genital and anal–genital sex. Eighty percent of the sample stated that they had used a condom at least once; 63% said they had in the last six months. Of these, 33% reported using a condom most or all of the time for anal sex. Condom use was less for oral sex. Those more likely to have used condoms included those who were better informed, more worried, knew someone with AIDS, had relations with more than one person, had been tested for the virus, or who claimed to have been influenced by the campaign. Respondents felt that the main advantage of condoms was that they helped prevent sexually transmitted diseases, but AIDS prevention and hygiene were also often cited. The main reasons that men gave for not using condoms was that they were monogamous or abstinent.

In general, perceptions of condoms were positive. At least two–thirds of respondents agreed that condoms were easy to use, the responsibility of both partners, appropriate for men, and should be part of the sexual routine. There was general disagreement with the ideas that condoms cause shame, take away romance, or that they are ineffective at preventing AIDS. A few men were concerned that proposing condom use would be offensive to others.

Forty–four percent said they were using condoms more now than in previous months. Over half claimed to have used condoms most or all of time in the last month. Some 80% thought that the total population should be using condoms, especially those practicing high–risk behavior (that is, those with multiple partners, gays, sex workers and drug abusers). However, only 16% had a condom with them at the time of the interview. Those more likely to be carrying condoms were those who stated that their attitudes and behavior had changed due to the threat of AIDS.

Researchers' Assessment of Effectiveness

The social marketers who completed this pilot project were pleased with their results. They felt that the educational campaign had had a positive effect: many respondents were aware of the campaign media, materials and messages propagated, many agreed with the suggestions of the message and a significant number claimed to have modified their sexual behavior in response to the information received.

The researchers recognized some limitations; risky behaviors continue, even among those claiming to have modified their behavior. Over 50% of respondents had had more than one partner in the previous four months, and 40% said they had had sex with people they had just met. Frequency of condom use had increased, but 37% stated that they had not used a condom in six months and 27% more used a condom only rarely in the last month.

Significantly, when reactions to the two posters were solicited, the same split in preference that had emerged in the focus groups re–emerged, with 49% preferring one presentation and 51% preferring the other.

Other stabilities in the data showed that the respondents also were split in another direction, for one group was more receptive and the other more resistant to AIDS prevention messages in general. The receptive population (including men who responded to either of the two poster messages) tended to be in their twenties, have some education, have accurate knowledge of sexually transmitted diseases and AIDS, be worried about AIDS, have been tested for HIV, know someone with AIDS, and be willing to limit their number of partners. In contrast, youths and those over 30, those with multiple partners or who seek relations with people they do not know, and those who do not believe AIDS is fatal, tended to be more resistant.

Follow–up Activities

On the basis of this pilot experience, CONASIDA specialists were able to make recommendations for continued AIDS prevention efforts in Guadalajara. The receptive group, now recognized and defined, can be targeted for continued support activities. For example, the tendency to use oil–based lubricants on condoms could be addressed by an informational campaign. However, since only about 33% of men claim to buy condoms, a further survey will be necessary to develop better understanding of how men acquire condoms so that projects can develop measures to increase control over their distribution. The resistant group can perhaps be subdivided (as by age) and reexamined to discover specific attitudes or concerns that can be addressed by a different communications approach.

A Social Marketing Perspective on This Pilot Project

This pilot serves as a useful teaching tool because it illustrates all the basic issues central to social marketing as summarized in the body of this chapter. The campaign was done in a politically friendly setting, in parallel with, though not in conjunction with, a national campaign. Several organizations shared data and collaborated on the project. Data from an initial KAP survey were used to identify need and to set goals, as well as to guide artists as they developed experimental communications concepts. In accordance with the need to be consumer–centered, researchers entered the gay community repeatedly. The fact that they could do this indicates that they were culturally sensitive and kept their political fences mended. The target population was invited to make choices about what messages most attracted them, and researchers accepted their choices as binding.

The multi–channel communications campaign was responsive to the target populations' attitudes and knowledge, and to researchers' expectations that people would be in different stages of "readiness" to receive the messages.

Support activities —in this case, the distribution of actual condoms— were built in to the project to help move the motivated toward trial and adoption of the new behavior.

A follow–up survey was built into the project to assess its effectiveness. On this basis, the population was better understood, gaps in knowledge were pinpointed, and recommendations were made for modifications of the campaigns.

SUMMARY

In sum, social marketing is more than advertising, more than communications, and more than public relations. It consists of an integrated strategy to encourage behaviors that marketers believe are in the interests of individuals or the society. It depends on the scientific collection and analysis of data on consumers' knowledge, attitudes and practices, linked to behavioral modification techniques, and applied in a context of marketer attitudes of concern for consumers and a desire to do no harm. The value of applying the social marketing approach to the prevention of AIDS is shown by its lengthening record of success at improving people's knowledge of AIDS and willingness to adopt preventive measures.

REFERENCES

M.C. Bateson and R. Goldsby. *Thinking AIDS, the Social Response to the Biological Threat.* Addison-Wesley, Reading MA,1988

R. Bayer *Private Acts, Social Consequences: AIDS and the Politics of Public Health* Free Press, NY., 1989

P. Biella "Design for a Latino AIDS Education Film." Oral Presentation to the American Anthropological Association, Phoenix,AZ, November, 1988. Mimeo.

R. Bolton*The AIDS Pandemic: A Global Emergency. Medical Anthropology 10(2-3)* special issue,1989.

S.G. Boodman "Clean Needles Don't Make More Addicts, Panel Told" *Washington Post* 4/25/89, p.A9

K. Carovano "Survey of AIDS Education Programs." Monograph prepared for AIDSCOM, Academy for Educational Development, 1989.

J.M. Carrier "Sexual Behavior and the Spread of AIDS in Mexico." *Medical; Anthropology 10(2-3):* 129-142,1989.

—— "Mexican Male Bisexuality." *Journal of Homosexuality* 11(3-4): 75-85, 1985.

—— "Cultural factors Affecting Urban Mexican Male Homosexual Behavior." *Archives of Sexual Behavior* 5(2): 103-124, 1976.

C.M. Cassidy, R. Porter, R. Feldman. "Ethnographic Survey of Nonpenetrative Sexual Behavior." Monograph prepared for AIDSCOM, Academy for Educational Development, 1989.

CONASIDA/AIDSCOM 1988 Mexico Project trip report, unpublished.

D. Crimp, ed. *AIDS, Cultural Analysis, Cultural Activism.* MIT Press, Cambridge, MA, 1988.

M. Debus Internal Memo, 2/21/89, Porter-Novelli, unpublished.

DOH (Philippines/AIDSCOM). Fall 1988 Philippines Project Trip Report, unpublished.

L.W. Frederiksen, L.J. Solomon, K.A. Brehony, eds. *Marketing Health Behavior, Principles, Techniques and Applications.* Plenum Press, NY., 1984

P. Fry and E. MacRae. *A que e a homossexual i dade.* Editora Brasiliense, Sao Paulo,1982.

D.V. Hart "Homosexuality and Transvestism in the Philippines, the Cebuan filipino Bayot and Lakinn-on." *Behavior Science Notes* 3(4:211-248), 1968.

P. Kotler and A. R. Andreasen. *Strategic Marketing for Nonprofit Organizations, 3rd edition* Prentice-Hall,Inc., Englewood Cliffs, N.J., 1987.

G.,M. MacDonald Helquist, W. Smith. "Reducing HIV Transmission,

Lessons from the recent Past." AIDSCOM, Academy for Educational Development, 1987.

R. Parker "Masculinity, Femininity, and Homosexuality: On the Anthorpological Interpretation of Sexual Meaning in Brazil." *Journal of Homosexuality 11(3-4):* 155-163,1985.

S.,R. Rosario Pareja, M. Butler de Lister. "Skills and Dexterity of Female Sex Workers of Santo Domingo in the Use and Handling of Condoms." AIDSCOM Report, Academy for Educational Development, 1989.

R. Shilts *And the Bank Played On, Politics, people, and the AIDS Epidemic.* Penguin Books, 1987.

C.L. Taylor "Mexican Male Homosexual Interaction in Public Contexts." Journal of Homosexuality 11(304):117-136,1985.

—— El Ambiente'Male Homosexual Social Life in Mexico City. Ph.D. Dissertation, University of California-Berkeley, 1978.

III. LESSONS FROM NATIONAL EXPERIENCES

Preface

Jaime Sepulveda

The following section of the book looks at the experiences of AIDS prevention programs in different regions of the world and from various perspectives. Of course, these lines of introduction are not intended to be comprehensive, but to point out different approaches to a health problem which stem from local epidemiological circumstances and cultural settings.

The chapter on Europe briefly describes the socio-cultural context of that region, which had, until recently, two major political systems. Among other factors, in the 1980s this recent change in European political reality increased the movement of people within Europe and with other areas of the world, which affects U.S. transmission patterns. Countries in Europe present diverse epidemiological patterns of AIDS transmission with more homosexual transmission in some areas while in others infection through intravenous drug (IV) use prevails. The responses to the AIDS epidemic therefore also vary, with approaches ranging from moralistic to technocratic, from pragmatic to emancipatory. Many lessons can be learned from this rich experience. The authors of this chapter propose that prostitution be decriminalized and sex workers be trained as peer educators, and give examples of effective needle-exchange programs. They also stress the fact that non-governmental organizations have and should continue to play a very important role in AIDS prevention in Europe.

In the United States, the epidemic took the public health system by surprise. The chapter on the United States explains most clearly the lesson that in AIDS prevention, knowledge does not automatically translate into behavioral change. Adequate information about AIDS is a necessary but not sufficient condition for the individual to adopt preventive measures or change behavior. In addition, the authors stress that information should come from sources which are considered credible by the audience of the intervention is aimed: peer education has proven most effective among those with high-risk practices. Furthermore, once behavioral modification is attained, it must be sustained. To do so, educational programs must be consistent, intensive and repetitive, with adequate evaluation. Some minorities are disproportionately represented in the AIDS epidemic in the United States. This means that educational programs must be culturally sensitive and linguistically appropriate to the target audience. This multi-cultural makeup is part of what leads the authors to stress that there is a limit to what governmental agencies can do directly to promote behavioral change. Non-governmental organizations sometimes have more credibility, access and information as to what interventions work best within their constituencies

The authors of the chapter on Africa address the problem of the overemphasis on the origin of AIDS; as they correctly affirm, at most it is only of historical interest. Their data show that an extremely high seroprevalence rate now exists in some regions and sub-populations of sub-Saharan Africa. This situation makes it poignantly evident that efforts must be maximized in regions where the AIDS epidemic is only starting, so that the epidemic can be contained, preventing its devastating spread to larger segments of the population. In reading this, as well as other chapters, one is left with the impression that there is a "threshold effect," and once infection rates reach a certain level, the epidemic spreads much more rapidly into larger populations. Commercial sex workers in Africa are a high-risk group for both acquiring and transmitting the disease. Some groups of commercial sex workers have participated in U.S./AIDS prevention programs, with striking responsiveness to education and willingness to implement preventive measures. Therefore programs designed to educate them on AIDS prevention are the most cost–effective, a central concern in a region where annual government health expenditure is patently insufficient.

The chapter on Brazil clearly illustrates the combination of "patterns" of AIDS transmission which exists in Latin America—heterosexuality, homosexuality, bisexuality, blood products and IV drug use are all factors in the Brazilian AIDS epidemic. It also focuses on the need to combat the "epidemic of prejudice" that often accompanies AIDS, both for humanitarian and practical reasons, as empowerment and self–affirmation have proven much more effective than fear and criticism in preventing transmission of AIDS. This chapter also communicates to the reader the marked importance non-governmental organizations have in the fight against AIDS in Brazil, with their combination of local research, incorporation of the target population in the creation and presentation of prevention programs and decentralization of AIDS–related services.

In Mexico, the response to the AIDS epidemic has evolved from an erratic approach in the early stages, followed by a well–planned, technocratic campaign, and, more recently, by a reactive response to external pressures. Compared to other places, the reaction from non–governmental organizations has, unfortunately, been insufficiently energetic, leaving governmental agencies fewer arguments with which to resist the pressure from right-wing groups. One lesson from the Mexican experience lays in the need for constant epidemiological and behavioral monitoring, because of the rapid changes that can take place in the AIDS epidemic.

The multiplicity of approaches and perspectives of national or regional experiences has to do not only with the variety of authors and writing styles, but the differences that exist in local epidemiological patterns and social responses to the epidemic. This diversity of approaches is therefore not only understandable, but actually desirable.

AIDS Education and Health Promotion in Brazil: Lessons from the Past and Prospects for the Future

Richard G. Parker

Since the earliest cases began to be reported in 1982 and 1983, AIDS has emerged as one of the most serious public health problems in contemporary Brazilian life. As in other nations, given the lack of a vaccine or a medical cure for HIV infection and AIDS, it quickly became apparent that education and health promotion would offer the only effective means of slowing the spread of the epidemic. Perhaps even more than in many other countries, however, not only the inherent complexities of AIDS itself, but also Brazil's immense social and cultural diversity seems to have raised a series of problems for the development of effective education programs. In this chapter, I will examine some of these problems, review the ways in which AIDS education activities have sought to respond to them on a variety of different levels, and look at the possible impact that these educational initiatives have had over the course of a number of years. On the basis of this discussion, I will evaluate the prospects for AIDS education in Brazil in the future, and offer some tentative suggestions about implications that the Brazilian experience has for AIDS education in other settings.

The Social and Epidemiological Context of AIDS in Brazil

Before turning to a more detailed discussion of the AIDS education activities themselves, it is worthwhile to situate this discussion within the wider social and epidemiological context of AIDS in Brazil. What is perhaps most immediately striking is the remarkable diversity of this context. Brazil is an immense country, with a territory of approximately 8500000 square kilometers, and a population of nearly 142 million people. Extensive regional differences cut across the bonds created by a common language, and social and cultural transformations play themselves out as much in space as they do in history. Nominally the largest Catholic nation in the world, Brazil might just as accurately be described in terms of the no less obvious presence of any number of Afro–Brazilian and spiritist religious traditions. It is perhaps best described, following Roger Bastide, as a "land of contrasts" in which the divisions of class, race and gender are evident during almost every moment of daily life, while tradition and modernity somehow seem to exist side by side.[1]

These basic contradictions in the character or quality of contemporary Brazilian life have become all the more evident over the course of recent decades, as the country has undergone a series of profound social and political changes. Unprecedented urbanization has transformed what was once an essentially rural society, stretching, and at times opening fissures in the basic fabric of social life. No less extensive economic transformations, linked to the complicated politics of both dependence and debt, have resulted in a series of deepening economic crises. Perhaps more importantly, twenty years of authoritarian military rule, followed by a gradual return to democratic government only in the early 1980s, have combined to undercut the basic legitimacy of both civil and state institutions, and have left a legacy of neglect and mismanagement in the public health and social welfare systems that has severely limited their ability to confront already existing health problems, let alone the problems posed by a new, emerging epidemic.[2]

It is within this context that the AIDS epidemic began to take shape in Brazil during the early 1980s, and both the ways in which it has developed as well as the ways in which Brazilian society has responded to it over the course of nearly a decade have been conditioned by this particular set of circumstances. Like Brazilian society itself, AIDS in Brazil has been marked, perhaps above all else, by its complexity and diversity. By July of 1989, with 7182 reported cases and 3572 known deaths (see Table 6-1), AIDS had clearly emerged as one of the most serious problems in contemporary Brazilian life. While the vast majority of these cases are found in large urban centers such as Sao Paulo (61.9% of the national total) and Rio de

---

[1] Roger Bastide, *Brasil, Terra de Contrastes* (Rio de Janeiro and Sao Paulo: Difel, 1978).
[2] Berber Daniel and Richard G. Parker, "The Third Epidemic: The Social Response to AIDS in Brazil," in *The Third Epidemic: Repercussions of the Fear of AIDS* (London: The Panos Institute, 1989); and Richard G. Parker, "Responding to AIDS in Brazil," in *Action on AIDS: National Policies in Comparative Perspective*, eds. David Moss and Barbara Misztal (Westport, CT: Greenwood Press, 1990 (In press).

Janeiro (14.5%), cases have been reported from every state and region of the country (see Table 6-2). Even greater diversity emerges in turning from its regional distribution to the specific modes of HIV transmission that have characterized the AIDS epidemic in Brazil. Whether looking at sexuality, the exchange of blood and blood products, or the use of intravenous drugs, the complexity and diversity that marks Brazilian life more generally can be found, as well, in virtually all of the specific contexts in which HIV infection has taken root and spread.[3]

Table 6-1. *Cases of* AIDS *and number of deaths by year, Brazil, 1980-1989.*[ab]

Year	No. of cases	No. of deaths
1980	1	1
1981	–	–
1982	7	5
1983	24	20
1984	116	93
1985	456	319
1986	905	565
1987	1 934	1 086
1988	2 781	1 157
1989[a]	958	326
Total	7 182	3 572

[a] Preliminary data through July 1, 1989.
[b] Data from Ministério de Saúde, Divisão Nacional de DST/AIDS, *Boletim Epidemiológico*, Ano II, No. 12, 1989.

While homosexual interactions have been particularly important in the spread of HIV, for example, the social and cultural organization of such contacts in Brazil seems to be especially complex, and multiple subcultures or sexual communities have developed over the course of recent years, at least in urban Brazil, in which same–sex sexual behaviors are linked to the construction of sexual identities in a variety of diverse ways.[4] Same–sex interactions do not always translate into the conscious elaboration of

[3] *Op. cit.* Richard G. Parker, 1990 (In press).
[4] Richard, G. Parker, "Acquired Immunodeficiency Syndrome in Urban Brazil," *Medical Anthropology Quarterly*, new series, 1(2) (1987): 155–75; and Richard G. Parker, "Youth, Identity, and Homosexuality: The Changing Shape of Sexual Life in Brazil," *Journal of Homosexuality*, 17(1/2) (1988): 267–87.

Table 6-2. *Number of cases and cases per million, by region and states, Brazil, 1980-1990.*[a][b]

Region State	No.	Cases per 1 000 000
BRAZIL	11 070	83.2
NORTH	90	11.2
Rondônia	8	11.5
Acre	7	20.1
Amazonas	18	10.7
Roraima	8	80.1
Pará	43	10.6
Amapá	5	24.0
Tocantins	1	1.1
NORTHEAST	805	20.9
Miranhão	50	11.0
Piauí	16	6.7
Ceará	112	19.3
Rio Grande do Norte	54	25.9
Paraíba	35	11.7
Pernambuco	229	34.3
Alagoas	46	20.9
Sergipe	29	22.4
Bahia	234	22.3
SOUTHEAST	9 133	208.7
Minas Gerais	374	26.0
Espírito Santo	82	36.4
Rio de Janeiro	1 593	127.1
São Paulo	7 084	244.5
SOUTH	747	36.6
Paraná	170	21.2
Santa Catarina	94	23.4
Rio Grande do Sul	483	57.7
CENTRAL-WEST	295	50.2
Goiás	89	20.4
Mato Grosso	57	39.9
Mato Grosso do Sul	55	35.0
Distrito Federal	94	61.7

[a] Through the first week of April, 1990.
[b] Data from Ministério de Saúde, Divisão Nacional de DST/AIDS, *Boletim Epidemiológico*, Ano II, No. 12, 1989; and Ano III, No. 9, 1990.

Table 6–3. *Number and percentage of cases of AIDS according to category of transmission and sex, Brazil, 1980–1990.*[ab]

Category of transmission	Males Number	%	Females Number	%	Total Number	%
Sexual transmission	7 752	69	353	30	8 105	65
Homosexual contact	4 583	41	–	–	4 583	37
Bisexual contact	2 167	19	–	–	2 167	17
Heterosexual contact	1 002	9	353	30	1 355	11
Blood transmission	2 272	20	654	55	2 926	24
IV drug use	1 580	14	395	33	1 975	16
Transfusion	379	3	259	22	638	5
Hemofilia	313	3	–	–	313	3
Perinatal transmission	109	9	102	9	211	2
Undefined or other	1 089	10	74	6	1 163	9
Total	11 222	90[c]	1 183	10[c]	12 405	100

[a] Through the second week of August, 1990.
[b] Data from Ministério de Saúde, Divisão Nacional de DST/AIDS, *Boletim Epidemiológico*, Ano II, No. 12, 1989, and Año III, No. 11, 1990.
[c] Proportional distribution by sex; male/female ratio:10:1.

homosexual or even bisexual identities, and the links between specific sexual practices and perceptions of risk are mediated by diverse social structures and cultural representations.[5] Perhaps not surprisingly, then, although homosexual contacts have accounted for 40.5% of the cases of AIDS reported in Brazil as a whole by July of 1989, bisexual contacts have accounted for another 19.3%, while cases linked to heterosexual interactions have risen to 8.9% of the national total (see Table 6–3).

Much the same complexity can be found, as well, in the exchange of blood and blood products in Brazil, where humanitarian values have always been less important than commercial interests. Blood has traditionally circulated from the poorest sectors of society, with the least access to adequate medical care, to the more well–to–do, and the commercialization

5 *Op. cit.* Richard G. Parker, 1987; and Richard G. Parker, "Sexual Culture and AIDS Education in Urban Brazil," in *AIDS 1988: AAAS Symposia Papers*, ed. Ruth Kulstad (Washington, D.C.: The American Association for the Advancement of Science, 1988), pp. 169–73.

of blood in Brazil has long resulted in high incidences of diseases such as *chagas*.[6] Not surprisingly, 9.1% of the reported cases of AIDS in Brazil have been linked to receipt of blood and blood products on the part of hemophiliacs and blood transfusion recipients (see Table 6–3), and even though important attempts have been made recently to regulate the blood industry, these efforts have often been fiercely resisted on a number of fronts, and have resulted in both the creation of a kind of black (or parallel) blood market, as well as in widespread uncertainty concerning the possible risks involved in both blood donation and the receipt of blood products.[7]

Finally, while intravenous (IV) drug use lagged behind other modes of transmission during the early years of the AIDS epidemic in Brazil, it has recently become the most rapidly expanding mode of transmission, and currently accounts for 11.8% of the cases reported in the country as a whole (see Table 6–3). In some areas, such as parts of the city and state of Sao Paulo where drug traffic routes have traditionally functioned, this percentage is significantly higher, and a variety of social and cultural configurations has made the problems raised by HIV infection and AIDS especially difficult to confront. When compared to the situation in some other nations, IV drug use in Brazil is less clearly defined as the focus for a unique, sharply bounded underworld. At the same time, however, IV drug use is high among some groups, such as female and transvestite prostitutes in many major urban centers, who are otherwise potentially at risk in the face of HIV infection, and the complicated overlapping of multiple risk factors raises a series of special problems in a variety of different settings.

Together with the basic social and economic problems faced by virtually all developing nations, the complexity and diversity of Brazilian life more generally, and the complicated social and cultural settings within which the AIDS epidemic has taken shape in particular, have raised a whole series of problems for AIDS education and health promotion in Brazil. These problems have been accentuated further still, in Brazil, as in so many other nations, by both pre–existing prejudices related to many of the groups and practices that have been linked to HIV transmission, as well as by fear and misunderstanding in the face of AIDS itself. The result has been a complicated and troubled situation in which some of the basic strategies and tactics developed for AIDS health promotion in other nations have been able to play an important role, while others have had to be developed in order to respond to the distinct social and cultural realities of contemporary Brazilian life. In the following section, I will try to outline some of the most important AIDS education materials and activities that have been developed

---

[6] ABIA (Associaçao Brasileira Interdisciplinar de AIDS), "The Face of AIDS in Brazil," presented at the IV International Conference on AIDS, Stockholm, Sweden, 1988.

[7] *Op. cit.* Richard, G. Parker, 1990 (In press).

thus far in Brazil, and to suggest some of the different approaches or strategies that seem to have guided planning and policy–making.

AIDS INFORMATION AND EDUCATION ACTIVITIES

In reviewing the development of AIDS education and health promotion activities in Brazil, it is perhaps best to think of a number of distinct levels, both in terms of sources, as well as in terms of types of information. These different levels can be distinguished both on the basis of their content as well as their specificity, and perhaps all involve rather different degrees of self–consciousness or reflection concerning the basic health promotion strategies that have been employed. Without claiming to have exhausted all of the sources of information on health promotion that have been available in Brazilian society, we can focus our attention on three areas that have been most significant in shaping wider views about HIV and AIDS, and that have most clearly offered an interpretation of the significance of these issues in relation to the population of individuals engaged in same–sex sexual behaviors: the mass media; the information and education campaigns mounted at a national level under the direction of the National AIDS Committee and the Ministry of Health; and the health promotion activities developed at the state and local level, largely through the work of nongovernmental AIDS service organizations.[8]

The role of the media in responding to AIDS in Brazil has been mixed at best. On the one hand, particularly during the earliest years of the epidemic, coverage of AIDS was extremely limited, and even when the media gradually began to focus increasing attention on AIDS–related issues, the result was often the production of highly distorted images of both the disease and its perceived victims. The early description of the epidemic, in Brazil as elsewhere, as a kind of "gay plague," clearly added to prejudice and discrimination against both perceived homosexuals, on the one hand, and people with AIDS, on the other.[9] Although sensationalist coverage has continued to mar at least some AIDS–related reporting, however, the broader response of the media in Brazil has generally become increasingly informed and responsible. Numerous articles in major newspapers and national magazines have focused on AIDS–related issues in relatively responsible ways, and public service announcements and special reports carried on major television networks have increasingly brought the discussion of AIDS into

[8] Richard G. Parker, Carmen Dora Guimaraes and Claudio J. Struchiner, "The Impact of AIDS Health Promotion for Gay and Bisexual Men in Rio de Janeiro, Brazil," presented at the World Health Organization/Global Programme on AIDS Workshop on AIDS Health Promotion Activities Directed Towards Gay and Bisexual Men, Geneva, Switzerland, 1989.

[9] *Op. cit.* Berber Daniel and Richard G. Parker.

the homes of more Brazilians than would have been possible through any other medium. Taken together, the printed media, radio and television have all contributed to the creation of what might be described as a kind of background of basic information—a background that has been crucial in shaping both attitudes and practices related to HIV infection and AIDS.[10]

The importance of television as perhaps the single most important medium for the transmission of information in Brazil has also provided a focus for the education activities of the Ministry of Health's National AIDS Program. As the communication medium that most clearly cuts across the major divisions of Brazilian society and unites the country's diverse geographical regions, television has emerged as the natural focus for broad based AIDS education and information campaigns that have been developed on a national level since 1986.[11] While posters, pamphlets and advertising billboards have all been employed in conjunction with television, the majority of the attention (as well as the financial resources) focused on AIDS health promotion since that time has been given over to a series of nationally broadcast public health announcements, developed for the Ministry of Health by commercial advertising agencies, emphasizing various aspects of the disease.[12]

The earliest materials developed for these national campaigns focused on the presentation of very basic information: how HIV is (and is not) transmitted, the role of sexual relations, IV drug injection, blood transfusions and the like. As the national campaigns have developed, a strategy has emerged in which new announcements are periodically introduced, successively shifting the focus of attention: an advertising campaign focusing on the potential risk involved in multiple sexual partners might be followed, some months later, for example, by a new announcement focusing on drug injection, and so on. Most recently, this series of advertisements has been superseded by yet another, using well–known public figures to discuss a range of AIDS–related issues as a means of raising AIDS awareness more generally.

At least in part because different commercial agencies have been involved in planning the advertisements used in these national campaigns, their underlying messages have sometimes seemed contradictory (ranging, for example, from the early slogan, "Love Doesn't Kill," to the more recent, "Don't Die From Love"), and have often drawn criticism from non–governmental AIDS service organizations. The underlying strategy behind these shifting announcements has nonetheless remained more or less consistent.

[10] Op. cit. Richard G. Parker, Carmen Dora Guimaraes and Claudio J. Struchiner.
[11] Lair Guerra de Macedo Rodrigues, "Brazil's Educational Programme on AIDS Prevention," World Summit of Ministers of Health Programmes for AIDS Prevention, London, January, 1988.
[12] Op. cit. Richard G. Parker, Carmen Dora Guimaraes and Claudio J. Struchiner.

As one way of responding to the social and cultural diversity of the country as a whole, they have sought to present basic information on different risk behaviors for a relatively general audience, while more clearly focused or controversial messages have largely been avoided.[13]

This is not to say that thought has not been given to a more careful identification of potential target groups. On the contrary, within its working plan for health promotion, the National AIDS Program has clearly targeted at least four broad audiences: health professionals; the public at large; groups engaging in high–risk behaviors; and adolescents.[14]

The third of these audiences, "groups engaging in high–risk behaviors," has been further broken down into "homosexual and bisexual men, intravenous drug users, and male and female prostitutes."[15] There has been considerable debate, however, concerning the most appropriate manner to develop materials for these different audiences, and groups as diverse as gay liberation organizations, on the one hand, and conservative sectors of the Catholic Church, on the other, have exerted pressure from a variety of directions that has clearly conditioned the development of government sponsored campaigns.[16] While central emphasis has been placed on promoting the use of condoms, for example, some voices within the Church have vigorously criticized this emphasis, and during at least one brief period references to condoms were taken out of government sponsored AIDS announcements in response to political pressure. Although the National AIDS Committee has worked closely with a wide range of concerned groups in developing its program, and has managed to achieve a certain degree of cooperation and collaboration, there is no doubt that a complicated set of political forces has limited its freedom of movement in a variety of ways.[17]

Many of the same forces that have limited the federal government's freedom in designing and implementing AIDS education programs have had a similar impact on the state and local level as well. When combined with the severe limitations of most state and local budgets, it is hardly surprising that little in the way of AIDS education and health promotion has emerged at the state and local level in most parts of Brazil. In some more well–to–do regions, such as in Sao Paulo, more available resources have made possible the development of relatively elaborate and innovative AIDS education programs that have drawn heavily on support from local communities. More commonly, however, as in financially hard–pressed Rio de Janeiro,

---

13 *Ibid.*

14 *Op. cit.* Lair Guerra de Macedo Rodrigues.

15 *Ibid.*

16 Hilary Regan, "Brazilian Bishops Split on Strategies to Control Spreading AIDS Epidemic," *Latinamerica Press* 19(14), (1987): 6.

17 *Op. cit.* Richard G. Parker, Carmen Dora Guimaraes and Claudio J. Struchiner; and *op. cit.,* Lair Guerra de Macedo Rodrigues.

an almost absolute lack of infrastructure and funding has made it difficult, at least until quite recently, for state and local public health officials to mount more than a minimal response. Even here, however, at the local level, important developments have begun to take place in recent years, particularly as a result of the formation of a growing number of voluntary associations and AIDS service organizations that have focused on AIDS education in a variety of different community contexts.[18]

While it is impossible, within the limited space available here, to review the activities of all of the different non–governmental organizations that have become involved in AIDS education activities in Brazil over the course of the past three to four years, even a brief discussion of the activities of a number of key groups can offer a sense of the role that non–governmental organizations and ASOS have begun to assume in AIDS education and health promotion activities in Brazil. Organized in Sao Paulo in late 1985, GAPA, the Support Group for the Prevention of AIDS, for example, was the first voluntary group in Brazil explicitly devoted to AIDS–related issues. Drawing its membership, at least initially, principally from the ranks of health care workers involved in the treatment of AIDS patients, on the one hand, and activists who had previously been involved in gay groups, on the other, GAPA was also the first non–governmental organization to become involved in AIDS health promotion. One of its earliest activities was the production of a controversial poster that drew on highly explicit and popular language to encourage safer sexual practices, particularly among men who have sex with men, and members of GAPA have continued to be involved in AIDS health promotion activities in variety of different contexts, though less through the publication of educational materials than through verbal presentations, debates and a range of other outreach activities. Over the course of nearly five years now, the group's activities have expanded rapidly, and essentially independent chapters of GAPA have been formed in other urban centers around Brazil. But its basic commitment to local level, community–based, and relatively focused health promotion activities has continued to direct the development of its program.[19]

Shortly after the formation of GAPA, intellectuals and activists from diverse backgrounds came together in Rio to form ABIA, the Brazilian Inter-disciplinary AIDS Association, which quickly developed into a highly sophisticated and professional organization that has played an important role both as a critic of AIDS–related public policy as well as a key producer of AIDS information and health promotion materials. For a number of years,

---

[18] *Op. cit.* Berber Daniel, and Richard G. Parker; and *op. cit.*, Richard, G. Parker, 1990 (In press); and *op. cit.*, Richard G. Parker, Carmen Dora Guimaraes and Claudio J. Struchiner.

[19] *Op. cit.* Richard, G. Parker, 1990 (In press); and *op. cit.*, Richard G. Parker, Carmen Dora Guimaraes and Claudio J. Struchiner.

ABIA's staff has been involved in developing a set of highly focused health promotion materials directed to a variety of groups within Brazilian society, and has supplied these materials to AIDS service organizations throughout the country. Particularly important projects have included educational videos developed for use with groups such as civil construction workers and street children as well as informational pamphlets developed for sailors and for gay–identified men. Less restrained than government officials by concerns about possible backlash from conservative sectors of Brazilian society, the materials developed by ABIA have been among the most direct and explicit available anywhere in Brazil. They have been distributed to groups working in AIDS education throughout the country, and, along with talks and presentations by ABIA's staff members for audiences as diverse as gay liberation groups, the employees of both state and private businesses, and a range of private and professional organizations, these activities have constituted what may be the most wide–reaching and influential AIDS education program developed by any non–governmental organization.[20]

Not surprisingly, this same emphasis on highly focused or targeted health promotion activities has also characterized a range of different groups and organizations that serve more clearly delimited clienteles. Gay organizations such as the Gay Group of Bahia in Salvador and Atobá in Rio de Janeiro have worked closely with a range of other AIDS service organizations as well as with government AIDS programs in developing a series of AIDS–related activities. While the number of gay groups in Brazil is quite limited, and their membership clearly does not include many men who may engage in homosexual behaviors without in any way developing a sense of homosexual identity, groups such as Atobá and GGB have played a key role in reaching out to this population, in distributing both educational materials and condoms, and in offering a range of other support services.[21]

Similarly, working within the Institute for Religious Studies (an ecumenical organization involved in social and human rights issues), a program focusing on the civil rights of prostitutes in Rio de Janeiro has developed a set of AIDS education booklets specifically targeted to female, transvestite and male prostitutes, and is currently involved in training members of these groups to act as health promotion workers in the specific areas where they work.[22] Prostitutes' associations in a number of different parts of the country have shown an increasing interest in AIDS education, as well as in the social and political issues that the question of AIDS has raised for perceived risk groups in Brazilian society. Together with the activities

20 *Ibid.*
21 *Ibid.*
22 Nani Rubin, "Prostitutas falam de AIDS as prostitutas," *Jornal do Brasil,* July 31, 1989.

of more general AIDS service organizations such as GAPA and ABIA, then, the emergence of specifically focused AIDS education activities rooted in local communities has perhaps been the most significant development in the field of AIDS education in Brazil in recent years. To the extent that this trend continues in the future, it offers the possibility of responding to a set of issues and concerns that may well be, for political reasons, beyond the reach of government AIDS programs, but that are clearly among the most urgent problems that must be confronted in response to AIDS in Brazil.

Ultimately, then, even if their development has been relatively unsystematic, a range of AIDS education and health promotion activities has gradually emerged in Brazil over the course of a number of years. For the most part, these activities have emerged independently, and, thus far at least, there has been relatively little in the way of collaboration or cooperation between different programs or organizations. Nevertheless, even if in largely unplanned and uncoordinated ways, general information available in the mass media, somewhat more specific messages developed in broad–based national advertising campaigns, and more focused or targeted information and education activities on the part of local level and community groups have all contributed to the discussion of AIDS in a variety of different contexts. Together, they have begun to respond, at least tentatively, to the complexity and diversity of Brazilian life more generally, as well as to the particular contexts within which the AIDS epidemic has had its greatest impact.

THE IMPACT OF AIDS EDUCATION

It is far easier to review the different AIDS education activities that have thus far been developed in Brazil than it is to fully evaluate their impact. Because none of the various educational programs described here have yet been systematically investigated through follow–up research, and it is impossible to adequately evaluate the relative efficacy of any particular strategy or source. Even in the absence of such data, however, it is nonetheless useful to seek to identify the kinds of criteria that must be taken into account in seeking to evaluate the impact of educational programs—the issues that they must address and the effects that they should produce. Having identified these criteria more adequately, it might then be possible, even on the basis of very limited data, to offer some preliminary observations on the initial impact of AIDS education in recent years, as well as some tentative suggestions concerning the prospects for AIDS education activities in the future.

Much of the discussion of AIDS education in general has naturally focused on the question of risk reduction in relation to HIV infection, and both the prospects and obstacles facing educational programs, as well as the definition of success and failure, have been analyzed and interpreted along these lines.[23] Clearly, in thinking about the educational response to HIV infection and AIDS, this question of risk reduction is central. At the same time, however, it must also be linked to a wider set of issues that, within a fuller definition of the AIDS epidemic, must also be addressed. As part of this broader definition, a range of issues linked to what has been described as "the third epidemic," the complex social response to both AIDS and people with AIDS, must also be confronted.[24] Indeed, it is possible that the question of risk reduction itself can be confronted only to the extent that this wider range of social issues is raised in the discussion of AIDS, and both AIDS awareness more generally as well as the specific questions of prejudice and discrimination should be taken, along with risk reduction, as key questions that must also be considered in evaluating the impact of AIDS education programs.

In turning to the very limited data that are currently available concerning these issues, the results thus far are clearly mixed, offering reason for both guarded optimism as well as realistic preoccupation. Data collected in 1987 and 1988 by Gallup International as part of an international survey on attitudes and opinions about AIDS, for example, found that Brazil was one of only two countries in which 100% of the individuals surveyed responded that they had heard of AIDS. No less impressive, 79% of the Brazilians surveyed pointed to AIDS as the most urgent health problem facing the country, the highest total in any of the countries surveyed. Although the question itself may be problematic, in responding to the perception of distinct "risk groups" the data collected seem to indicate a high correlation between information and education activities, on the one hand, and perceptions of risk, on the other: of those individuals who responded to the survey, 95% indicated that AIDS is likely to become an epidemic among homosexuals, 95% mentioned people who need blood transfusions, and 92% pointed to IV drug users, while 67%, an unusually high number, saw AIDS as a potential epidemic among the general population. And, again, in turning from perceived risk groups to the more important question of risk–related behaviors, 97% pointed to HIV transmission through blood transfusions and needle sharing, 88% mentioned intimate sexual contact with a person of the same sex, and 84% pointed to intimate sexual contact with a person of the opposite sex.[25]

[23] Harvey Fineberg, "Education to Prevent AIDS: Prospects and Obstacles," *Science* 239 (1988): 592–6.

[24] Jonathan Mann, "Global AIDS: Epidemiology, Impact, Projections and the Global Strategy," World Summit of Ministers of Health Programmes for AIDS Prevention, London, January 1988.

In spite of this relatively impressive degree of AIDS awareness on the part of the general population, as well as relatively accurate perceptions of risk, only 14% of the individuals who responded to the Gallup International survey in Brazil indicated that they had made any changes in their behavior as a response to AIDS. Just as troubling, only 69%, a relatively low percentage, in comparison to many of the other countries surveyed, indicated that people with AIDS should be treated with compassion.[26] AIDS awareness, at least on the part of the general population, has thus not necessarily translated into risk–reducing behavioral change with any degree of frequency. While the nature of the survey's research design makes it impossible to evaluate the specific reasons for this particular configuration, the relatively low expression of concern for people with AIDS themselves may indicate that ingrained prejudices and pre–existing forms of discrimination in Brazilian society have had an important impact in creating an attitudinal climate that continues to inhibit a more positive response to AIDS–related risks. It may well be the case, in light of this, that addressing questions of prejudice and discrimination will be as crucial as the question of risk itself in seeking to stimulate risk reduction on the part of the general population.

As in a number of other countries, in turning from the general population to somewhat more specific groups within this population, once again very limited evidence offers some reason for hope that important changes in both attitudes and behaviors are taking place as a result of AIDS education activities in Brazil. Given the importance that virtually all sources of AIDS information have placed on the use of condoms as a means of reducing risk, it is important to note, for example, that one limited study conducted by a Sao Paulo newspaper found that condom use had increased from 6% to 27% among young people between the ages of 15 and 25 between December of 1985 and February of 1987. The same study found that condom use had increased from 17% to 49% among self–identified homosexual and bisexual adult males—the groups that have had perhaps the greatest access to targeted or focused health promotion materials from a number of different sources.[27]

Similar results have been reported as well in a recent study based on a limited number of extended interviews with gay and bisexual men in Rio de Janeiro, which linked a combination of concern, knowledge and information, and personal experience with HIV infection and AIDS to relatively exten-

[25] Norman L. Webb, "Gallup International Survey on Attitudes Towards AIDS," in *The Global Impact of AIDS*. eds. Alan Fleming *et al*. (New York: Alan P. Liss, Inc., 1988): 347–55.

[26] *Ibid*.

[27] "Pesquisa revela medo de contrair AIDS," *Folha de Sao Paulo*. February 22, 1987; and Luiz Mott, "A Penetração do Preservativo no Brasil PÓSAIDS," BEMFAM, *Publicações Técnicas*. No. 14 (1988).

sive behavioral change: fully 96% of the informants interviewed reported changing their habits in response to AIDS, 86% reported using condoms on a regular basis, and 58% reported reducing the number of their sexual part-ners. Rates of both active and passive anal intercourse have fallen from 4% to 10%, while the practice of mutual masturbation rose by 24% among those individuals interviewed, indicating a significant change not only in partner relations but in the very dynamics of sexual practice as a response to perceived risks. Again, however, the diversity of the target population has been emphasized, and researchers have underlined the need for caution in extending these findings, based principally on interviews with gay–identi-fied men, to the wider population of men who have sex with men but do not identify themselves as homosexual or bisexual.[28]

While such studies have been extremely limited, they nonetheless suggest that more focused AIDS health promotion activities can have a powerful impact in stimulating both behavioral and attitudinal change among specific populations with a heightened perception of risk. They would suggest that, just as increasing emphasis should be given in the future to addressing questions of AIDS–related discrimination and prejudice, greater attention should also be given to smaller–scale, increasingly focused health promotion activities developed for and by specific commu-nities. As in a number of other countries, the model of health promotion taking shape within, and in relation to, the gay community or homosexual population offers a useful model that might ultimately be extended to other communities confronting the risks of HIV infection and the problems posed by AIDS.[29]

Finally, it is important to emphasize the urgent need for research aimed at providing fuller data on the current situation and at evaluating more effectively the impact of specific interventions and educational programs. None of the limited studies carried out thus far has been sufficiently linked to any specific health promotion activity to really evaluate its impact or to establish causal links. At best, they offer very limited approximations of what may be occurring, and of why it may be taking place. It is important to stress the urgent need for more carefully formulated research aimed at the evaluation of health promotion interventions and AIDS education programs. Even as we await the kinds of data that will make it possible to come to truly informed decisions concerning these issues, it is nonetheless possible, on the basis of the discussion developed here, to offer a number of prelimi-nary suggestions concerning the most reasonable approaches. In closing, then, I would like to turn briefly to some of the specific policy implications

[28] *Op. cit.* Richard G. Parker, Carmen Dora Guimaraes and Claudio J. Struchiner.

[29]. Charles F. Turner, Heather G. Miller and Lincoln E. Moses, eds., *AIDS, Sexual Behavior, and Intravenous Drug Use.* (Washington, D.C.: National Academy Press, 1989).

that emerge from this discussion, and to look at the prospects for AIDS education in the future in Brazil.

LESSONS FROM THE PAST AND PROSPECTS FOR THE FUTURE

In looking back at the history of AIDS education in Brazil over the course of nearly a decade, it is clear that a number of developments have taken place that offer hope for the future. As data from the Gallup International survey seem to indicate, there has emerged a widespread conviction on the part of the general public that AIDS is the most potentially serious health problem currently facing the country, and this conviction clearly opens the door for the kind of commitment to AIDS education that will ultimately be necessary if Brazil is to respond effectively to the epidemic. Perhaps more importantly, there has been widespread agreement at all levels concerning the importance of AIDS education as the real key to confronting the epidemic. Finally, a range of AIDS education and health promotion activities have already been implemented, and a significant amount of expertise has been acquired along the way that provides a foundation for even more sophisticated and effective activities in the future.

As significant as these developments are, however, it is important to underline the fact that there is only limited evidence to indicate that they have translated into the kinds of behavioral changes that will ultimately slow the spread of HIV transmission in Brazil. Even among particular groups such as self–identified homosexual men, evidence for some important changes in behavior cannot yet be generalized to the wider population of men who have sex with men. In Brazil, as in other countries, it seems clear that information, in and of itself, is not enough to stimulate risk–reducing behavioral change, and that a range of other issues will ultimately need to be addressed in developing more sophisticated and effective health promotion programs in the future.

As an extension of this point, it may be that the most basic goals of AIDS education programs cannot all be met through the kinds of relatively general educational programs that have been most pronounced thus far in Brazil. The evaluation of education programs in settings where diverse activities have been undertaken over a period of time has suggested, for example, that behavioral change is in fact most effectively stimulated through highly specific or targeted health promotion activities, while more generally oriented activities are better suited to the maintenance of changes over time.[30] Once again, the Brazilian case would suggest that while

---

[30] Patricia E. Evans *et al.* "Does Health Education Work? Publicly Funded AIDS Education in San Francisco, 1982–1986," IV International Conference on AIDS, Stockholm, Sweden, 1988.

widespread public service announcements can have an important impact in raising the general level of AIDS awareness, they may well have little impact on the actual reduction of risk–related behaviors. Just as information alone is not enough, unfocused educational materials are not adequate, in and of themselves, to bring about risk–reducing behavioral change.

These points clearly offer implications for future AIDS education activities, both in Brazil and elsewhere. While focused or targeted materials have been developed by local level and non–governmental organizations, which have generally had more freedom of movement in this area, they have been the most recent, and most limited, of the AIDS activities carried out in Brazil thus far. During much of the past decade, the largest portion of available resources has been given over to more widespread and generally oriented media campaigns. While these campaigns have achieved some degree of success in constructing what might be described as a kind of general background of knowledge about HIV and AIDS, and while this background is no doubt crucially important as a foundation for behavioral change in the future, it would appear that it is not enough to bring about such change on its own.

On the basis of these facts, it seems reasonable to suggest that the prospects for effective AIDS education in the future in Brazil will be greatest to the extent that it is possible to direct resources to more clearly focused health promotion activities, and to draw on the experience and personnel of the growing number of local level organizations already involved in AIDS health promotion activities. Thus far, only limited collaboration has emerged between the educational activities of the National AIDS Program and the non–governmental organizations involved in AIDS–related activities. Both a fuller partnership, and a commitment to providing necessary financial resources should be taken as important goals for the future. The kinds of widespread media campaigns that have dominated AIDS education activities in the past will continue to have an important role to play in the future, both in reaching the hard to reach (the individuals and groups that may, for a variety of reasons, not respond effectively to more focused materials), as well as contributing to the maintenance of behavioral change where it has already taken place. But the key impact of small–scale, local level activities in more effectively stimulating such change in the first place should be recognized and acknowledged in the development of complex policy initiatives.

Finally, in addition to rethinking the basic educational strategies that should guide AIDS education activities, careful consideration must also be given to the range of issues that must actually be addressed as AIDS education in Brazil moves into the 1990s. Attention must continue to focus not only on AIDS itself, but on the wider social context within which AIDS takes place and the wider social responses that ultimately shape the climate of risk–reducing behavioral change. Just as some settings stimulate and encourage health–promoting change, others discourage it, and addressing the issues of injustice, prejudice and discrimination that might ultimately inhibit a positive response to AIDS must become an even higher priority in years to come. In Brazil, as in other countries, AIDS education activities must therefore respond not only to the epidemics of HIV infection and AIDS, but also to the epidemic of fear and prejudice in the face of AIDS, and it is only by struggling with these issues that it will be possible to build on information by constructing an environment that is truly capable of nurturing risk–reducing behavioral change in the face of HIV and AIDS.

Achieving these goals, of course, will by no means be an easy task. In Brazil, as in other parts of the world, the AIDS epidemic will almost certainly get worse before there is any hope that it will get better. Confronting it, above all else through education and health promotion, will require collaboration and cooperation on a scale that has not yet emerged in relation to any other social issue. It will require a far greater commitment of human and financial resources than have thus far been made available. The dedicated work of a growing number of men and women, from a wide range of professions and disciplines, along with the tentative steps forward that have been taken over the course of recent years, offers hope for the future. The challenge will be to transform hope into reality.

Support for research on the social dimensions of AIDS in Brazil has been provided by the Wenner–Gren Foundation for Anthropological Research and the Fundaçao de Amparo a Pesquisa do Estado do Rio de Janeiro.

Prevention Through Information and Education: Experience from Mexico

Jaime Sepulveda

On December 7, 1989, the Mexican Attorney General's office received a lawsuit from *Pro–vida* —an ultra–conservative, "pro–life" civilian group with ties to the Catholic Church— against the National AIDS Committee (CONASIDA). They pressed charges for promoting promiscuity by advocating condoms as a preventive measure against AIDS. *Pro–vida* also called for a massive march to protest against the AIDS campaign (in progress in the mass media and the metropolitan subway system), which would culminate at the gates of the Ministry of Health with an act of condom burning.

This was the climax of a long–standing controversy between CONASIDA and radical right–wing groups. Previous negotiations with these groups and representatives of conservative segments of the Catholic Church had only postponed the final confrontation. An aggressive, explicit and humorous AIDS prevention campaign in the metropolitan subway system—the second largest in the world, with five million users daily—elicited their most vigorous response.

The attempt to silence the mass media information campaign about AIDS transmission and prevention not only failed, *but* backfired. After careful analysis of the charges, the Attorney General threw the lawsuit out of court, deciding there was no crime to prosecute. The march, on the other hand, was attended only by a handful of followers and received little attention. Support for the AIDS campaign from vast segments of society appeared promptly. Intellectuals, artists, non–governmental organizations and academic institutions expressed their indignation to such intolerance in newspaper advertisements. Hundreds of newspaper articles, editorials and cartoons endorsed the need for clear information and satirized the new inquisitors and "guardians of morality."[1]

When this sad episode was over, the only possible winner was AIDS. It is true that the heated controversy produced more newspaper inches than any press campaign could have imagined achieving. Enormous amounts of press coverage were generated, fostering public debate and awareness. But it also distracted the attention and energies of public health officials. The real fight is against AIDS, and it is difficult enough as such.

This chapter describes the demographic and epidemiological context of AIDS in Mexico. The various phases of the information and communication campaigns against HIV are discussed, along with their failures, their successes and the public reactions to them. Finally, some reflections on lessons learned from health promotion for AIDS prevention and control in Mexico are included.

SOCIO–DEMOGRAPHIC CONTEXT

The population of Mexico is close to 90 million; it ranks as the eleventh most populated country and the largest Spanish–speaking country, in the world. Geographically speaking, Mexico belongs to North America, a fact that is frequently ignored. Culturally and historically, however, it is more closely bound to Central and South America.

The distribution of the Mexican population through out its territory (two million square kilometers) is not uniform. The capital city and three other metropolitan areas concentrate almost a third of the population. On the other hand, there are over 100 000 rural dispersed localities. In the 1980 census, 92% of the respondents claimed to profess the Catholic religion.

At present, the gross national product (GNP) per capita is the equivalent of 2 361 U.S. dollars. This figure represents an eight percent decrease as compared to 1980 data. A very significant proportion of the GNP is allotted to the payment of the foreign debt.

An overview of the health situation in the country shows a protracted epidemiological transition profile. That is, diseases of the modern world coexist with diseases related to poverty. Chronic and degenerative diseases and injuries are now the main causes of death, but diarrheas and respiratory infections still cause an unjustifiable number of deaths, particularly among children.[2]

---

[1] *La Jornada* and other Mexican newspapers with national circulation; January 1990.

[2] G. Soberon, M.A. Gonzalez and J. Sepulveda, "The health care reform in Mexico: Before and after the 1985 earthquakes," *American Journal of Public Health* 76 (6) (1986): 673.

This incomplete epidemiological transition is further challenged by the emergence of old and new diseases. Measles, for example, which had been controlled in the past, is resurfacing with great force. Dengue was eradicated three decades ago and has re–emerged as a fluctuating epidemic for the last ten years. Even more recently, AIDS appeared in the health scenario as a truly emergent disease.

The border between Mexico and the U.S. is three thousand kilometers long. It has been said that the two countries are "distant neighbors" because of their differences in historical roots, social values, foreign policy and economic strength, among other factors. Be that as it may, the fact is that there is an intense flow of population between these two nations. In 1989, for instance, over one hundred million people crossed the U.S. —Mexican border, with forty–nine million at the Tijuana— San Diego gateway alone.[3] It has been estimated that there are close to four million Mexicans in the U.S. of which approximately 1.5 to 2.0 million are undocumented workers. Texas and California, two of the states with the highest number of AIDS cases, are also the recipients of the largest share of agriculture workers from Mexico. Of all reported Mexican AIDS cases by July 1988, 10.4% had resided in the U.S. sometime in the previous five years.

International travel has obviously facilitated the spread of HIV worldwide. In this regard, Mexico offers conditions that promote rapid HIV spread, since it has good air travel communications. There are thirty–five international and forty–one national airports in the country. During 1988, a total of 16 million passengers travelled through the major airports, which has undoubtedly contributed to the spread of HIV within the country.

EPIDEMIOLOGY OF AIDS CASES IN MEXICO

The first case of AIDS in Mexico was diagnosed in 1983, in a Haitian student. His first symptoms had surfaced in 1981. All 17 Mexican cases reported in 1983 were rather affluent homosexual males who had travelled and engaged in sexual activities abroad. The cause of AIDS had not been discovered yet, and a parallel epidemic of stigmatization against homosexuals developed. By the end of 1986, 250 cases had been reported (Table 7–1), with the majority of cases still associated with homo/bisexual activities. Early on, it became evident that bisexual behavior is quite common in Mexico, accounting for more than a quarter of all cases.[4]

[3] Jorge A. Bustamante and Wayne A. Cornelius, eds., *Flujos migratorios mexicanos hacia Estados Unidos* (Mexico City: Fondo de Cultura Economica, 1989).

[4] Jose Luis Valdespino, Jose Antonio Izazola and Blanca Rico, "AIDS in Mexico: Trends and Projections," *Bulletin of the Pan-American Health Organization* 23 (1-2)(1989): 20-4.

Transmission through blood products was already unusually high in 1983, with seven percent of the cases. At that time, up to one–third of the 700 000 blood unit supply in the country came from paid blood donors. In many of the private blood and plasma collection centers, elementary hygienic measures were not taken; evidence of reuse of blood collection instruments (syringes, catheters, saline solutions) prompted the closure of these private centers.[5] In one specific commercial plasma center located in an underprivileged area bordering Mexico City, cumulative HIV seroprevalence increased from 6.3% to 9.2% in five months. Of the 281 seropositive donors, 62 (22%) had documented seroconversion during those five months. A case control study demonstrated that frequency of plasma donation was strongly related to the risk of becoming seropositive, with no other risk factors associated. A survey of employees disclosed the frequent reuse of disposable blood collection equipment.[6]

Table 7–1. *AIDS cases in Mexico, 1986–1990.*

Date	No. Cases	Duplication Time	Sex Ratio	Risk Factors Hetero	Bisex	Homo	Blood	Perinatal
Dec. '86	250	5 mo.	20:01	4	30	60	7	0
May '87	500	7 mo.	14:01	11	26	48	14	0.5
Dec. '87	1 000	12 mo.	14:01	11	26	48	14	0.5
Dec. '88	2 000	15 mo.	6:01	20	23	37	20	1
Mar. '90	4 000	17 mo.	5:01	24	21	26	26	2
Aug. '91	8 000		5:01	24	20	33	20	2

In Mexico 1987 was a year of rapid growth in the AIDS count. A monthly epidemiological bulletin on AIDS was first published in March, with 344 cases accumulated. By then, homosexual and bisexual men accounted for three–quarters of AIDS cases, with the rest divided between heterosexuals and blood transfusion recipients, and a few perinatal cases appearing on the scene. By the end of the year more than 1 000 cases had been reported.

Serological surveys started early on in relation to the epidemic, concentrating on homosexual men in Mexico City. In 1985, the first study showed 5% seroprevalence, which steadily rose to 23% in 1986, 33% in 1987 and

5 Jaime Sepulveda, Maria Lourdes Garcia, Jose Luis Dominguez Torix and Jose Luis Valdespino, "Prevention of HIV Transmission through Blood and Blood Products: Experiences in Mexico," *Bulletin of the Pan-American Health Organization* 23 (1-2) (1989): 108-14.
6 C. Avila, H. Stetler, J. Sepulveda *et al.*, "The epidemiology of HIV Transmission among paid plasma donors, Mexico City, Mexico," *AIDS* 3 (1989): 631-3.

38% in 1988. As is true everywhere, this level of seroprevalence has to be taken with caution, since not a single survey was based on probability samples, and therefore no inferences to the homosexual community as a whole can be made. Sentinel seroprevalence studies were conducted in other specific groups. From 1987 to 1989, HIV prevalence studies in female prostitutes were carried out in 18 cities. Although the prevalence of infection among this group is lower in Mexico than in other countries, an increase has been recently observed in Mexico City. HIV transmission among prostitutes in Mexico occurs mainly through sexual activity; intravenous drug addiction is almost nonexistent in this group. Prevalence rates have ranged between 0.2% and 1% in most cities and reach 5.2% in Mexico City. Male prostitutes, however, reached 16% seroprevalence rates in the capital.

All cases found in Mexico are HIV–1; no HIV–2 infection has been detected. Partial studies regarding HTLV–I have also been conducted, with only a few cases confirmed in Tijuana among prisoners.[7]

As with all epidemics, the acceleration of growth is not sustained over time; eventually the rate of transmission decreases, and consequently the same occurs with disease incidence. The curve of growth, which was exponential during the first years, has become damped exponential. Therefore, it now takes about 15 months for cases to duplicate. Along with the slowing of the growth of the epidemic, the years 1988–1990 showed a shift in the proportion of cases according to risk factors. The 650 cases reported during the first quarter of 1990, for example, are fairly equally distributed in four categories of risk: male homosexual (26%), bisexual (21%), and heterosexual contacts (24%) and recipients of blood or blood products (26%).

The rapid change in the sex ratio of cases, with increasing numbers of women contributing to the morbid count, has two causes. First, women of reproductive age in Mexico receive blood transfusions far more frequently than men. Second, the large pool of bisexuals in Mexican society makes a bridge of transmission to the heterosexual community. Mainly as a result of the former, rather than by heterosexual contact with bisexual men, women became infected and started to give birth to infected children. The number of perinatal AIDS cases is still relatively low (two percent), but has been growing steadily.

Making projections is a slippery business. Early estimations, assuming sustained exponential growth, described a catastrophic situation. Current mathematical models provide less somber estimates: by the end of 1991, about 20000 accumulated cases will have been reported, but we have to take subregistration and delay of registration into account. Heterosexual transmission will play a larger role and consequently perinatal transmis-

---

[7] F. Güereña, H. Gomez, M.A. Vaca *et al.*, "HIV-1 prevalence in selected Tijuana Sub-populations," sent for publication to the *American Journal of Public Health*.

sion will increase. Cases associated with blood transmission, before the HIV screening regulations rendered the blood supply safe, will reach a peak in 1991 or 1992 and will then progressively diminish. More cases will come from rural areas, both as a consequence of spread from large metropolitan areas to less populated towns, and of infected migrant workers returning home from the United States. Within a decade of the first reported case in the country, the profile will have shifted from an epidemic of affluent homosexual men to an endemic of the underprivileged.

Responses to the AIDS Epidemic in Mexico

In order to make this section more readable I have analyzed the responses of government, non–governmental organizations and the mass media separately, each one of which has three periods of observation: the early years (1985–1986), the intermediate phase (1987–1988) and the current years (1989–1990). Non–governmental organizations are by no means uniform in their response. Two polarized views from liberal and ultraconservative groups are briefly documented, in order to cover more ground and a wider perspective (Table 7–2).

Table 7–2. *Responses to the AIDS epidemic in Mexico: government, non–governmental and mass media.*

Government Response	Non–Government Response		Mass Media Response
	Gay and Liberal NGOs	Pro–vida and Right–wing groups	
I.Erratic, Medicalized 1985–1986	Silence	Slight Opposition	Alarmist
II. Planned, Technocratic 1987–1988	Anger, Protest	Strong Opposition	Reactive only to "sensational" news
III. Reactive, Participatory	Protest, Participation	Lawsuits, Marches	Fatigue

GOVERNMENT RESPONSE

Erratic, Medical Approach (1985–1986)

In 1985 isolated actions geared towards preventing HIV/AIDS were undertaken. Few cases of AIDS had been reported, but public concern about the disease existed, particularly because of international news. The Pan American Health Organization (PAHO) called for a meeting in December of 1985 to provide guidelines for every country in the region for the creation of national programs to combat AIDS.

In February of 1986 the Secretariat of Health informally created the National Committee for AIDS Prevention (CONASIDA). The purpose of this committee was to assess levels and trends of HIV/AIDS in the country; establish criteria for diagnosis, treatment and prevention; and coordinate the adoption and evaluation of appropriate standards, guidelines and control activities. To these ends, CONASIDA established five subcommittees: epidemiological surveillance, health promotion, clinical aspects, blood control and legal advice. Almost all the members of the committee were medical doctors from the public health sector. It comes as no surprise then that theirs was a medical approach.

One of CONASIDA's first actions was to include mandatory screening of all blood and plasma units in the General Health Law in May, 1986. An immediate consequence of this fortunate action was the detection of astonishing levels of HIV seroprevalence among paid blood donors. The evidence of high seroprevalence rates among this group (7.2%) as compared to voluntary blood donors (0.02%) allowed for further legal modifications a year later.

The AIDS case definition of the US Centers for Disease Control was implemented in Mexico. Monitoring of cases all over the country soon followed, with reports from most states. Early attempts to prevent blood transmissions in large hospitals emphasized donor screening and training of blood bank employees. Distribution of pamphlets and brochures with questions and answers for the general public about AIDS, along with some materials for gay/bisexual men, began. By then, ELISA tests were commercially available, and CONASIDA organized the first serological surveys among homosexual men. An erratic information campaign started, conveying either macabre messages (a picture of the feet of a corpse, with a tag showing the number of AIDS cases hanging from the toe) or humorous details, such as the distribution of match boxes with a condom and the slogan, "I don't play with fire."

Planned, Technocratic Approach (1987–1988)

A Mexican monthly AIDS bulletin came out for the first time in March 1987. The publication aimed to inform health officials about new developments in the epidemic and to give feedback to epidemiologists from all over the country. It also attempted to provide the press with regular information; reporters called every other day for the latest AIDS case count before the bulletin came out. In addition to the usual tables containing epidemiological information, this bulletin provides editorial comments and scientific news, which has made it the main source of AIDS information for health personnel in the country, with a monthly circulation of 12 000.

The most important legal contribution of CONASIDA, without a doubt, has been the prohibition of the commercial blood market (Table 7–3). This was not easy, since one–third of the blood supply in the country came from paid blood donors, and some institutions in the health sector derived their entire supply from that source. There were immense commercial interests in this industry, and the National Chamber of Hospitals opposed the measure. The legal initiative had to be approved by Congress; in May of 1987, the Health Law was amended to make blood commerce illicit, with a grace period of six months before becoming effective. This period enabled the health sector to make provisions to avoid a shortage of blood. A large mass media campaign took place to stimulate altruistic blood donations. The much feared blood shortage never occurred.

Table 7–3. *Legal reforms to the General Health Law about AIDS.*

May 1986	Mandatory Screening of Blood and Plasma Units
Nov. 1986	AIDS Included in the List of Diseases Subject to Epidemiological Surveillance
May 1987	Prohibition of Commercialization of Blood
Aug. 1988	Creation by Presidential Decree of the National Councilfor AIDS Prevention and Control (CONASIDA) as a Decentralized Unit of the Secretary of Health

By this point, the CONASIDA team felt confident in moving into a new phase of the campaign, one that would be carefully planned and aimed at addressing the specific information needs of the population. With that purpose in mind, in April of 1987 a survey on knowledge and attitudes about AIDS in the general public was conducted through a questionnaire enclosed in major newspapers, asking readers to complete and return it. Admittedly, respondents may not have been representative of readers, and these in turn do not represent the population at large, but it was a quick, inexpensive way to cover a large, if unrepresentative, segment of society. This action was complemented by a random telephone survey and a survey among subway users, both in Mexico City.

Based on the information collected, it became evident that although many people had heard of AIDS, many misconceptions prevailed. The mass media campaign was specifically designed to address these misconceptions, by informing about modes of HIV transmission and prevention measures, and by combating myths. The campaign used various channels to reach the general population and people with risky sexual behavior, and was supported by interpersonal communication so as to have a larger impact. Evaluation of impact was an important consideration. Technocracy suggested a quasi–experimental study to test hypotheses and to measure levels of change in knowledge and behavior immediately before and after the campaign. Knowledge, attitudes and practice (KAP) surveys have been used since the 1960s in fertility surveys. The rationale behind KAP surveys lies in the theoretical concept that knowledge is a required previous and conditioning step for changing attitudes, and that these two together determine practices. Therefore, in order to modify behavior the first step is to provide information. This concept certainly made a lot of sense then. As we will see later, information is a necessary condition, but is not sufficient to modify behavior.

The late 1987–early 1988 radio and television campaign against AIDS was aggressive; the word condom was mentioned for the first time ever in the mass media. The spots on television used cartoons to give information on modes of HIV transmission and to combat myths prevalent at the time (the belief that casual contact and mosquito bites can transmit AIDS, for example), while promoting monogamy as the best preventive choice and condoms as an alternative. The impact of the campaign can be partially evaluated by the results of the May, 1988 KAP survey. The television spots were run for several months, with 17 856 repetitions on private and state channels. They were aired at no cost; the commercial cost would have been over ten million US dollars.

A large–scale KAP study was planned for September of 1987 and May of 1988, before and after the campaign. The population studied comprised five groups of particular interest: the general population, university students, health personnel, homosexual men and female prostitutes. Six large metropolitan areas were selected to conduct the study: Mexico City, Guadalajara, Monterrey, Acapulco, Tijuana and Merida. The minimum sample size for each group was 100. Five groups in six cities surveyed two times gave 60 separate surveys to analyze. More than 8 000 individuals were interviewed.

Four hypothesis were tested in the "before and after" study. Statistics included comparisons of means and proportions and analyses of variance. The knowledge indicator was measured as the number of correct answers to 30 questions on etiology, transmission, myths, preventive measures, existence of vaccine or drugs, and perception of risk and groups at risk, among other topics. The attitude indicator was constructed with 22 variables, the answers to which were assigned a negative or positive value according to whether the response was in favor of or against the adoption of preventive measures. Use of condoms in the last four months (last month for female prostitutes) was utilized as a proxy indicator of safer practices.

Hypothesis 1: The general population will be better informed about AIDS and will have more positive and compassionate attitudes after the campaign. Overall, the level of knowledge increased from 70.8% of correct answers to 75%, a statistically significant difference. The main changes in knowledge were related to etiology, forms of transmission and prevention methods. However, myths persisted about AIDS as an exclusively homosexual disease and the possibility of casual contact. In contrast to what was expected, attitudes did not become more positive or compassionate, and in fact in some regards worsened. Therefore, the first premise of the hypothesis proved correct, but not the second.

Hypothesis 2: There will be a significant increase in condom use after the campaign in all populations studied. Important differences were found in age structure, education level and marital status among the groups, which obviously influenced both the access to information as well as the public health need of a condom. Students, gay men and prostitutes were younger and more often single. Education level was highest among students, gays and health personnel, and quite low for prostitutes. The proportion of prostitutes who used a condom in the last month increased significantly from 44% to 57% and within this group of users, condoms were more frequently used (by ten percent) in every single sexual encounter after the campaign. The proportion of homosexual men who reported condom use in the last four months increased from 37% to 43%, also a statistically significant difference. Among users, the frequency of condom use in every sexual act increased only five percent.

The other groups did not increase their use of condoms significantly. However, the vast majority of non–condom users said they were monogamous; one–half of the students interviewed had not initiated sexual activity. Therefore, the hypothesis was only valid for the groups at highest risk of HIV infection.

Hypothesis 3: Groups with high–risk practices will be better informed about AIDS and will have more favorable attitudes toward adoption of preventive measures than the general population. Of all the groups, female prostitutes had the lowest level of information about AIDS (81% of correct answers) while homosexual men had the highest (87%). This is most likely a result of the much lower educational level of prostitutes which conditions access to and use of information. It was of interest that 85% of prostitutes identified homosexuals as a group at high risk of HIV infection but only 79% considered themselves to be at risk, while gay men considered prostitutes as a high risk group 84% of the time while considering themselves at risk in 82% of circumstances.

Generally speaking, attitudes were more compassionate towards people with AIDS in both groups than in the rest. In gay men, this might be related to the fact that 16% knew at least one seropositive person or someone with AIDS. More positive attitudes in these groups were also evident in the will-ingness to use a condom in the next sexual relation (85% of prostitutes, 82% of gay men). These data support the hypothesis that attitudes towards people with AIDS and AIDS prevention are more favorable in prostitutes and gay men.

Hypothesis 4: Health personnel will have more positive and compassion-ate attitudes toward HIV–infected people. Surprisingly, health personnel perceived AIDS as a health problem less often (24%) than the general popu-lation did (36%). More worrisome is the fact that 30% of health personnel thought AIDS could be transmitted by casual contact. A higher proportion (51%) in this group said they would reject a friend if he or she had AIDS than the general population (ten percent). Therefore the hypothesis cannot be accepted.

Conversations with the National Actors Association brought their partici-pation in the campaigns. A very popular actress and singer filmed a spot in which a song of hers was used to advocate condoms. In a provocative atti-tude, a pack of condoms in hand, she said, "Enjoy love. Do it responsibly." Before its release, the spot was presented at a press conference by the Secretary of Health, along with other artists that would support the campaign with other messages. The morning of the press conference (April 18, 1988) all the newspapers ran a full one–page ad with the heading "prophylactic or condom: the name doesn't matter, what matters is that it helps save lives." This strategy had the intention of removing the vulgar, almost secretive connotation of the word "condom", and to substitute the use of a lesser known word such as "prophylactic" for a more common one. It was felt that in a fight against a sexually transmitted disease, sexual matters and preventive measures had to be discussed openly. The ad ended with the slogan "AIDS is not a moral problem, it is a public health problem of the greatest importance."

The reaction of the political right was immediate. The Secretary of Health was accused of "starting the sexual revolution in Mexico" and "inducing promiscuity." Controversy was immense, with more than 1500 newspaper articles, both for and against the campaign.

The private television network refused to air the spots and hinted at sanctions against artists involved. The campaign was stopped dead.

After the shock and frustration of not being able to provide the information that was so vitally necessary, more conciliatory messages were tried. Still using well–known personalities, this time the best soccer player in the country, the new television spot warned, after he scored a goal, that AIDS was incurable and offered the lukewarm slogan "Get more information" while giving the AIDS hotline number. The spot was so mediocre and unexplicit, that viewers were left wondering what was the message about.

For the last few months of 1988, public attention was concentrated on the national presidential elections. In terms of AIDS–related health promotion in mass media, silence was the norm.

Reactive, Participatory Approach (1989–1990)

The new administration faced enormous social and economic challenges. CONASIDA spent the early months of 1989 evaluating past experiences with the media and debating new approaches. CONASIDA moved toward changing the top–down attitude in designing AIDS campaigns. To this end, a large public–consultation forum took place in May, 1989, to learn what society felt was needed. A wide spectrum of community groups accepted CONASIDA's invitation to participate in the debate. Academics, artists, gays, public officials, civil libertarians, prostitutes, priests, leftists and conservatives heatedly discussed such topics as the roles of government and the media, sex education in schools, discrimination and human rights, among others.

CONASIDA was severely criticized by both liberals and conservatives; the former focused on insufficient presence of AIDS information, and the latter maintained that the promotion of condoms induced sexual promiscuity. The few who applauded the campaigns were accused of being pro–government, which was considered an insult by both the left and the right. Three recommendations resulted from the forum, influenced by the larger presence of liberal groups:

1) AIDS is a public health issue, not a moral one.
2) Information should be explicit.
3) Non–governmental organizations must assume a more active role.

The Secretary of Health ordered immediate action which resulted in an "intermediate" campaign consisting of 18 radio and T.V. spots. The first part of the "intermediate" campaign outlined new epidemiological trends, lessening emphasis on groups that were stigmatized by previous campaigns. The second part was aimed at recognizing and encouraging public involvement in the fight against AIDS. For this we used testimonials by an opposition party community organizer, adolescents, HIV infected individuals, a top–level manager from a multinational corporation, a rock group, etc., all ending with the phrase: "This is what I am doing: and you.... what are you doing?"

While the intermediate campaign was going on, CONASIDA was preparing new messages that would be positive, prevention oriented and colorful. The launching pad for the new campaign would be the Mexico City Metro, the second largest subway system in the world, providing transportation for more thamfive million daily users.

For our campaign theme, we chose a popular Mexican lottery game, played by Mexicans of all ages. The lottery game consists of a board and cards representing different characters —the lady, the macho, the drunk, the mermaid, the dandy, death— and is played like American bingo.

The lottery characters were selected to represent groups at risk, and along with humorous popular sayings, appear in 21 different posters which were displayed in subway cars, in corridors, and on train platforms. Some of the posters answered basic questions about AIDS prevention, others were directed at groups at risk, stressing the fact that information is the best weapon against AIDS. Particular attention was focused on women, underlining the fact that females are the group where AIDS is advancing most rapidly now in Mexico. Women were encouraged to insist that their partners use a condom. Two T.V. spots were aired, emphasizing that everyone can be at risk and the same slogan was used for the whole campaign: AIDS is not a matter of luck, but of life or death.

The materials were pre–tested in focus groups composed of passengers from different subway stations. Results showed that the concepts were largely accepted and understood. Some messages were adjusted according to the reactions of the focus groups. The campaign was inaugurated on December 1, 1989. A week later, I was sued and the legal process mentioned at the beginning of this chapter took place.

This year, 1989, a total of 29524 spots repetitions were aired including the three T.V. campaigns.

NON–GOVERNMENTAL RESPONSE

Gay and Liberal Groups

With the idea of being more objective about the views and actions of gay and liberal non–governmental organizations in their fight against AIDS, various leaders of those organizations were asked to contribute to this chapter. What follows in this section are excerpts of their written material, with the only bias being my translation and style editing.

Since 1983, existing gay associations have been concerned about AIDS, but because of a lack of clarity about the dimensions and significance of the epidemic, an almost total lack of resources and all sorts of organizational limitations, non–governmental organizations involved in the fight against AIDS were not effective against the advance of the epidemic. An effect of the governmental concept of the disease was the treatment of AIDS by non–governmental organizations (as well as CONASIDA) as a purely medical problem in the early years. The erratic quality of the actions of non–governmental organizations and society in general coincided with the erratic approach of the governmental actions during the same period (especially from 1985 to 1986).

Heterosexuals in Mexican society were far from considering AIDS their problem in the early 1980s, something which still occurs today. The history of AIDS in Mexico would have been a different one if gay and heterosexual organizations like those in the U.S. Australia, Holland and other countries had existed. In addition, non–governmental organizations in many countries received private, public and international funding which we have only begun to receive in the first half of 1990.

The technocratic planning period (1987–1988) in governmental action against AIDS corresponds to a time of pluralistic tendencies in the actions of non–governmental organizations: the Mexican Foundation for the Fight Against AIDS was born, and the work of various groups was reoriented. The first marches of mourning in memory of those who died of AIDS, and in support of people with HIV and AIDS took place in the mid–1980s as well. Outside of Mexico City, except for Guadalajara, Tijuana and Merida, the activities of non–governmental organizations were very limited until the very end of the 1980s.

A group of investigators from various public universities began to produce critical and analytic written material with the aim of promoting a national, political debate about AIDS instead of purely scientific advances. This effort produced the book, *AIDS in Mexico: The social effects.* Journalists, social researchers, gay militants, heterosexuals whose consciousness about the seriousness of the problem had been raised, students and people with HIV/AIDS all added their grain of salt to the creation of a non–medical, non–bureaucratic understanding of AIDS. The central idea was that AIDS is everyone's problem we have to fight it with all means available to us, from science to sexual education, from culture to mass media and politics. Specialization has no place in this fight, because in this struggle we all have a part to play. From this experience an autonomous research project was created, an information network was set up and the creation of an office for the defense of human and civil rights associated with AIDS was proposed, which is underway.

During the period from 1989 to 1990 non–governmental organizations and the government coincide once again: this is a reactive/participatory phase for both. Of importance during this period is a new environment of mutual recognition and respect between CONASIDA and non–governmental organizations. The Confederation of Non–Governmental Organizations: Mexicans Against AIDS, with 12 member organizations but no financial resources, was formed at this time. The birth of the Confederation coincided with the celebration of the First Social Participation Congress, organized by CONASIDA in May of 1989. Because disagreements on strategy, pacing of political actions and interpretation of the political moment in relation to AIDS, four important members of the Confederation left the organization a short time later. These organizations then formed the Mexican Network of Non–Governmental Organizations, which currently includes about fifteen groups.

It appears that 1990 will be a year of consolidation for the liberal, democratic non–governmental organizations. Now that we have undergone the important transition from conceiving AIDS as an exclusively health–related problem to understanding that the formulation of public policies is basic to the fight against AIDS, we can begin to reach other goals. We should take the lead in the struggle to create a social policy against AIDS. People who are HIV positive and people with AIDS, who have thus far been the objects of the good intentions of many non–governmental organizations and the government, must join this struggle, and do so under the same conditions that exist for activists who are "well." Funding, organization, administrative and financial transparency, clearly defined goals, public negotiation skills, imagination, daring, dedication and solidarity are all factors which are not easily coordinated in tasks of the magnitude of the fight against AIDS. It seems that this government and the liberal, democratic non–governmental organizations agree in principle. Now we have to make this common interest reality.

Right–wing Groups

Ultra–conservative groups have been congruent in their position about AIDS throughout the epidemic. The only possible change has been the intensity of their opposition to the campaigns, but not the arguments. In the early years (1985–1986), when there were very few organized informative actions by the government or liberal groups, they remained relatively quiet. After the press conference of April 12, 1988 in which a new phase of the campaign was announced, they did not hesitate to react. Archbishops and Catholic groups protested and in their own press conferences denounced that by advocating condoms, the Secretary of Health was "encouraging homosexuality, prostitution and promiscuity." Later on, they requested extramarital sex and homosexuality be penalized, and the creation of rehabilitation centers for homosexual men so they could be "cured" of their sexual preference.

With the change of administration, these groups exerted new pressure to have condoms removed as part of the strategy to combat AIDS. They claimed that every new case of AIDS was the responsibility of CONASIDA, by promoting a product (condoms) with a high failure rate.

Five demands were made in a public manifesto on November 8, 1989, signed by the National Union of Parents, a small but vocal group:

- Monitoring of the correct use of the health sector's budget, with no expenditure on condoms;
- Cancelation of all campaigns advocating condoms;
- Legal prosecution of health officials for certain crimes, such as moral offenses, apologetics for vices and minor corruption;
- Education of youth in "universal values";
- Promotion and protection of the family as the basic building block of society.

The attacks concentrated on top CONASIDA officials, myself, among others, asking for their resignation. Later on, when the subway campaign started, they sought penalization: resignation was not enough.

THE RESPONSE OF THE MASS MEDIA

The behaviour of the press has varied considerably in its treatment of the AIDS epidemic in Mexico. For clarity, the three phases used above to classify the governmental education efforts are mentioned here as a reference frame , although the presentation of AIDS in the mass media is divided into two phases, alarmist and reactive to information.

During the governmental AIDS education program's erratic, medical phase (1985–1986), the behavior of the Mexican press, as in most countries, was characterized by sensationalist, stigmatizing and anti–homosexual articles, with the presentation of gays as the only people affected by the new disease. This could be called the "alarmist" phase of the mass media which greatly misinformed the population.

In the second, technocratic phase of government programs (1987–1988), news articles became less sensationalist, increased in quantity and the type of information presented changed. Some information about modes of transmission, methods for prevention and biomedical aspects was included. This phase is basically "reactive to information" provided by international news agencies or epidemiological information about the development of the epidemic produced by the Secretariat of Health. During this phase the average number of stories about AIDS published daily in the Mexican press was ten, and on the days after events such as press conferences, the National AIDS Information Day or the inauguration of a new phase of an education campaign, the number reached 15 to 20 articles. During this phase, the press emphasized the discussion between the government, conservative and gay and liberal groups, and continued to neglect information about the disease itself

The present phase, which corresponds to the reactive–participatory period of governmental action, is again a reactive phase for the mass media, as was the previous, technocratic period. The number of daily articles averages seven to ten, with considerably more articles published after events such as the inauguration of the subway poster campaign and the lawsuit against top CONASIDA officials. In general, articles continue to be those received from the international news agencies, or about the current number of AIDS cases, which has always been a rather morbid fascination of the press (besides which the statistics used are frequently incorrect). In spite of the constant presence of information about AIDS in the mass media, specific aspects of the disease are not addressed, so that collective, accurate knowledge of AIDS is not generated nor is a participatory discussion promoted. Only some television and radio networks made an effort to promote a participatory discussion, in live programs, with interviews to guests and with an open telephone–line to recieve questions and comments from the audience. Most of them invited both CONASIDA and NGOs representatives with a less than satisfactory result: more was discussed about adequateness of strategies, than about the AIDS epidemic, prevention and other specific issues.

Lessons Learned

1. The use of the mass media in AIDS prevention can contribute to an increase in knowledge and can help combat myths and stigmas quite effectively. Television and radio are useful in the solution of contradictions and doubts about AIDS, as well as for their capability of reaching illiterate people.

2. The use of fear in prevention campaigns produces rejection and is counterproductive because it reinforces the negative attitudes and stigmas of the general population and produces denial among high–risk groups.

3. The dissemination of information about AIDS is useful for changing

attitudes of stigmatization and rejection towards groups with high–risk practices.

4. Participation of members of target groups such as youth, homosexuals, seropositive people and prostitutes as educators in campaigns is an efficient way to gain acceptance of information.

5. The combination of quantitative and qualitative studies is optimum for the identification of audiences, messages and communication channels to be used.

6. Increased knowledge and emphasis on changing attitudes does not produce changes in high–risk practices. However, the design of materials through focus groups which aim to change the perception of risks and benefits can achieve behavior change.

7. Educational campaigns directed at health care workers require, besides information about AIDS, a normative, technical and material infrastructure. After an initial information campaign, the institution of preventive measures related to occupational exposure and regulation of fair treatment of persons with HIV and AIDS is necessary.

8. Collaboration with non–governmental groups is indispensable for more efficient prevention campaigns.

Many people contributed in various ways to this chapter. Mario Bravo, Francisco Galvan, Lourdes Garcia, Luis Gonzalez de Alba, Blanca Rico and Jose Luis Valdespino generously lent ideas and written material. Edith Velasco typed, with a perennial smile, several drafts of this manuscript. In particular, my special gratitude goes to Betania Allen, who expertly edited the chapter, with equal grace and patience.

Targeted AIDS Intervention Programs in Africa

Peter Lamptey
Sharon Weir

THE CULTURAL CONTEXT OF AIDS IN AFRICA

The 55 nations of Africa cover an area three times the size of Europe and are inhabited by almost 650 million people who speak more than 1 000 different languages. The diversity of its geography, natural resources, peoples, governments, infrastructures, indigenous and colonial heritages, and religions make generalizations about the culture of Africa or its ability to combat AIDS difficult if not impossible.

In a continent, however, where the average per capita gross national product is usually less than U.S. $600 and the average per capita budget for health and education is almost always less than U.S. $60,[1] countries do share some of the same obstacles in the development and maintenance of health programs. In these countries, health programs often fare poorly when competing with much-needed agricultural, transportation and educational programs. When health programs are developed, weak infrastructures in communication, transportation, and electrical power can make the delivery of health care services unreliable or unavailable to most people who live in rural areas. Under such circumstances, morbidity and early mortality prevented in other regions of the world continue to bring suffering to

[1] Nafis Sadik, *The State of the World's Population 1990* (United Nations Population Fund, 1990).

145

Africans and result in an average life expectancy of only 53 years, compared to 67 years in Latin America and 76 years in Northern Europe.[2]

It is also clear that the AIDS epidemic in Africa will challenge its leaders in ways that other epidemics and other diseases have not. Smallpox, for example, was eradicated by health immunization teams armed with injections in heroic mass immunization campaigns. Yaws was also brought under control by special health teams. Primary health care systems are currently tackling diarrhea through the creation of diarrheal disease programs that bring health education and oral rehydration therapy to women with children. No similar efforts have been marshalled for the treatment or prevention of sexually transmitted diseases (STDS) even though such diseases are endemic in several areas and the sequelae can be just as serious. The social stigma that accompanies sexually transmitted diseases has handicapped educational and prevention efforts for gonorrhea, syphilis, chanchroid and other sexually transmitted infections. Rather than developing health promotion or disease prevention programs for sexually transmitted diseases, most countries have come to rely on clinical management at a few isolated STD clinics or at general medical outpatient clinics, often inappropriate or inadequate self–medication, and traditional treatment regimens. The historical neglect of the prevention and treatment of sexually transmitted disease and a well–established reliance on self–medication are contributing to the unique difficulties that many countries share in developing AIDS prevention programs in Africa.

While the appearance of a well–publicized, incurable sexually transmitted disease such as AIDS offers new challenges for ministries of health, lessons can be learned from the African experience with family planning programs. These lessons include the importance of reaching youth through family life education in the schools; of training staff to communicate articulately in a non–judgmental manner and to maintain client confidentiality; of providing a range of method choices for different lifestyles and preferences; of monitoring non–compliance; and of reaching out to populations not likely to attend a traditional family planning clinic such as adolescents, the unmarried and men.

Pragmatic political lessons on how to reduce barriers to family planning have proven especially relevant to AIDS prevention. These lessons are being learned from the struggles of family planning programs such as the program in Kenya, which was initiated in 1967 and had almost no effect on the birth rate for fifteen years, although there was a significant drop in infant mortality and significant increases in primary education during the same period.[3] A drop in the fertility rate did not occur until there was high-

---

[2] *Ibid.*
[3] *Ibid.*

level and continued policy backing for the program, until services were expanded to reach a greater proportion of the population, and until improvements were made in program management.

The challenge for policy leaders in Africa will be to apply the relevant lessons from family planning, primary health care and infectious disease control and to develop new strategies for the prevention of sexually transmitted diseases, including AIDS. The epidemiology of HIV infection in Africa indicates the necessity of targeted programs among the most likely to be infected where the epidemic is still in its early stages and more widespread community–based programs where the infection is well entrenched. The salient issues will be how to mobilize politically disenfranchised groups who are at increased risk of infection, such as prostitutes, to consistently use condoms; how to cost–effectively educate and re–educate people who cannot be reached through access points such as workplace or school settings; how to improve the acceptability of condoms for STD control as well as family planning; how to effectively identify and use resources already available in a community to combat AIDS; and how to improve communication and negotiation skills of both men and women in regards to condom use.

In conclusion, by 2025, Africa could account for nearly one–fifth of the world's population; Nigeria alone could have 500 million inhabitants, as many as are currently in all of Africa.[4] Even though Africa's high fertility rate will in some ways overshadow the impact of the premature loss of lives due to AIDS, the immediate development of AIDS intervention programs must be ensured to limit the number of people who will suffer as a result of AIDS.

AIDS IN AFRICA

It is difficult, if not impossible, to determine precisely when and where the AIDS epidemic started. The debate regarding the origin of HIV has been emotional and unscientific, with most of the early hypotheses based more on conjecture than on sound epidemiological and other scientific evidence. At this point in the epidemic, the origin of AIDS is irrelevant, as are the origins of other diseases like syphilis, smallpox and gonorrhea. What is important is that HIV is present in virtually every country in the world. Current evidence, especially from hospital records in Africa and from Africans in Europe, strongly suggests that the epidemic of AIDS in Central Africa, the most seriously affected area in Africa, began to spread during the late 1970s

---

[4] P. Piot, M. Carael, "Epidemiological and sociological aspects of HIV–infection in developing countries," *British Medical Bulletin* 44 (1) (1988): 68–88.

and early 1980s—about the same time the epidemic started in the U.S. and Haiti.[5]

The number of AIDS cases reported to the World Health Organization Global Programme on AIDS (WHO/GPA) has been used to follow the spread of the epidemic to different parts of the world. As of February 1989, nearly 22000 cases of AIDS had been reported from the African continent.[6] This number represents 12% of the total number of AIDS cases reported worldwide. The number of reported AIDS cases, however, is a poor surveillance tool for a number of reasons. The poor quality of reporting in many developing countries; the deliberate official falsification of case numbers; the difficulties in standardizing the diagnosis of AIDS cases among countries with different levels of medical resources; and difficulties in the clinical diagnosis of AIDS in children are some of the reasons why the number of reported cases has not been very accurate, and is therefore of limited usefulness. The WHO/GPA estimates the cumulative number of cases in Africa in 1988 to be 200000 and projects that a total of one million cases will have occurred by 1992.[7]

Most of the cases of HIV infection in Africa are caused by HIV–l, but HIV–2 has been detected in most countries of West Africa, as well as in Mozambique and Angola. Preliminary data suggest that five percent of the general population in the Cape Verde islands and some countries in West Africa are HIV–2 antibody positive.[8] The pathogenicity of HIV–2 has not been clearly defined and there is still debate whether it is as infectious as HIV–l.

The major route of HIV infection in Africa is bi–directional heterosexual transmission[9] with a female to male ratio of approximately one to one. Anal intercourse has not been shown to be a significant mode of transmission. A number of hypotheses may account for the relatively rapid heterosexual spread of HIV in some parts of Africa. Behavioral factors such as multiplicity of sexual partners, frequent contact with prostitutes, and lack of cultural factors such as circumcision, have been identified as important risk factors. The high prevalence of STDs, especially those such as chancroid,

[5] World Health Organization, *Update: AIDS Cases Reported to Surveillance, Forecasting and Impact Assessment Unit* (Geneva: Global Programme on AIDS, 28 February 1989).

[6] J. Chin, P. Sato, J. Mann, "Estimates and Projections of HIV/AIDS to the year 2000," (Geneva: World Health Organization, May 1989).

[7] B. Bottiger et al., "Prevalence of HIV–l and HIV–2/HTLV–IV Infection in Luanda and Cabinda, Angola," *Journal of Acquired Immune Deficiency Syndromes* 1 (1988): 8–12; and P.M. Flutz, et al, "Seroprevalence of HIV–l and HIV–2 in Guinea Bissau in 1980," *AIDS* 2 (1988): 129–132; and P.J. Kanki, "West African human retrovirus," *AIDS* 1 (1987): 141–5.

[8] R. De Lays, B. Vanderborght, A. Van Geel, H. Hewerswyn, J. Hursman, G. Van der Groen, P. Piot. "Innogenetics N.V., Antwerp, Belgium, CLB, Amsterdam Netherlands Institute," Abstract 552, IV International Conference on AIDS. June 1988, Stockhom, Sweden.

[9] P. Piot, M. Carael, J.K. Kreiss et al., "AIDS virus infection in Nairobi prostitutes: spread of the epidemic to East Africa," *New England Journal of Medicine* 314 (1986): 414–8.

syphilis, and herpes that cause genital ulcers, appear to be a major contributory cofactor in the spread of HIV in Africa.[10] It is believed that STDs promote HIV transmission by increasing the infectivity of seropositive individuals or by enhancing the susceptibility of their contacts or both.[11] Several sources of data have confirmed the importance of diseases causing genital ulcers as important cofactors in the sexual transmission of HIV.[12] The treatment, control and prevention of STDs may, therefore, represent one of the most effective means of decreasing the heterosexual transmission of HIV.[13]

With the high seropositivity rates in the general adult population, perinatal transmission has become the second most important mode of transmission of HIV. Seropositivity rates as high as 20% have been reported in women seeking prenatal care in urban areas of East Africa.[14] It has been estimated that from 30–65% of infants born to infected mothers became infected.[15] The WHO/GPA projects that by 1992, 200000 AIDS cases will have occurred in children from 0 to 14 years old (20% of all cases in Africa). HIV is most prevalent in children under one year and in sexually active adults from 20 to 40 years old.[16] This pattern confirms the heterosexual transmission of HIV and the perinatal transmission of HIV from mother to child.

The third most important route of HIV transmission in Africa is through blood transfusion. A large transfusion demand is created by high rates of blood loss from malaria, abortion and child delivery, as well as from malnutrition. Blood banking facilities exist in most major urban centers, but are rudimentary or nonexistent in most rural areas.

The recent availability of blood screening capabilities in most countries in sub–Saharan Africa may have significantly reduced transmission of HIV through infected blood and blood products in some urban areas. In Zimbabwe, for example, nearly 100% of the blood and blood products are screened for

[10] P. Piot, M. Carael, J.M. Simonson et al., "HIV infection among men with sexually transmitted disease: Experience from a center in Africa," The New England Journal of Medicine, 4 August (1988): 274–8; and D.W. Cameron, F.A. Plummer, N. Simonsen et al., "Genital ulcer disease and female–to–male heterosexual transmission of HIV," IV International Conference on AIDS. June 1987, Washington, D.C.; and K. Holmes and J. Kreiss, "Heterosexual transmission of HIV: Overview of a neglected aspect of the AIDS epidemic," Journal of Acquired Immune Deficiency Syndromes 1 (1988): 602-610; and J. Pepin et al., "The interaction of HIV infection and other STDs: An opportunity for intervention," AIDS 3 (1989): 3–9; and C.P. Hudson et al., "Risk factors for the spread of AIDS in rural Africa: Evidence from a comparative seroepidemiolgical survey of AIDS, Hepatitis B and Syphilis in Southwestern Uganda," AIDS 2 (1988): 255–60.

[11] Op. cit. D.W. Cameron, F.A. Plummer, N. Simonsen et al.

[12] Op. cit. D.W. Cameron, F.A. Plummer, N. Simonsen et al.; and op. cit. J.M. Simonson et al.; and Op cit, C.P. Hudson, et al.; and L.J. Da Costa, F.A. Plummer, et al., "Prostitutes are a major reservoir of STD in Nairobi, Kenya," Sexually Transmitted Disease 12 (1985): 64–7.

[13] Op. cit. K. Holmes, J. Kreiss; and Op cit, J. Pepin et al.

[14] B. N'Galy et al., "Epidemiology of HIV infection in Africa," Journal of Acquired Immune Deficiency Syndromes 1 (1988): 551–8.

[15] Op. cit. P. Piot, M. Carael.

[16] Ibid.

HIV,[17] and in Kenya and Cameroon blood screening equipment and reagents are available in virtually every district and provincial hospital in the country. In some centers, attempts have been made to reduce the number of unnecessary blood transfusions and to reduce blood donation by individuals who are at high risk of being HIV–infected.

AIDS is predominantly an urban problem in most countries in Africa[18] but in some countries, such as Uganda, relatively large rural outbreaks have been reported.[19] Table 8–1 shows the HIV seroprevalence rates in urban and rural Rwanda. The rate in a sample of rural blood donors was 4.5% in contrast to a rate of 18.0% in urban donors. Urban clients of prostitutes had a rate of 28% and urban prostitutes a seroprevalence rate of 88%.[20]

Table 8–1. *HIV Seroprevalence in Rwanda.*

Population	HIV Prevalence Rate %
Adults (R)	3.0
Blood Donors (R)	4.5
Blood Donors (U)	18.0
Prostitute Clients (U)	28.0
Prostitutes (U)	88.0
R=Rural, U=Urban	

There is limited information on the HIV seroprevalence rate in the general population in most countries in Africa. Serosurveys of general populations carried out in 1986 showed a seroprevalence of 1% in Cameroon, four percent in the Central African Republic, 5% in the Congo, and 15% in Uganda.[21] WHO/GPA estimates that 2.5 million people were infected with HIV in the African region by 1988.[22]

The most accurate estimates of the distribution and number of cases of HIV infection in a country would be obtained by national seroprevalence surveys. However, large seroprevalence surveys have proven expensive and difficult to implement. Surveillance of sentinel groups of both high —and low— risk populations is a more practical and affordable method, not only of

[17] Personal communication: Jean Emmanuel, Blood Transfer Center; Harare, Zimbabwe, 1989.
[18] *Op. cit*. C.P. Hudson *et al*.; and *op. cit*. B. N'Galy, *et al*.
[19] *Op. cit*. P. Piot, M. Carael.
[20] *Op. cit*. J. Chin, P. Sato, J. Mann.
[21] *Op. cit*. B. N'Galy *et al*.
[22] *Op. cit*. J. Chin, P. Sato, J. Mann.

assessing the magnitude of the epidemic but also of following its progress. While some epidemiologic data are available from some countries including Zaire, Kenya, Senegal, Uganda and Rwanda, there are many African countries with little or no available data.[23] Most of the data that do exist are from certain high–risk groups, especially prostitutes, in large urban centers and, to a limited extent, from selected groups in the general population such as women attending prenatal clinics, hospital in–patients and blood donors. Many of these studies, however, contain serious methodological flaws and biases and comparability is further limited by the use of different methods in testing for HIV. However, in the absence of more reliable data, these studies provide very useful information on the extent of the infection in some sentinel groups and may serve as indicators of the spread to the general population.

A comprehensive review of the available literature on the seroepidemiology of HIV in prostitutes in 28 countries in sub–Saharan Africa demonstrates a wide range of different patterns of HIV infection among different countries and an often equally wide range of patterns within countries.[24]

The lowest reported rates of HIV infection in prostitutes are found in the Anglophone countries of West Africa, namely Nigeria, Sierra Leone, Ghana, Liberia and Gambia, all with rates of less than ten percent (Table 8–2). Moderately high rates of HIV infection are found in prostitutes in the Francophone countries of West Africa. Limited data available from countries in this area generally show very low HIV rates in the general population but disproportionately high rates of HIV in prostitutes. Cameroon has the lowest rate of HIV infection in prostitutes at 7.1% in the capital, Yaounde, but rates among prostitutes in the rest of the Francophone West Africa region range from 40 to 60% in cities in Togo, Senegal, Burkina Faso, Mali, Ivory Coast and Guinea Bissau. The highest rates of infection in prostitutes are found in the urban areas of East and Central Africa. Rates of 50 to 90% are common among prostitutes in the major urban centers of Tanzania, Uganda, Malawi, Congo, Rwanda, Burundi, Kenya, Zaire and the Central African Republic.

The HIV seroprevalence data in prostitutes closely parallels that of the severity of the AIDS epidemic as determined by the number of AIDS cases reported to WHO/GPA (Table 8–3). The relatively high rates of infection in prostitutes in countries such as Senegal, Cote D'Ivoire and Togo, could be partially explained by the frequent travel between the Francophone coun-

---

[23] *Op. cit.* B. N'Galy, *et al.*; and P. Piot *et al.*, "Acquired immune deficiency syndrome in heterosexual population in Zaire," *Lancet*, 2 (1984): 65–9; and P. Piot *et al.*, "Retrospective seroepidemiology of AIDS virus infection in Nairobi populations," *Journal of Infectious Disease* 155 (1987): 1108–12.

[24] W. Carswell, B. Janowitz, "The Current HIV Epidemic and Prostitution: Review of Seroepidemiology." Working paper WHO/GPA and FHI. 1988.

tries of Africa and the relatively more prosperous urban economies making
prostitution more profitable.

Table 8–2. *Number of reported AIDS cases and HIV seroprevalence in
prostitutes in sub–Saharan Africa.*

Country	No. of Reported AIDS Cases[†] February 1989	HIV Seroprevalence in Urban Prostitutes* 1986–1988 (%)
West Africa		
Nigeria	13	1.2
Ghana	227	2.1
Cameroon	62	7.1
Burkina Faso	26	11.0
Togo	2	31.0
Ivory Coast	250	51.0
Central/East Africa		
Congo	1250	34.0
Rwanda	987	30.0
Malawi	2586	56.0
Uganda	5508	67.0
Tanzania	3055	75.0
Kenya	2732	85.0

[†] Source: World Health Organization, *Update: AIDS Cases Reported to Surveillance, Forecasting
and Impact Assessment Unit,* (Geneva: Global Programme on AIDS, 28 February 1989).
* Highest reported seroprevalence rate from most recent study of prostitutes. Sample sizes
range from 67–773.

Table 8–3. *AIDS cases in sub–Saharan Africa.*

Age Group	Cumulative 1987 AIDS Cases Reported	Cumulative 1992 AIDS Cases Projected
Children (0–14 years)	46 000	200 000
Adults (15–60 years)	105 000	800 000
Total	151 000	1 000 000

Source: J. Chin, P. Sato, J. Mann, "Estimates and Projections of HIV/AIDS to the year 2000"
(Geneva: World Health Organization, May 1989).

There is a paucity of data on the prevalence of HIV in the partners of prostitutes. Some useful data, however, are available on clients of STD clinics, who are likely to be partners of prostitutes. In Nairobi, most of the clients of the Pumwani STD clinic admit to frequent sexual contact with prostitutes and an estimated 20% of patients with chancroid are HIV positive.[25]

The epidemiology of HIV infection in Africa is complicated by the great heterogeneity of cultures and environments. In many ways this diversity is far greater than the diversity found in North America and/Europe.[26] Further epidemiological and behavioral research is needed in different subpopulations in order to develop appropriate intervention programs.

RATIONALE FOR TARGETING AIDS INTERVENTIONS

The pattern of response to the AIDS epidemic in African countries has been no different than the response in other countries. In most of Africa, an initial period of denial was followed by a period of inaction, based on the rationale that the magnitude of the problem was exaggerated. The next phase was to undertake the "soft," noncontroversial interventions such as blood screening, and to begin very limited information, education and communication campaigns. The rationale for focusing on blood screening is that the technology is available, although it is expensive; it is safe and acceptable to everyone; and it is a relatively easy way to achieve a sustainable, demonstrable impact.

By early 1987, AIDS public education campaigns had been launched on every continent, featuring an extensive range of radio, television, and press discussion about "safe–sex" practices.[27] In Africa, some of these public education campaigns have included the use of popular traditional music and adaptation of folklore. The quality of the programs varies from country to country as does the content of these messages.[28] Some of these messages have been described as too vague while others have been criticized for being too specific and for condoning casual sex.[29]

These information, education and communication campaigns have experienced several problems. Most of them were put together hurriedly with limited planning. Very little baseline research was done to deter-

---

[25] L.J. Da Costa, F.A. Plummer et al., "Prostitutes are a major reservoir of STD in Nairobi, Kenya," Sexually Transmitted Disease 12 (1985): 64–7.

[26] Op. cit. B. N'Galy et al.

[27] J.P. Baggaley, "Perceived effectiveness of international AIDS campaigns," Health Education Research Theory and Practice 3 (1) (1988): 7–17.

[28] J.H. Hubley, "AIDS in Africa: A challenge to health education," Health Education Theory and Practice, 3(1) (1988): 41–7.

[29] Op. cit. J.P. Baggaley.

mine appropriate messages and most of the messages were not pretested adequately. Programs lacked adequate financial and technical resources so that most of the campaigns were short–lived. Evaluation of the impact has been the exception rather than the rule.

In the absence of evaluation, it is difficult to assess the impact of these public education programs. The continuing spread of HIV among high–risk groups and to the general population suggests that these programs may not, by themselves, be adequate in reducing behaviors that promote the spread of HIV infection.

In order to have an impact on the sexual transmission of HIV in Africa, we need programs that reach those most at risk of acquiring or transmitting the infection. Mathematical modeling suggests that individuals with the highest rate of partner change and/or number of partners contribute disproportionately to the acquisition and transmission of STDs including HIV infection.[30] High rates of partner change and high numbers of partners are particularly important in the spread of infection among high–risk groups such as prostitutes and their partners.[31] Groups that are at high risk of HIV infection in Africa include sex workers of various types (prostitutes, barmaids, etc.) and their partners, STD clinic clients, truckers, military personnel, sailors, street children and young unmarried persons living in urban areas.

Prostitutes constitute the largest easily targetable high–risk group in Africa but they are relatively few in number compared to the general population of sexually active individuals. There are several reasons why high–risk groups such as prostitutes are priority target groups for interventions. They constitute an important reservoir of STD in some parts of Africa.[32] Sex workers are at high risk of acquiring HIV infection and transmitting it to their customers. The clients of sex workers are also a priority target group for the same reasons. Sex workers can be identified and reached with intervention programs. The clients of sex workers are usually more difficult to reach, but may be relatively easier to reach than the larger and more dispersed group of sexually active individuals who eventually come into contact directly or indirectly with the clients of prostitutes.

Mathematical modeling of HIV also helps us to compare the impact of alternative interventions, to allocate resources, and to advise on policy formulations. Models that have looked at prostitution suggest that inter-

[30] B. Auvert, M. Moore, W. Bertrand, A. Beauchet, P. Aegerter, D. Lusamba, K. Tomba Diong, J. Kinowski, "Dynamics of HIV infection and AIDS in a central African city," (Unpublished); and R.M. Anderson, R.M. May, "Epidemiological parameters of HIV transmission," *Nature* 333 (1988j): 514–9.

[31] *Op. cit.* B. Auvert, M. Moore, W. Bertrand, A. Beauchet, P. Aegerter, D. Lusamba, K. Tomba Diong, J. Kinowski.

[32] *Op. cit.* L.J. Da Costa, F.A. Plummer *et al.*

ventions directed at prostitutes and their partners could have a dramatic and cost–effective impact on HIV transmission.[33]

The lower rates of HIV infection in European and North American prostitutes could be partly explained by the early adoption of safer practices such as non–penetrative sexual stimulation, the use of condoms, and utilization of opportunities for diagnosis and treatment of STDs.[34]

In countries that are in the early phases of the epidemic, programs designed to reach the high–risk groups are the most rational and cost–effective approach. Such interventions aim at preventing individuals with multiple partners from becoming infected or at containing the infection within the relatively small populations and preventing spread to larger segments of the population. These targeted interventions have to be undertaken quite early in the epidemic in order to have maximum impact. The rapid spread of HIV in the gay communities in Europe and the U.S. in the prostitute population of Central and East Africa[35] and in the intravenous (IV) drug using population of Bangkok[36] are excellent examples of the need to reach these high–risk groups early.

As the epidemic progresses and spreads into the general population, targeting of these priority groups may no longer be sufficient by itself to substantially reduce the number of individuals infected via the sexual transmission of HIV. Several African countries have already reached a stage where infection rates in the urban populations of blood donors and pregnant women are as high as 20%.[37] When conditions reach this level of infection, the priority target population for intervention must extend beyond individuals with multiple partners. There is a very large group of people who may not have multiple partners and who do not have sex with prostitutes but are at equal risk of HIV infection because their regular partners are infected. The definition of the target population has to be broadened to cover this much larger group. Even during this stage, however, targeting of prostitutes and their clients remains important because of the increased opportunity for the spread of information about infection among this group.

[33] Op. cit. B. Auvert, M. Moore, W. Bertrand, A. Beauchet, P. Aegerter, D. Lusamba, K. Tomba Diong, J. Kinowski.

[34] Op. cit. K. Holmes, J. Kreiss.

[35] P. Piot et al., "Epidemiological and sociological aspects of HIV infection in developing countries," British Medical Bulletin 44(1) (1988): 68–88.

[36] Bangkok Post, August 3, 1989.

[37] P. Lamptey, A. Neequaye, S. Weir et al., "Pilot program to reduce the risk of HIV infection among prostitutes in Accra, Ghana" (Unpublished).

TARGETING PRIORITY GROUPS

Only a few programs targeted to prevent the sexual transmission of HIV among high–risk behavior groups have been implemented in Africa. Progress has been slow, primarily due to a variety of political factors. Decision makers and program managers have been reluctant to develop and implement interventions for those on the fringes of society whose behavior is considered unacceptable to the mainstream. In some countries, the fear that acknowledging AIDS and implementing interventions will harm the tourist industry has been a factor. It is more difficult to understand the reluctance of governments to implement programs for groups such as the military, a high–risk group that is relatively noncontroversial, powerful and vital to the defense of these countries, but also at considerable risk for HIV infection.

The AIDSTECH Project of Family Health International (FHI), funded by the United States Agency for International Development, has developed a strategy to create and implement intervention programs targeted at various high–risk behavior groups. AIDSTECH provides technical assistance and financial support to national AIDS control programs designed to reach high risk groups in ten countries in Africa.[38] A four–part intervention program seeks to offer a comprehensive and integrated approach to the prevention of the sexual transmission of AIDS. First, an AIDS education program reaches priority target groups with important information about how AIDS is transmitted and how to reduce the risk of infection. Second, a condom distribution program gives these groups the means for reducing their risk of infection. Third, strengthening STD services reduces the additional risk of HIV infection associated with STDs that cause genital ulcers. Fourth, a system of program monitoring, evaluation and planning for long–term sustainability of the program provides managers with the information needed to improve the program, document its success for policy makers and funding agencies, and plan for meeting long–term program resource needs.

THE EDUCATIONAL PROGRAM

Goals, Objectives and Strategies
The goal of the education program is to modify the behavior of high–risk groups and their partners in ways that will reduce the sexual transmission of HIV. The objectives of the education program are the following:

[38] AIDSTECH Semi Annual Report to the Agency for International Development, June 1989.

- To inform high–risk groups about AIDS, particularly that it is a sexually transmitted disease.
- To motivate high–risk groups to change their behavior in order to reduce their risk of infection.
- To motivate high risk groups to use condoms correctly and consistently.
- To teach high–risk groups how to obtain, store, use, and dispose of condoms properly.
- To teach high–risk groups how to recognize common symptoms of STDS and understand the importance of obtaining prompt treatment.

The strategies for achieving these objectives depend on the nature of the high–risk groups and how well they are organized, whether there is an STD clinic available to be the focal site for a program, and what personnel are available to work with the program. The three basic strategies that may be adapted for local use include the use of peer health educators, the use of STD service providers, and the use of other community–based programs.

The peer health educator strategy has been used in Ghana, Cameroon, Mali and Burkina Faso and will be used in a number of other countries including Kenya, Zimbabwe and Nigeria. The client outreach strategy is being be used in Kenya, Zimbabwe and Cameroon. The STD Clinic strategy is being used in Kenya.

Peer Health Educators
The peer health educator strategy features the identification and recruitment of natural leaders of the high–risk group to be health educators and condom distributors to their peers. Where possible, existing organizations of the group are used to identify leaders and to involve the target population in the planning and implementation of such programs.

The criteria for selection as a peer health educator include acceptance by other members of the group, being an opinion leader in the target group, and exhibiting a concern for one's peers and a willingness to be trained and to work with the program. Those selected receive special training in how to educate their peers and how to distribute condoms.

The effectiveness of peer health educators can be enhanced by other health education and condom distribution efforts. Supportive interventions should be included whenever possible, such as periodic community meetings led by peer health educators where dramatic presentations, condom demonstrations and educational lectures can be given to a large group; and on–site AIDS education and condom distribution programs in places where prostitutes and clients are present, such as bars, night clubs and hotels. Workshops with hotel and bar managers can help to sensitize them to the danger of AIDS to their customers and employees and can help to develop employer–assisted AIDS prevention programs.

STD Clinic Education

The STD clinic AIDS education strategy features the use of current STD service providers, outreach workers and contact tracers to educate individuals at risk of HIV infection as they come to the health facility for treatment of STDS. This strategy uses the available infrastructure to reach a variety of individuals at high risk of acquiring STDS, including HIV, and is particularly useful in countries where prostitutes are required to visit an STD clinic regularly.

Components of the STD clinic–based strategy include improving the attitudes of STD clinic staff toward all clients, but especially toward prostitutes; educating health care providers about AIDS and how to promote condom use; training clinic staff to educate their clients to recognize symptoms of common STDS; and developing educational materials for use in the STD clinic.

Development and Implementation of Education Programs

No matter which educational strategy or strategies are selected, KAP surveys and/or focus groups are useful to develop the educational program and make sure messages are culturally appropriate. Focus groups provide a mechanism for using prostitutes and clients as resource persons in the development of materials, serve as a forum for the exchange of ideas, promote understanding about the need for behavior change, and improve the acceptability of the intervention program. Focus groups can be repeated to serve as a forum to discuss the long–term acceptability of the program, provide feedback to program staff, and to assess perceived changes in condom demand. Along with development of the educational message itself, the means of communicating the message is developed based on an analysis of the most appropriate media (i.e. posters, pictorial brochures, video), whether printed information should be completely pictorial or not, and whether translation into local languages is needed. The prototype materials are then designed by local experts so as to be culturally appropriate and are pretested among the target population, modified as needed, and finalized for distribution. The content of the message usually includes:

- Facts about AIDS, including that it is transmitted sexually and is more likely to be transmitted if genital ulcers and other STDS are present.
- The fact that a healthy–looking sexual partner can transmit the AIDS virus without even knowing that he or she is a carrier.

- The strong recommendation that prostitutes quit prostitution or, if that is not possible, require their clients and other partners to use condoms consistently.
- The message that individuals practicing high–risk behavior, especially prostitutes and their partners, should be checked regularly for the presence of genital ulcers or other STDs and treated if necessary.

Educators are trained to use the AIDS education materials and instructed to teach the proper use of condoms. Condom instructions include how to tell the inside of a condom from the outside, how to place it on the penis, how to squeeze the air out of the tip, how to unroll it, how to remove it, and how to dispose of it. In addition, individuals are taught not to store condoms close to a heat source or to re–use condoms.

Even though AIDS is a deadly disease and the content of the messages is very serious, educators are encouraged to use humor in presenting educational messages and to role play how male clients could be convinced to use condoms.

Where HIV testing is available, educators are taught that a negative test for HIV infection does not imply immunity to infection and negative test results should not be used to assure sexual partners that unprotected intercourse is safe. In Cameroon, some prostitutes who were tested and found to be free of HIV infection asked for a card indicating that they were free of infection that they could show to their clients. Such requests should be anticipated and resisted.

Condom Marketing and Distribution Programs
The goal of condom marketing and distribution programs is to increase condom accessibility to individuals at high risk of HIV infection and their partners. The objectives of a condom marketing and distribution program are to develop and implement a targeted marketing system to increase condom demand and use among prostitutes and high–risk groups; to implement a system that will provide easy access to affordable condoms for members of target population; and to assure sustainability of condom distribution programs. There are several strategies for condom distribution, including distribution:

- by peer health educators;
- by trained STD clinic staff;
- through condom cost recovery strategies such as a condom social marketing program;
- by an employer–assisted work–site distribution program;
- and through the family planning network.

In each case, issues must be resolved regarding the management and implementation of the condom distribution program including:

- storage and distribution of condoms from a central storehouse to the STD clinic or health educator to the prostitutes and their partners;
- training of condom distributors'
- coordination of education and condom distribution efforts;
- monitoring of the number of condoms supplied to and distributed by each condom outlet; and
- whether condoms will be sold, at what price, and by whom.

It should be noted that even though STD clinic staff can be trained to promote condom use and should have supplies of condoms available to provide to patients, STD clinic staff cannot be relied upon to be the sole supplier of condoms to members of high–risk groups as they only see patients who come to the clinic.

Cost–recovery Strategies

Condoms are the most expensive component of AIDS intervention programs for prostitutes and their partners. Therefore, efforts must be made to help members of high–risk groups recover at least part of the cost of the condoms, for example, through strategies such as subsidization of the costs of condoms and condom distribution by employers, bar and hotel owners, or unions. Every program could benefit from a study to assess the feasibility of a condom cost–recovery program. Initially even if condoms are provided free of charge as part of a marketing strategy to increase demand, an effort should be made later to determine whether men and women are willing to pay for condoms and at what price.

One very promising cost–recovery strategy is the development and implementation of a condom social marketing program. Condom social marketing programs use the retail market to distribute and sell low–cost condoms. In Zaire and Cameroon, the following activities are being under-taken as part of a condom social marketing program targeted at the general population as well as prostitutes. Assessment of current condom prevalence is the first step. Next, city–wide market surveys are made to verify preliminary information on retail distribution patterns, pricing, packaging, promotion, sales volume and velocity, attitudes of retailers toward low–cost condoms, trade practices, and purchasing patterns of wholesalers and retailers. This results in the identification of potential local collaborating firms and institutions. The development of brand names, packaging graphics, a pricing structure (to wholesaler, retailer and consumer), and estima-tion of revenue potential to the project follows. Finally, a marketing plan with detailed strategies for sales, distribution, advertising and promotion, and evaluative research is implemented.

Strengthening STD Services

The goal of the STD services component is to reduce STDS as a cofactor of transmission for individuals at high risk of HIV infection. The objectives of the STD services program are improvement of STD prevention activities (e.g. health education and condom distribution) and improved diagnosis of STDS, affordable treatment of STDS and confidential test results, and implementation of sentinel surveillance of STDS.

Thus far, the strategy for reaching these objectives has been the strengthening of current programs at general health facilities or at designated STD clinics. Development of a program usually includes a needs assessment of the related STD health facility in terms of supplies and equipment, training, educational programs and counseling. Next, a plan is developed for implementing activities to meet the needs designated as the highest priority.

A strategy to diagnose and treat STDS outside of a health care facility may be implemented in Calabar, Nigeria. In Calabar, local program managers are planning to periodically arrange meetings of prostitutes in sites such as brothels where they usually receive health education regarding AIDS. After a meeting to discuss AIDS and the need for early recognition and treatment for STDS, an opportunity will be provided for the women to be examined and tested for STD infection. The specimens will be taken to Calabar for testing and the results given to the women at a follow–up meeting.

Finally, where possible, the STD component of the intervention program includes STD testing and monitoring of the prevalence of infection to provide program managers with information about disease trends and insight into the effectiveness of the intervention program.

Program Evaluation, Monitoring and Planning for Sustainability

Program evaluation, monitoring and planning for sustainability include estimation of program impact, identification of program strengths and weaknesses, and identification of resources needed to sustain the program. Monitoring and evaluation of intervention programs must not be burdensome to the implementing group and should provide a meaningful and practical assessment of how well the program is meeting its objectives.

Several strategies exist for evaluation of the effectiveness of interventions. The most persuasive outcome indicator is a demonstrated decrease in HIV incidence that can be linked to the program. This indicator, while the most persuasive, is the most costly and time–consuming to obtain. Obtaining valid estimates of this indicator can involve following a cohort of prostitutes exposed to the intervention and a control group of prostitutes not exposed to the intervention and estimating the difference in their seroconversion rates over time. This can require a significant amount of data collection and can be extremely difficult to implement with highly mobile individuals such as prostitutes. It is also nearly impossible to implement where initial rates of HIV infection are extremely low.

Family Health International has chosen to rely instead on two different indicators of behavior change: changes in reported condom use and changes in STD incidence. Changes in reported condom use are based on pre and post–knowledge, attitudes and practice (KAP) surveys of prostitutes exposed to the intervention and, where possible, a comparison group of prostitutes not exposed to the intervention. Activities necessary for implementation of KAP surveys include development of the survey protocol, pretesting the questionnaire, training interviewers, editing and coding questionnaires, preparing data for analysis and subsequent analysis of data. Validation of reported condom use, where possible, is recommended.

In addition to changes in condom use, estimates of changes in STD incidence among the target population can be used to evaluate programs. Where possible, programs should include baseline and follow–up examinations of a sample of women for evidence of gonorrhea, syphilis, and genital ulcer disease.

Where the program is clinic–based, programs are also evaluated by means of pre and post surveys of knowledge and attitudes among STD clinic staff and through monitoring STD clinic statistics on the number of patients seen, tests provided, condoms distributed and women counseled.

It should be noted, however, that the success of a program may be related to variables that are difficult to quantify. Success in accessing the prostitute community and in obtaining their cooperation is clearly essential but difficult to measure. Success can also depend on the quality of the interaction between prostitutes and health providers. Qualitative information from focus groups of program participants and staff can be used to interpret KAP and STD incidence data.

Because fiscal assistance is usually limited to the start–up years of a program, an integral part of interventions should involve planning for the management of the program and developing a plan for sustaining the program for the next five years. Activities designed to improve the management and implementation of the program include the performance of relevant needs assessments and the collection of baseline data (via interviews, focus groups, informal interviews, participant observation, demand studies, etc.) on condom supplies, staff requirements, need for vehicles, need for STD treatment equipment and supplies, need for educational materials, training and other budget requirements. Planning meetings are also needed to clarify objectives, define institutional responsibilities, select sites, prepare a program time frame, prepare the budget and identify funding sources. Another necessity is the implementation of systems to identify and hire program staff, purchase materials, equipment, and supplies, train and retrain staff, and to monitor supply and distribution of condoms, educational materials and STD equipment. The performance of a recurrent cost analysis to measure the ongoing costs of the program and to develop and promote a financial plan for meeting these costs should be included in the program design. The costs which will burden the program over the long term should be specified (i.e. equipment maintenance, utilities, building costs). Finally, an assessment of the potential involvement of other interested groups to provide personnel support or funding—i.e. local AIDS committees, women's groups—is very useful.

CASE STUDIES OF TARGETED INTERVENTIONS

A number of targeted intervention programs for prostitutes have been implemented in Ghana, Cameroon and Kenya. These programs will be described briefly to illustrate the different approaches, their successes and some of the problems encountered.

Kenya

The first AIDS education program targeted at prostitutes in Africa was initiated in Nairobi, Kenya in early 1985. Almost 600 prostitutes were registered in a study of the epidemiology of STDs at the Special Treatment Clinic in Nairobi.[39] As part of the study, a community–based health education program was developed in the community in which many of the prostitutes lived. A research group made up of members of the research team and elected members of the prostitute community set program priorities and served as a forum for communication between the prostitutes and the researchers. The elected representatives also served as health educators and condom distributors to their peers.

The study population was divided into three groups: an "intensively followed group" that came to the STD clinic every two weeks for follow–up; a "non–intensively followed group" and later another control group of newly recruited prostitutes. Health education was provided to the "intensively followed group" through individual counseling sessions at the clinic

[39] Op. cit. P. Piot, M. Carael, and J.K. Kreiss et al.; and Ngugi E.M. and Plummer, F. "Health Outreach and control of HIV infection in Kenya," Journal of Acquired Immune Deficiency Syndrome 1 (1988): 566–70; and E. Ngugi, F.A. Plummer et al., "Prevention of HIV transmission in Africa: Effectiveness of condom promotion and health education among prostitutes," Lancet, 15 Oct. 1988: 887–90.

and through *barazas*, general community meetings. The "non–intensively followed" group and later the newly recruited control group were free to come to the clinic at any time, could meet with the health educators, and could attend the *barazas*. The intensively followed women were counseled and provided condoms as they came to the clinic. The 15–30 minutes of counseling included the facts about AIDS as well as the results of their HIV test if available. The *barazas* were held approximately every six months and were open to all women in the community, whether or not they were enrolled in the study. The educational messages conveyed during the *barazas* were the following: that sexually transmitted diseases including HIV infection were prevalent in the prostitute community; that those with HIV infection were likely to transmit it to their clients; that women with STDs were more likely than others to become infected with HIV; and that uninfected women who continued to practice prostitution were at great risk of becoming infected. Women were encouraged to cease prostitution if at all possible. However, if ceasing prostitution were not possible, the women should insist that their clients use condoms. The messages were conveyed at the *baraza* via skits, role playing and songs.

The educational program was effective in increasing condom use. Prior to enrollment in the program, baseline condom use was ten percent or less for each of the three groups. By November, 1986, at least occasional condom use had increased to 80% for the "intensively followed" group, to 70% for the "non–intensively followed" group, and to 58% for the control group of new recruits. Analysis of factors associated with increased condom use among women in the control group showed that women in the control group who attended a *baraza* on their own were more likely to use condoms than those who had not attended a *baraza*. In all three groups the reason given most frequently for condom use was concern for personal health, and in particular, a desire to avoid getting HIV infection and AIDS.

The program was able to document that any condom use resulted in a three–fold reduction in the risk of seroconversion.[40] This is remarkable, given the high exposure to HIV infection, and might reflect a multiplier effect of condom use due to reduction of other STDs that might have increased susceptibility to HIV. Although *barazas* were the only educational measure associated with increased condom use, counseling and individualized instruction served a valuable purpose by answering specific questions and providing a confidential atmosphere for discussion of HIV test results. The study also showed that positive HIV status did not influence the subsequent use of condoms among the women. This is felt to be at least in part due to the women's concern about infecting their clients and possibly due

[40] OR = 0.34, p<0.05, 95% CI=0.13-0.92

to the impact on the general population, including the clients of prostitutes, of the broader AIDS health education programs implemented by the Ministry of Health.

Ghana

The goal of the Ghana Pilot Study was to evaluate a strategy to limit the spread of HIV infection by training a selected group of prostitutes as health educators to teach their peers about AIDS and motivate them to use condoms and/or spermicidal foaming tablets regularly with their customers.[41]

The pilot program was initiated in June, 1987 under the direction of Dr. Alfred Neequaye, Chairman of the Ghana Technical Committee on AIDS, and jointly funded by the American Foundation for AIDS Research and FHI.[42] Seventy–two prostitutes in Accra were tested for evidence of HIV infection, educated about AIDS, motivated to use condoms to protect themselves from HIV infection, and supplied with condoms and spermicidal foaming tablets containing nonoxynol–9 for clients who refuse to use condoms. Prevalence of HIV infection at baseline was 4.2%. The 72 women enrolled in the program were divided among the six health educators. Each health educator met with each woman in her group at least once every two weeks to reinforce the educational messages and deliver condoms. An educational brochure developed with the assistance of a Ghanaian artist was also distributed by the health educators and reviewed with the women. The brochure was pictorial and carried the simple messages that AIDS is a sexually transmitted fatal disease and that a woman should use condoms every time she has sex to reduce her risk of infection.

The pilot program was successful in increasing the use of condoms and spermicides among prostitutes during a six–month period. In June, prior to the implementation of the program, only 13% of the 72 women reported regularly using condoms or spermicidal tablets. Three–month and six–month follow–up surveys of the women were conducted to estimate the impact of the educational program. The response rate was 63% at three–months and 58% at six months. Most of the women who were not interviewed were traveling outside the city during the follow–up interviews. During both follow–up surveys, all of the women interviewed reported regular use of condoms or spermicides with their customers. When asked during the three–month interview specifically about their use of condoms and spermicidal foam tablets in the past week, 54% of the 268 sexual acts reported by the 47 women re–interviewed were protected by condoms alone, 13% by tablets, 27% by both condoms and tablets, and 6% by neither.

[41] A.R. Neequaye, G. Ankra–Badu, J.A. Mingle *et al.*, "HIV infection in Ghana," 2nd. International symposium on AIDS in Africa, October 1987, Naples, Italy S4.4: 50.

[42] *Op. cit.* P. Lamptey, A. Neequaye, S. Weir *et al.*

30% of the women interviewed had never used condoms prior to program initiation. During the six–month interview, 72% of the sexual acts reported were protected by condoms alone, 23% by tablets alone and 6% by both condoms and spermicides.

Unfortunately, even though the reported use of condoms with customers increased significantly, regular condom use with husbands or boyfriends remained around 20 percent throughout the six months of the study. Lack of protection with boyfriends is potentially just as dangerous as failure to use condoms with customers because the boyfriends often were originally customers.

Insight into some of the problems encountered with condoms was also obtained from the follow–up surveys. Two–thirds of the women reported condom breakage as a problem. 40% reported that customers object to using condoms and 11% named other problems such as the fact that using condoms delays the customer's orgasm, that the condom can irritate the vagina, that customers do not perceive themselves at risk of getting AIDS, and that customers often have no experience using condoms.

A fourth of the women reported that customers never initiate use of condoms and almost half said that customers initiate use less than half of the time. To motivate a customer to use a condom, two–thirds of the women said that they tell the customer that condoms offer protection from AIDS.

When asked what her response is when customers refuse to use a condom, over half said that they refuse to have sex with the customer and about a fourth said they use a foaming tablet. Nine percent said that they would accept the customer without a condom.

Based on the success of the pilot program in Accra, similar programs were implemented in Cameroon and Mali. The success of the pilot study has also served as the impetus for the development of an expanded self–sustaining program in Accra that will reach more than 600 women. Not only does the expanded program promise to save many lives through the prevention of HIV infection, but it also offers the opportunity of addressing several important issues raised by the pilot program regarding condom acceptability, evidence of HIV–2 infection, and program sustainability that are critical for the development of successful programs in other countries.

Cameroon

In 1987 only 35 clinical cases of AIDS had been diagnosed in Cameroon when the Ministry of Health under the direction of Dr. Lazare Kaptue–Noche, Dr. Roger Salla, Dr. Marcel Monny–Lobe and Dr. Leopold Zekeng decided to implement a prevention program similar to the program initiated among prostitutes in Ghana.[43] Baseline seroprevalence data of the 125 prostitutes enrolled in the program showed that the rate of infection (7.1 percent) was indeed significantly higher than the rate among the general population (0.5 percent).

The goal of the study was to test an intervention model that would slow the transmission of HIV infection among urban prostitutes in Yaounde. In early 1988, eleven prostitutes were selected from hotels, bars and night-clubs throughout Yaounde. They were trained to educate their peers about the danger of AIDS and other STDs, to motivate their peers to practice safer sex including the use of condoms and spermicidal foaming tablets, and to distribute condoms and tablets to the prostitutes enrolled in the program.

According to data collected during a baseline survey, most of the women were in their twenties, had been born in or near Yaounde, had never been married, and went into prostitution for financial reasons. Almost one–fourth of those who had heard of AIDS had not changed their behavior since hearing of AIDS because they did not know what they could do to protect themselves. At baseline, less than 30% of the women said that they used condoms with customers more than half of the time.

Mid–point and follow–up data showed that the program was successful in improving knowledge of AIDS among the prostitutes and in increasing their use of condoms. Seven months after program initiation, almost two–thirds of the women reported using condoms with more than half of their customers. One year after program initiation, 52% of the women still reported using condoms more than half of the time. The women who did not use condoms reported having problems with condoms, including pelvic irritation and reduced pleasure; clients who did not want to use condoms; and condoms not always being available. According to the women, clients who refused the use of condoms said that AIDS did not exist, that they were healthy and not afraid of getting AIDS or any other STD, that condoms broke often and/or that condoms reduced their pleasure.

After one year of experience with the program, the Ministry of Health developed and is implementing an expansion of the model intervention program. The expanded program will target prostitutes in three cities: Yaounde, Douala and later Maroua. In addition, clients of the prostitutes and patients with sexually transmitted diseases in those cities will be

[43] M. Monny–Lobe, L. Zekeng, D. Nichols et al., "An AIDS targeted intervention for prosti-tutes in Yaounde, Cameroon" (Unpublished); and M. Monny–Lobe, D. Nichols, L. Zekeng, R. Salla, L. Kaptue, "The use of condoms by prostitutes in Yaounde, Cameroon," Poster W.D.P.87 presented at Vth. International Conference on AIDS. June 1989, Montreal, Canada; and M. Monny–Lobe, D. Nichols, L. Zekeng, R. Salla, L. Kaptue, "Prostitutes as health educa-tors for their peers in Yaounde: changes in knowledge, attitudes and practices," Oral presenta-tion W.G.0.21 at Vth. International Conference on AIDS. June 1989, Montreal, Canada.

targeted. As part of the program, an ethnographic study to gain additional information about prostitutes and their clients is now underway.

The expanded program has also complemented the efforts of the prostitute health educators to distribute condoms through the development of a condom social marketing program. This social marketing program will advertise and sell condoms to prostitutes, to their partners and to the general public. Programs such as these improve the acceptability of condoms among the general population, increase condom availability and recover some of the costs of the program. By targeting groups at increased risk of infection relatively early in the epidemic, the Ministry of Health in Cameroon may be effective in curtailing the epidemic.

LESSONS LEARNED FROM GHANA, CAMEROON AND KENYA

Several important lessons can be learned from these pilot programs. It is evident that the strategy of community–based peer health education can be used effectively over the short term to improve the knowledge of AIDS and use of condoms among high–risk behavior populations such as prostitutes. When the danger of HIV infection is clearly explained to people who practice high–risk behaviors, and the means of reducing their risk of infection, i.e., condoms, are provided at an affordable price, a substantial proportion will change their behavior. Prostitutes may not change professions, but they may significantly increase their use of condoms, and may be more selective in their recruitment of clients. Further studies are needed to ascertain whether increased condom use can be sustained and whether improved knowledge about the modes of transmission of the virus and its other characteristics, such as the relation between HIV infection and the existence of other STDs, will be retained.

Finally, it is clear that reaching high–risk communities is not necessarily easy. The program coordinator and all program staff must treat the target populations with respect and earn their trust. Staff must also recognize that sub–groups of prostitutes and other marginal populations exist and that the age, education level and ethnic backgrounds of high–risk groups may vary greatly. Any pre–existing organizational structures should be recognized and utilized in developing educational and condom distribution program so that the programs are acceptable and sustainable.

CONCLUSION

The AIDS epidemic and the need to change the sexual behavior and practices of those at high risk of HIV infection has revealed the inadequacy of our knowledge about sexuality. Despite widespread acceptance and use of barrier contraceptives, such as condoms, that have resulted from family planning programs, these same programs have made very few attempts to understand the sexual behavior and practices of clients. Most programs have deliberately avoided discussions of sexual behavior in order to maintain the privacy of the individual or couple and to avoid offending them.

With the onset of the AIDS epidemic, several programs have been initiated that aim to change sexual behavior and practices that we know very little about. Some of the unanswered questions that affect the success of programs include: What is the extent and magnitude of polypartnerism and prostitution in different cultures? What is the extent of the interaction between partners during sexual encounters and how does this affect the adoption of new behaviors? What are the triggers to behavior change and how can behavior change be sustained? How often is sex planned or impulsive and how do behavior–modifying drugs, such as alcohol, influence the application of learned behavior?

Condoms have become the mainstay of "safe sex" to prevent the transmission of HIV. However, are there other choices in sexual practices in different cultures? Our knowledge of the use of condoms has gaps such as the specific characteristics of use occasions, breakage rates (real or imagined) under different use conditions, the characteristics of the successful condom user and the obstacles to compliance.

These are only some of the questions that need to be answered in order to design and implement intervention programs that will have the desired impact. However, the urgency of the AIDS epidemic requires that interventions be started immediately, monitored closely and evaluated. Programs must be modified later, based on new knowledge and lessons learned, and the relevant applied behavioral research must be conducted in order to fill in the gaps in our knowledge.

The biggest obstacle to interventions with priority target groups has been the reluctance (after outright refusal) of decision makers and program managers to approve interventions to reach these high–risk groups. Several years ago, the authors visited a number of African countries in an attempt to develop projects to reach prostitutes. A few decision makers with foresight were willing to try innovative programs to reach a target population that they had never before considered seriously. However, most decision makers refused, with the explanation that there were no prostitutes in their country and therefore there was no need for such a program. The HIV seroprevalence rates in prostitutes in those countries where there have been no interventions now range from 50–90%.

It took nearly three decades to get decision makers to understand and accept that excessive population growth is a detriment to development in

African countries. Even a decade is too long for decision makers to undertake programs to prevent AIDS; the HIV seroprevalence of prostitutes in Nairobi increased from 4% to 85% in less than seven years.

A second major problem in implementing high–risk group interventions is the difficulty in reaching these populations. It has not been too difficult to identify the visible high–risk groups such as prostitutes in bars or night –clubs. The major difficulty is reaching the submerged part of the iceberg— women who have multiple partners, but who do not consider themselves sex workers. The problem is further compounded by the belief of politicians and law enforcers that prostitution can be prevented by periodic police raids, by persecution of prostitutes and by invoking legal, bureaucratic and ethical reasons to discourage prostitution.

Some high–risk groups can be reached through limited targeted projects, but the vast majority can be reached only through nationally supported programs that reach all segments of the population.

A third major obstacle to behavior change is the difficulty in reaching the partners of high–risk groups. One can classify the African target population into two groups: The primary high–risk groups include prostitutes, clients of prostitutes and intravenous drug users. Secondary high–risk groups are the partners of the primary group—i.e. the non–paying partners of prostitutes and other partners (spouses, girlfriends and boyfriends) of clients of prostitutes and partners of intravenous drug users. This secondary high–risk group constitutes a very large section of society that serves as the bridge for infection to the rest of the population.

A number of model programs, such as those in Ghana, Kenya and Cameroon, have already demonstrated that interventions designed to reach prostitutes are ineffective unless an attempt is made to change the behavior of the clients as well.

Programs designed to reach potential clients of prostitutes include interventions aimed at truckers and the military as well as AIDS education and condom social marketing programs targeted at clients in bars and night–clubs. Preventing the infection of the unsuspecting sexual partners of the primary high–risk group has proved extremely difficult.

There is a tendency for men to label sex with a prostitute as relatively unsafe but sex with their regular partners as safe. It may therefore be difficult to convince such a man, who may already be infected, to practice safe sex with his spouse. The situation is further complicated by the fact that in order for the primary high–risk group to practice safe sex with their regular sexual partners, they may have to admit to them that they have had other sexual partners. Further research is required to determine the best way of reaching these very different subpopulations.

The economies of most countries in sub–Saharan Africa have been struggling for the past decade, and health programs have suffered because of the inadequacy of resources. The situation has been further compounded by the AIDS epidemic which has required considerable human and fiscal resources both from national and international sources. The international response has been remarkable but inadequate to meet the needs of the AIDS epidemic.

Even if we are successful in convincing decision makers to support programs to prevent sexual transmission of HIV by promoting behavior change in those individuals who practice high–risk behavior, we will be faced with a problem of not having enough resources to implement these programs. Despite the fact that sexual transmission is the major route of HIV infection in Africa, woefully inadequate resources have been allocated to the programs aimed at reducing sexual transmission through behavior change.

Table 8–4 shows an analysis of the condom requirements for programs targeted at prostitutes.[44] The model assumes a cost of five cents per condom, two sexual encounters per day for each prostitute, and a prostitute population of 61 per 10000. The total cost of condoms for prostitutes of African cities with populations greater than 100000 is estimated to be $8.6 million per year. The total budget for the WHO Global Programme on AIDS (GPA) is only $90 million dollars for 1989, an amount that is manifestly insufficient for providing education, STD services and condoms to the general population.[45] Even if this entire amount were spent solely on Africa, it would represent only 14 cents per sexually active person per year and would be insufficient to purchase three condoms for every adult. Clearly, with so few resources available, targeting high–risk populations for interventions is currently economically as well as epidemiologically sensible.

Finally, policy makers and program implementers who choose to develop intervention programs targeted at groups that practice high–risk behavior, such as prostitutes, must not permit those groups to become scapegoats for the epidemic. Sensitivity to the lifestyles of individuals and a commitment to help and serve others are as important as condoms to the success of prevention. It is time that more than a tiny fraction of Africa's high–risk population be reached by an AIDS education and condom distribution program.

[44] A. Bhat, B. Muskovitz, D. Sokal, M. Potts, "Condom supplies for high–risk behaviors: strategies, status, costs and future prospects" (Unpublished).

[45] "AIDS: Prevention, policies and prostitutes," *Lancet* 20 May 1989; 1(8647): 1111.

Table 8-4. *AIDS containment model for surb–saharan Africa" cities over 100000 in Population.*

Assumption:
Prostitute Population: 0.0061 Per Capita
Number of encounters per prostitute: 2 Encounters per day
Cost of condom and international transport: $0.05 per Condom
Total cost of condoms: $8 604 080

Country	City	1989 Population Estimates	1989 Est. Prostitute Population	Number of Condoms Needed	Cost of Condoms Per City	Cost of Condoms Per Country
Burkina Faso:						
	Bobo Dioulasso	230425	1406	1012027	$50,601	
	Ouagadougou	407971	2489	1791810	$89,590	$140191
Cameroon:						
	Douala	1411781	8612	6200544	$310027	
	Yaounde	765386	4669	3361574	$168079	$478106
Congo:						
	Brazzaville	730222	4454	3207137	$160357	
	Point Noire	365006	2227	1603105	$80155	$240512
Cote d'Ivoire:						
	Abidjan	2799892	17079	12297125	$614856	
	Bouake	536324	30272	2355536	$117777	$732633

Ghana:					$857013
Accra	2315875	14127	10171324		$508566
Kumasi	1082261	6602	4753292		$237665
Sekondi-Takor	504470	3077	2215633		$110782
Kenya:					$569,249
Kisumu	393010	2397	1726102		$86305
Mombasa	606309	3698	2662907		$133145
Nairobi	1592890	9717	6995973		$349799
Malawi:					$98990
Blantyre-Limb	450775	2750	1979805		$98990
Nigeria:					$4478701
Ibadan	2426741	14803	10658247		$532912
Kano	1143176	6973	5020827		$251041
Lagos	3039437	18541	13349209		$667460
16 other cities	13785459	84091	60545760		$3027288
Rwanda:					$52629
Kigali	239657	1462	1052575		$52629
Togo:					$94968
Lome	432461	2638	1899369		$94968
Uganda:					$281023
Kampala	1279705	7806	5620463		$281023
Un. Rep. Tanzania:					$580065
Dar es Salaam	1404679	8569	6169350		$308467
Mwanza	322974	1970	1418500		$70925
Other cities	743351	4535	3264802		$200673

REFERENCES

J.P. Duran, Merlin, M., Josse, R., Garrigue, C., Kaptue–Noche, L. *et al.* "AIDS Survey in Cameroon." III International Conference on AIDS. June 1987, Washington, U.S. Poster WP 78, p. 123.

Global Diseases Surveillance Report. Global Epidemiological Working Group, Fort Detrick, MD, 21701.

L.G. Gurtler, Zoulek, G., Frosner, G., Deinhardt, F. *et al.* "Prevalence of HIV 1 and HIV 2 in a selected Malawian population." Third International Conference on AIDS. June 1987, Washington, D.C., THP 93, page 179.

L. Kaptue, Monny–Lobe, M., Zekeng, L., Lamptey, P., Potts, M., Douglas, N. "HIV–l infection among prostitutes in Yaounde (Cameroon)." 3rd Int. meeting on AIDS in Africa. September 1988/Arusha, Tanzania. WP 47, p. 66.

G. Leonard, Gershy–Damet, G.M., Sangare, A., Verdier, M., Rey, J.L., Denis, F. "Cohort and periodic cross sectional studies of HIV and HTLVI seroprevalence in Ivory Coast." 3rd. Int. Symposium on AIDS in Africa. September 1988, Arusha, Tanzania. TP 17, p. 74.

Minstre de la Sante de Burkina Faso. *Projet Sida, Plan a court terme.* August 1987.

P. M'pele, Itoua–Ngaporo, A., Rosenheim, M., Eozenou, P., Yala, F., Makuwa, Gluckman, J.C., Gentilini, M. "HIV antibodies in prostitutes, Brazzaville and Pointe–Noire (Congo)." 3rd. Int. meeting on AIDS in Africa. October 1988, Naples, Italy. TH 30, p. 87.

N. Namaaran, Plummer, F.A. "Cross sectional study of HIV infection in Southwest Uganda." Second International Conference on AIDS and Associated Cancers. October 1987, Naples, Italy. Poster TH 37, p. 91.

Ministry of Health. *AIDS Programme.* Cameroon, Feb. 1988.

W.M. Nkya, Howlett, W.P., Assenga, C., Nyombi, B., Kiwelu, I., Maembe, A., Mbirigenda, M. 3rd. International Conference on AIDS in Africa. September 1988, Arusha, Tanzania. Poster TP 9, p. 70.

P. Van de Perre, N. Clumeck, Carael, M., Mzabihimana, E., Robert–Guroff, M., De Mol, P., Freyens, P., Butzler, J–P., Gallo, R.C., Kanyamupira, J–B. "Female prostitutes: a risk group for infection with HTLV III." *Lancet,* (1985): ii, 524–7.

The Role of Behavioral Sciences and Health Education in HIV Prevention: Experience at the U.S. Center for Disease Control

Mark L. Rosenberg
Dennis D. Tolsma
Lloyd J. Kolbe
Fred Kroger
Marcie L. Cynamon
G. Stephen Bowen

Researchers first recognized the AIDS epidemic in the United States in June and July 1981, when the Center for Disease Control (CDC) published two short reports regarding unusual clusters of Pneumocystis carinii pneumonia and of Kaposi's sarcoma among gay men. In September 1982, in the first published use of the term "acquired immune deficiency syndrome" and of the acronym "AIDS", the CDC reported on 593 AIDS case reports it had received. By September 1989, exactly seven years later, the CDC had received case reports on 107 308 persons with AIDS, 63 836 of whom had died. Today, an estimated one million Americans are infected with the human immunodeficiency virus (HIV), and virtually all will ultimately develop AIDS.

The continued increase in AIDS cases led to an unprecedented research and prevention effort. The two principal modes of HIV transmission among adults were quickly identified: sexual transmission and sharing of needles among IV drug users. Both methods depend on behavioral choices by individuals, and as a result, as stated in a report by the National Academy of Sciences, "education will be a central preventive public health measure for this disease under any circumstances."[1] The purpose of this chapter is to discuss the CDC's approach to AIDS education in the United States and the lessons we have learned from that experience.[2]

THEORETICAL BASIS FOR EDUCATION AND COMMUNICATION INTERVENTIONS

The HIV epidemic caught the US public health system ill–prepared to mount a major prevention effort. Without vaccines to prevent HIV infection or effective drugs to treat infection once it occurred, the public health service needed to develop educational programs to prevent infection by changing those behaviors through which HIV was spread. The interventions were primarily educational, but they required building a new and firm behavioral science base to complement the microbiology and epidemiology bases that had long been a cornerstone of US public health efforts.

Focusing on the behavioral science model that underlies these educational efforts should not obscure the many other changes that were required for these efforts to be effective. These necessary changes included increasing the availability of addiction treatment services; increasing the quality and availability of services for family planning and sexually transmitted disease prevention and treatment; increasing access to health care services, especially for minorities; and providing adequate training to and addressing the fears of health care professionals.

When the epidemic was beginning, few operating public health agencies had been able to agree on what constituted the behavioral sciences or how to best use them. Today, we can broadly define the behavioral sciences as scientific approaches to understanding and changing behaviors. The traditional social and behavioral science disciplines that can contribute to HIV prevention include psychology, anthropology, sociology, demography, education, criminology, economics and political science. These disciplines are not usually well established, appreciated, or even represented in public health agencies. In addition, when behavioral or social scientists work in public health, they frequently are involved in statistical or epidemiologic analysis rather than in the specific discipline for which they were trained.

Additional barriers to the utilization of behavioral and social sciences include lack of training in behavioral sciences for the medical scientists and managers who administer and conduct most public health research, and a bias against research in the behavioral sciences ("soft") as opposed to laboratory and bench sciences ("hard"). Medical scientists and the tradi-

[1] Institute of Medicine, *Confronting AIDS: Directions for Public Health, Health Care, and Research* (Washington, D.C.: National Academy Press, 1986).
[2] Centers for Disease Control, *Strategic plan for Prevention of Human Immunodeficiency Virus (HIV) Infection, 1990s and Beyond* (Atlanta, GA: CDC, 1990).

tional cadre of public health workers often have felt that the concepts and constructs of the social sciences are simply plain common sense and are well within the grasp of any reasonable and well-educated individual, and that social and behavioral scientists tend to complicate their writing with needless jargon. Yet when public health researchers in the laboratory sciences have discussed AIDS prevention, they frequently have shown a lack of appreciation for those "common sense" social science concepts, for example, by failing to differentiate among behavioral determinants, behaviors and health outcomes.

The behavioral epidemiology model underlying CDC's HIV prevention strategies addresses health outcomes as the product of behaviors, and those behaviors, in turn, as the result of determinants that affect those individual behaviors.[3] This model has been expanded to include determinants that may be demographic, social, psychological (cognitive or emotional), physiological or environmental. An important implication of this model is that interventions should be designed to influence specific behavioral determinants.

This model is based on the premise that to help effect a change in behavior, one must first determine why people behave in a certain way and then try to influence those factors that make them behave that way. For example, to reduce the HIV infection rate (health outcome) by reducing the number of sexual partners that a specific individual might have in a year (the behavior), one must find out what factors (determinants) affect that individual's decision to have multiple partners. Some psychological determinants may be cognitive, such as the extent to which individuals believe they can become infected as a result of a risk behavior. Other psychological determinants may be emotional and relate to feelings such as loneliness, isolation, or desire for intimacy. Physiological determinants may be related to testosterone levels or to the physical pleasure of a sexual encounter. Social determinants may relate to group norms such as the perception that being an accepted member of a group requires a certain type and frequency of sexual contact. Additional determinants may be environmental, such as the absence of social settings which promote psychological or emotional intimacy without sexual contact. Environmental factors can include those economic forces involved in the exchange of sex for drugs, or sex for money. Environmental factors also include the availability of tax dollars to support HIV expenditures, the availability of drug addiction facilities, the availability of STD diagnosis and treatment facilities, and the integration of HIV counseling and testing into primary care facilities.

[3] L.J. Kolbe, "Behavioral epidemiology of AIDS: an organizing model," in *AIDS 1988: American Association for the Advancement of Science Symposia Papers*, ed. R. Kulsted (Washington, D.C.: American Association for the Advancement of Science, 1989), pp. 217–223.

Another example could involve reducing the frequency of HIV infection among infecting drug users (health outcome) by decreasing the sharing of infecting drug needles (behavior). The model suggests that an effective intervention would have to be based on understanding the factors (determinants) that lead intravenous (IV) drug users to share needles. A psychological factor might be the practice of sharing infecting drug needles as a way to establish social networks among IV drug users; environmental factors might be an inadequate number of "slots or vacancies" in a drug treatment program or treatment that is ineffective or that frequently leads to recidivism (reversion to previous behaviors) and long waiting periods, discouraging many IV drug users from even seeking treatment. A campaign to change this behavior might aim to change the way that IV drug users form social relationships and to increase access to effective addiction treatment programs.

LESSONS LEARNED FROM BEHAVIORAL AND SOCIAL SCIENCES

Knowledge alone is not enough to change behavior. Even though a correlation may exist between knowledge and behavior change at the individual or group level, one cannot assume a direct causal relationship.[4] Information about HIV transmission is a necessary but not sufficient condition for changing behavior.

To achieve a desired outcome, it is necessary to both change the target behavior and maintain the new behavior. Because recidivism is very common and can result in exposures to HIV, successful programs must aim to change behavior and sustain those changes over a long period. This suggests that modification in behavior may be more effective and realistic than total elimination of undesired behaviors.[5] Reinforcement of desired behaviors must be built into any program that attempts to change behaviors to achieve public health outcomes. Recidivism should be expected, and reinforcements for desired behaviors should be part of every program.

Some individuals' behavior may be much harder to change. There are three implications from this. First, large–scale efforts to change behaviors must recognize this variability and include special programs targeted to specific population segments. Second, a small group of recalcitrant individuals could pose a continued risk to the broader population if special efforts are not made to address them. Third, some individuals may avoid high-risk behaviors in certain settings—such as having sexual intercourse or

[4] National Research Council Committee on Risk Perception and Communication, *Improving Risk Communication* (Washington, D.C.: National Academy Press, 1989).

[5] M.H. Becker, J.G. Joseph, "AIDS and behavioral change to reduce risk: a review," *American Journal of Public Health* 78(4) (1988): 394–410.

sharing needles with strangers—but engage in high–risk behaviors in other settings, such as having sex or sharing needles with regular partners.

A heterogeneous population will include a variety of cultural subgroups, and one cannot assume that findings from one subgroup will apply to another. For example, interventions that are successful among white, middle–class, homosexual males may not be applicable to heterosexual adolescents or socio–economically disadvantaged individuals of racial or ethnic minority backgrounds. Demographically diverse groups may share common risk behaviors that have different determinants of those behaviors; they may also engage in different risk behaviors.

Working through governmental organizations to promote a particular set of behaviors in areas that are controversial and highly stigmatized presents numerous difficulties. There will probably be a need for non–governmental organizations to help effect change. In addition, the help of political scientists can be critical in understanding and overcoming barriers to change.

To be effective in modifying behaviors, educational programs must be consistent, intensive, systematic and combined with other strategies. As community–based interventions to reduce other behavioral risk factors have repeatedly shown, HIV information and education must be reinforced repeatedly.[6] The dictum "multiple channels, repeated multiple times," is a simple but direct lesson learned anew in HIV prevention. Educational materials and behavior change interventions must be culturally and linguistically relevant, sensitive and specific to the population of persons at risk.

Information must come from credible sources and be reinforced by social and reference group norms. People use information from the media to help support their behaviors when that information corresponds to prior beliefs and values. Personal networks, opinion leaders and trust in information sources are important. In some communities, for example, a local athlete, a politician, or even ex–addicts or former "street kids" may be more credible sources than a university professor or physician. An effective intervention must therefore be based on an understanding of the network and sources of effective information dissemination within particular subgroups and communities.[7] This understanding can frequently be gleaned from ethnographic studies.

The likelihood that an intervention will be effective increases when members of the target group or community feel they had a significant role in identifying the problem and in designing, implementing, and evaluating that intervention. Both community leaders and peers must be part of this

---

[6] D. Nelken, "AIDS and the social sciences: review of useful knowledge and research needs," *Review of Infectious Disease* 9 (5) (1987): 980–6.

[7] *Ibid.*

process. Mistrust of government officials or "experts" can lead people to discount or totally ignore information from particular sources. For this reason, peer education may be most effective with high–risk populations whose social norms differ most significantly from the general social norm, such as drug users and prostitutes. The chance of effecting change is greatest when individuals believe that outcomes result not from fate but from specific causes and that they themselves have the ability to determine these outcomes by affecting those causes. Individuals who believe they can make a difference, do make a difference. This notion, described as the internal locus of control for individuals and as empowerment for communities, is also true for organizations and countries.[8]

The perception of risk is influenced by many factors, and the perceived risk may be quite different from the true risk. Risk perception is heavily influenced by community norms and attitudes. People tend to underestimate familiar risks and overestimate unfamiliar and potentially catastrophic risks.[9] In addition, when risks and their negative consequences are perceived as inevitable, people tend to deny their abilities to effect successful change.

THE IMPORTANCE OF BEHAVIORAL SCIENCE FOR PUBLIC HEALTH PROGRAMS

Changing even relatively simple behaviors can be difficult. Changing behaviors related to the spread of HIV is much more complex for several reasons: these behaviors are highly personal, stigmatized, and often addicting, individuals perceive the subjective risks as being quite uncertain, and the illness is life–threatening. In addition, those groups that are disproportionately infected are often socially and economically disenfranchised.

Our experience suggests that rapid progress in understanding the relevant behaviors and in developing effective interventions demand a scientific approach that can achieve two goals: a) separate empirical findings (data) from value judgments and doctrine; and b) use scientific methods to test hypotheses and to design and evaluate interventions. An established body of knowledge and set of scientific methods in the social and behavioral sciences can be very useful in this effort.

THE MEASUREMENT INSTRUMENTS

To put HIV education and prevention programs on a firm base, we need data to answer five key questions:

8 W. Foege, "Alexander Langmuir annual lecture," CDC, Atlanta, GA, April 25, 1990.
9 *Op. cit.* D. Nelken.

- How do people behave? (behavioral surveillance);
- Why do they behave that way? (research into determinants of behaviors);
- What are the outcomes of these behaviors in health, social, and economic terms? (outcomes);
- How can these behaviors be changed? (program design and implementation);
- How effective are our efforts to change these behaviors? (program evaluation).

The following section addresses the first two questions: How do people behave? (behavioral surveillance) and Why do they behave that way? (research into determinants of behaviors).

Behavioral surveillance is the application of general epidemiologic surveillance to behaviors. In 1988, CDC defined epidemiologic surveillance as follows:

> The ongoing systematic collection, analysis, and interpretation of health data essential to the planning, implementation, and evaluation of public health practice, closely integrated with the timely dissemination of these data to those who need to know. The final link in the surveillance chain is the application of these data to prevention and control. A surveillance system includes a functional capacity for data collection, analysis, and dissemination linked to public programs.[10]

Long experience with surveillance has shown that collecting information about a public health problem is critical to assessing the extent of the problem, identifying the populations at greatest risk, developing interventions and evaluating the effectiveness of these interventions. Many behaviors that are risk factors for specific preventable adverse health outcomes, such as failure to use seat belts, alcohol consumption, smoking, lack of exercise and poor nutrition, have been monitored through surveillance systems.

Surveillance of behaviors is both similar to and different from surveillance of adverse health outcomes such as AIDS or HIV infection. Both types of surveillance require clear, operational case criteria (i.e. case definitions) and uniform reporting systems. Surveillance of behaviors is more complicated, however, because, to some extent, how a question is asked may influence the answer. Although observational data (where specific behaviors are observed and recorded) are more reliable than self–reported data, observational studies may be very difficult to conduct when the behaviors in ques-

[10] S.B. Thacker, R.L. Berkelman, "Public health surveillance in the United States," *Epidemiology Review* 10 (1988): 164–90.

tion, like sexual and drug use behaviors, are stigmatized, highly private and frequently illegal.

The goal of any behavioral surveillance program must be to develop a coordinated approach to asking about and compiling information on these behaviors. Surveillance staff must identify those specific behaviors of greatest importance —both risk behaviors to be discouraged and preventive behaviors to be encouraged and maintained— and create operational definitions for those behaviors. Another goal is to collect the behavioral data that are needed for program evaluation. Behavioral data are needed to evaluate the impact of interventions because biological data, such as HIV infection rates and AIDS case reports, can indicate progress in prevention efforts in the aggregate but are an impractical way to measure the effectiveness of specific interventions.

The following steps should be taken to develop a behavioral surveillance system:

1) Create an inventory of past, current, and planned activities to collect information about sexual and drug use behaviors.

   a) For your own agency, describe the types of data collected, data sources, how the data are used and costs of data collection. Describe these data collection systems with respect to usefulness, cost, sensitivity, specificity and predictive value positive, representativeness, timeliness, simplicity, flexibility and acceptability.

   b) For other agencies, including the World Health Organization (WHO), state and local health departments and non–governmental organizations, review the general types of data they currently collect or plan to collect, and identify areas where coordination of efforts would be productive and where they would be duplicative.

2) Assess the types of behavioral data that are needed to design, implement and evaluate interventions to prevent HIV transmission.

   a) Explain why these data are needed, and describe how they will be used by health agencies and by non–governmental organizations to prevent HIV transmission.

   b) Review needs for data representative of the national population as a whole as well as data focusing on specific target populations and/or geographic areas.

3) Examine data needs within the political context.

   a) Review the obstacles and barriers to design, implementation and analysis.

   b) Review data collection instruments in terms of political acceptability and sensitivity of behavioral data.

4) List and describe the gaps between currently available data and data that are needed for program planning, implementation and evaluation. Rank the data gaps by their importance for AIDS prevention, program planning and evaluation.

5) Describe the methodologies for information collection and management technologies available for behavioral surveillance, assessing the relative advantages of various modes of data collection.

   a) List a variety of options for obtaining and coordinating the needed data with estimated costs and time requirements for each option.

   b) Discuss how sensitive questions and data could be reviewed and approved by advisory boards at local, state or national levels.

   c) Describe each option with respect to reliability, validity, cost, efficiency, effectiveness and acceptability.

Our knowledge of the determinants of sexual and intravenous drug use behaviors was limited and deficient in many areas. The last attempt at a systematic and comprehensive survey of sexual behaviors in the US was done by Kinsey more than 40 years ago. That study was limited in scope and had significant methodological limitations. Knowledge of the determinants of drug use behaviors was similarly limited. The controversial nature of both sexual and drug use behaviors probably resulted in decreased funding for research in these areas and impeded the accumulation of critical knowledge.[11]

Knowledge, attitudes and beliefs are cognitive determinants of behaviors. Because AIDS was a newly identified disease, public health officials felt that the lack of knowledge about HIV infection and how it was transmitted might have played a significant role in determining HIV–related behaviors. Public health personnel thought that such knowledge was probably necessary (though certainly not sufficient) for affecting behavior change. The National Health Interview Survey (NHIS) was used to assess and subsequently track changes in knowledge, attitudes and beliefs about AIDS. NHIS is

[11] C.F. Turner, H.G. Miller, L.E. Moses, eds., *AIDS, Sexual Behavior and Intravenous Drug Use.* (Washington, D.C.: National Academy Press, 1989b).

a continuous, cross–sectional household interview survey conducted by CDC's National Center for Health Statistics (NCHS). Each week, a national probability sample of the civilian, non–institutionalized population is interviewed by Bureau of the Census personnel to obtain information on health, demographic and other characteristics of each household member.

To collect information for developing and targeting new education programs, the NHIS began in August 1987 to include specific questions to assess the public's knowledge about HIV transmission and prevention as well as awareness and utilization of the HIV–antibody test.[12] Since August 1987, AIDS knowledge and attitude questions have been administered to one randomly chosen adult at least 18 years of age in each sample household. About 3 800 interviews are conducted each month.

The first NHIS AIDS Knowledge and Attitudes Survey was conducted from August to December 1987, and provisional survey results were published monthly. From January to April 1988, the NHIS AIDS questionnaire was revised to include questions about the brochure, *Understanding AIDS*, which was mailed to every U.S. household in May and June 1988. The current questionnaire contains items on self–assessed knowledge about AIDS, HIV transmission, perceived effectiveness of various preventive measures, experience with blood donation and testing, and self–assessed likelihood of being seropositive.

In comparing August 1987 questionnaire responses to August 1988 responses, we found the most substantial increase in knowledge was related to transmission of HIV. The marked increase in the percentages of adults who considered it "very unlikely" or "definitely not possible" to transmit HIV through various forms of casual contact reflected important gains in knowledge.

The overall gain in knowledge about HIV and AIDS coincided with the national multimedia public awareness campaign as well as with increased support for CDC—funded state and local public information efforts.

Changes in attitudes, knowledge and behavior among specific groups have been documented, but whether these changes are linked causally to specific educational interventions is not clear. We lack basic knowledge about risk behaviors, and we need valid and comprehensive studies. There is a great need for new instruments and methods to measure accurately the determinants and patterns of sexual behaviors and intravenous drug use. Despite the acknowledged importance of information on sexual behaviors and intravenous drug use, there may be many significant barriers to collecting this information.[13]

[12] Centers for Disease Control, "Guidelines for effective school health education to prevent the spread of AIDS," *Morbidity and Mortality Weekly Report* 37 (Suppl. S–2) (1988).

[13] C.F. Turner, "Research on sexual behaviors that transmit HIV: progress and problems," *AIDS*, 3 (1989a): 563–71.

Interventions

Education to prevent the spread of HIV began early in the epidemic and was concentrated in the few large cities where larger numbers of cases accumulated quickly. Health departments in San Francisco and New York were among the first governmental units to conduct educational efforts. Voluntary or social organizations in the gay community, however, were responsible for most of the initial campaigns launched and for much of the educational materials produced. For the federal fiscal year 1984, the U.S. Congress earmarked ten million U.S. dollars for health education/risk reduction programs in high-HIV–incidence communities. In subsequent years, the federal appropriations for national and state educational interventions rose significantly. By fiscal year 1989, about $100 million was appropriated for information and education programs, exclusive of funding to support counseling, testing, referral and partner notification activities.

As the epidemic progressed, the PHS developed a plan, subsequently published as the March 1987 "Information and Education Plan to Prevent and Control AIDS in the United States."[14] The PHS plan focused on four basic target populations: the general public; school– and college–aged populations; persons at increased risk of infection or already infected; and health workers. A number of intervention strategies have since been undertaken to inform and educate each of these target groups.

The General Public

An informed and educated public provides the foundation on which comprehensive prevention programs can be built. In a democratic society, individual as well as community and corporate decisions are best made on the basis of current and accurate information. Decisions based on fear, prejudice, or disproven theories are not likely to provide satisfactory results.

In 1986, CDC awarded funds to state and local health departments to educate the general public (as well as persons at increased risk of infection). In that same year, the Surgeon General published his report on AIDS. Systematic efforts to inform and to educate the general public in the United States through a national information campaign began in October 1987, with the launching of a public service advertising campaign entitled America Responds to AIDS. Using television, radio and print advertisements, the initial phase of the campaign sought to humanize the disease. Persons with diagnosed AIDS, families and friends of persons with AIDS, and professional health care workers providing services to persons with AIDS were featured in the ads.

[14] Centers for Disease Control, "Guidelines for AIDS Prevention Program Operations," (Atlanta GA: CDC, October 1987).

All of the advertising materials also included the National AIDS Hotline (NAH) phone number, as the final "call to action." The NAH is a 24–hour, toll–free information and referral service that uses live operators to answer callers' questions anonymously. The hotline now has services for English and Spanish speaking callers, as well as TTY services for the hearing–impaired. For the past two years, NAH has handled an average of 1.7 million calls per year, the largest call volume ever reported by a health–related telephone service.

Beginning in January 1988, the National AIDS Information Clearinghouse (NAIC) became the principle distribution center for printed materials on human immunodeficiency virus infection and AIDS. During its first year of operation, NAIC distributed more than 43 million pieces of printed information. Equally as important were the clearinghouse's extensive services and materials data bases. By linking those data bases with NAH, NAIC enabled callers to the hotline to receive specific referrals to a wide range of services in communities throughout the nation. Health professionals can obtain information on educational programs and materials that have been developed by others and that address many of the various target populations.

In June 1988, the United States became the seventh nation to distribute a brochure on AIDS to all households. The brochure contained information on the nature and cause of AIDS, its transmission and prevention, and how to obtain additional information about AIDS. The brochure, *Understanding AIDS*, was mailed to 107 million households, with additional distribution to overseas military installations, prison systems and shelters for the homeless. Copies of the brochure were developed in English, Spanish, Laotian, Mandarin Chinese and Braille, and an audiotape version of the brochure was produced.

The brochure was intended to cover six key issues:

- ways in which HIV is transmitted;
- how condoms can be effective in preventing HIV transmission;
- when to get tested;
- how you won't contract HIV infection through casual contact;
- how to discuss AIDS with children; and
- information on the blood supply and donating blood.

The brochure was developed in cooperation with a private advertising agency. CDC received advice from persons working on AIDS prevention at national and local levels, persons with AIDS, religious organizations and community groups. The draft brochure was tested on 12 different focus groups in six cities. These focus groups included minorities, young people, women, single persons and parents, representing a wide range of income levels.

The brochure's ultimate goals were to prevent the transmission of HIV, to create a positive climate for the care of the individuals infected with HIV, and to reduce the frequency of high–risk behaviors. The brochure's contribution to these outcomes was not assessed because the brochure was only one of many programs that have attempted to reach these goals. Evaluation, therefore, focused on short–term indicators of the brochure's impact, such as changes in knowledge, attitudes and particular behaviors such as seeking counseling and testing, and teaching children about AIDS. This evaluation used the National Health Interview Survey (NHIS).

On May 4, 1988, the brochure was officially released by Health and Human Services Secretary Otis R. Bowen, M.D., at a press conference, with copies provided to national leaders, state health officers and the media. Copies were not distributed to the general public until May 26. Distribution continued through June 15, 1988. Thus, the first three weeks in May, when the population was unexposed to the educational campaign, were compared with the period from the last week in May through the end of July, when the population had been exposed. NHIS data were used to answer three questions: Who received the brochure? Who read it? What impact did it have?

The brochure was reported to have been received by 63 percent of all interviewed individuals, suggesting that the brochure was received by approximately 111 million individuals. More whites than blacks reported having received the brochure. With passing time, the percent of the individuals who recalled receiving the brochure decreased. Almost eight out of ten individuals who received the brochure (86.9 million people) read at least some of it, with five out of ten (55 million people) reading most or all of it. The overall readership was about equal among all adult age groups and among whites and blacks, but readership was greater among better educated individuals.[15]

Measurements of brochure impact suggested that three out of ten individuals who read the brochure said that it gave them new information. Those individuals most likely to get new information or to have questions answered were the most difficult to reach: young people, blacks and those with less than a high school education. Specifically, more blacks than whites reported that the brochure gave them new information or answered questions that they had about AIDS. Females were much more likely than males to have read the brochure carefully and to feel that it gave them new information.

[15] National Center for Healt Statistics, D. A. Dawson, AIDS Knowledge and Attitudes for May and June, 1988, Provisional Data from the National Health Interview Survey. Advance Data from Vital and Health Statistics, No. 160. DHHS Pub. No. (PHS) 88-1250. Public Health Service, Hyattsville, MD.

Almost four out of ten individuals who received the brochure discussed it with other family members. Of those persons with children aged 10–17, 30 percent reported higher levels of knowledge about AIDS than did persons who had not read the brochure. It could not be assumed, however, that those persons were better informed because of the brochure.

We also measured how the brochure's distribution might have affected the demand for certain services. The experience of selected state–operated AIDS hotlines and the National AIDS Hotline during June were analyzed first. Overall, hotline calls in the selected states increased more than 120 percent in the first week of June, 30 percent in the second week, and ten percent in the third week. The number of calls decreased for the remainder of the month. There was an increase of more than 200 percent in the average daily number of calls to the National AIDS Hotline during June. Through July 12, the National AIDS Information Clearinghouse distributed an additional 15 million copies of the English version and nearly four million copies of the Spanish version of the brochure. The number of clinic visits to counseling and testing sites in selected areas was also examined. Analysis showed increased attendance in some areas and no change in others.

Some questions could not be answered with the data currently available. One issue was how to measure the efficacy of the brochure in a controlled setting and population as opposed to the overall effectiveness in the population at large. It was not possible to separate the effects of the brochure since it was one component of a multifaceted information and education campaign. In any similar future effort, an assessment of the brochure in terms of cost–benefit or cost–effectiveness analysis would be helpful and would require stating specific measurable objectives for the brochure as well as extensive planning from the very first stages of brochure development.

This brochure represented the largest distribution of health information ever attempted in the United States. *Understanding AIDS* was the single most widely read publication in the United States in June 1988, with 86.9 million readers. *The Readers Digest* was second, with about 48 million readers. Twenty–six million people learned something new. The data showed significant improvement in the percentage of people who understood how HIV is transmitted. The brochure reached less educated, young and minority populations. Questions about the effectiveness of this brochure remain unanswered; in future efforts, more evaluation will be needed. A more extensive evaluation process would be complex and expensive, but if it were designed early in the education process, it would be possible.

In October 1988, a third phase of the information campaign was launched. It targeted women at risk and sexually active adults with multiple sex partners. This phase of the campaign sought to provide populations at increased risk of infection with specific information on preventive behaviors.

The fourth phase of this continuing effort was launched in May 1989 and was targeted to parents and young people. It was designed to encourage dialogue between adults and youth, especially parents and their children. This campaign brought to the attention of the U.S. news media that a large proportion of AIDS cases were probably contracted by persons in their teen years.

Whereas the triad of public service announcements, hotline, and clearinghouses have formed the U.S. information program's core, an additional aspect of the general public education strategy has been to forge ties with numerous health, education, business, labor, religious and voluntary organizations. A special emphasis has been placed on establishing links with organizations that are composed of and serve racial and ethnic minority populations. These organizations develop and/or deliver educational materials and programs which are uniquely appropriate for their constituent populations and are consistent with the national prevention agenda. Additional materials and programs have been developed by state and local health departments.

Data gathered since August 1987, through the NHIS, enable the Centers for Disease Control to monitor trends in what the general public knows and believes about HIV/AIDS, over time. In general, knowledge about the actual routes of HIV transmission have reached nearly peak levels (95 percent to 97 percent). Erroneous notions about transmission through casual contact with infected persons, while changing slowly, suggest that the need for comprehensive, accurate health communications will be ongoing.

Beginning with the fifth phase of the information campaign, launched in the summer of 1990, an in–house staff of research and evaluation specialists conducted context and formative evaluations of campaign materials and strategies. They have also performed efficacy, process and effectiveness evaluations, with an emphasis on behavioral impact. Formative evaluation of campaign materials will utilize the voluntary organizations with which CDC has developed close working ties, especially those organizations that serve racial and ethnic minority populations.

Building an information delivery infrastructure that requires modern communications technology, strategies and strategists has been a learning experience for all persons involved; however, most of the lessons learned from the U.S. experience have been drawn from the experiences of other nations and other programs (e.g. chronic disease and family planning). Unrelenting demands to implement programs rapidly, on a scale unprecedented in U.S. public health history, while recruiting adequate numbers of staff with requisite skills, often have hampered our opportunities for learning truly new lessons. As our program efforts mature, quality staff are added, and a more supportive social environment is established, we expect our opportunities for advancing new understanding will increase.

School–and College–aged Persons
Childhood and adolescent development includes the establishment of attitudes and behaviors that directly and indirectly influence the future health of youth. Early behavior choices, in areas such as sexual behavior, substance abuse and safety practices, directly influence the current health status of young people.

The 1987 National Adolescent School Health survey was the first national survey since the 1960s to measure several critical adolescent behavioral risks and their perceptions of the risks. A random sample of eighth and tenth grade students reported engaging in behaviors that increased health risks. For example, 56% of the students indicated they had not worn a seat belt on their most recent trip. About 25% of boys and 42% of girls indicated that they had seriously considered suicide at some point in their lives. Among eighth–graders, 51% said they had tried smoking tobacco, 77% said they had used alcohol, and 15% said they had tried marijuana.

The results of this survey indicated that most adolescents studied had correct perceptions of sexual risk factors for HIV infection, and smaller majorities understood sexually transmitted disease signs. Unfortunately, the results also told us that many of these young people were unsure or had incorrect perceptions about HIV.

Fewer than one percent of U.S. AIDS cases occur in the 13–19 age group. The much larger number of AIDS cases in persons in their 20s and the lengthy time between infection and emergence of symptoms, however, suggest that many of these HIV infections actually occurred during adolescence. Therefore, if infection is to be avoided, the knowledge and skills needed to avoid risk must be learned before or during adolescence. A primary means to accomplish this is through AIDS education programs in the nation's schools.

Because 48 million children and teenagers attend school daily, schools have great potential to promote health. Domestically and internationally, school health education is viewed as an essential part of education and of school health more generally.[16] While many states have general policies encouraging school health education, not all have specific health education requirements for high school graduation (in 1987, only 27 states had such requirements).

Education in schools can produce knowledge, attitude and practice

[16] L.J. Kolbe, "International policies for school health programs," *Hygiene: International Journal of Health Education* 6(3) (1987): 711; and J.O. Mason, G.R. Noble, B.K. Lindsey *et al.*, "Current CDC efforts to prevent and control human immunodeficiency virus infection and AIDS in the United States through information and education," *Public Health Report* 103(3) (1988): 255–60.

changes. Data have shown that well-conceived, well-executed school health education, carried out with fidelity to the curricula and by appropriately trained teachers, can improve health knowledge and influence attitudes and behaviors. In a major quasi–experimental evaluation of four different curricula, educationally significant improvements were observed at a three–year follow–up. As expected, producing knowledge gains with only few hours of instruction was easy, but these curricula also accomplished positive changes in health behavior and health attitudes.

Recent research documents the promising potential of school health education. In the evaluation described above, one prominent curriculum used in the United States and abroad was implemented and assessed. Smoking behavior in experimental groups that received fifth and sixth grade units of the curriculum were compared with control groups that did not receive them. This comprehensive kindergarten through seventh grade curriculum addresses tobacco within a broader health behavior framework. At follow–up in the seventh grade, the smoking rate in the study group was 37% lower than in the control group. In another study, an innovative South Carolina program called "School and Community Program for Sexual Risk Reduction among Teens" combined specific educational messages and skills with broad community involvement, which included parents, teachers, representatives of churches and community leaders. Three control counties experienced net increases in the estimated pregnancy rate, but overall, the study population reduced its pregnancy rate by 54%.

These and other data can be used to argue for a comprehensive, ongoing approach to school health education, in preference to one–time or single–subject approaches. A comprehensive approach must be planned and sequential, and it must introduce concepts and materials at developmentally appropriate points in the child's growth. Moreover, the term "comprehensive" means more than including all appropriate topics or all grades from kindergarten through 12, although both are features of a sound approach. In particular, comprehensive school health curricula should provide opportunities to develop needed skills and qualities (e.g. decision–making and communication skills, resistance to persuasion, and a sense of self–efficacy and self–esteem).

Integrating HIV content into a comprehensive program of school health is endorsed by the CDC, the Presidential Commission on the HIV Epidemic, and leading educational organizations such as the National Association of School Boards and the National Association of State Boards of Education.

Although many individual school systems had begun their AIDS education efforts earlier, AIDS education in schools expanded significantly in 1987 with the launch of a new national program that provided financial and technical assistance to state and large city school agencies. By 1988, all states and 17 cities were participating in the program. These education agencies are now responsible for assisting all school systems in their state or city to develop, implement and evaluate AIDS education approaches and to progress toward a more comprehensive health education approach to AIDS education (as well as education about other sexually transmitted diseases). In addition, the funds help to support periodic surveys of student knowledge, attitudes and behaviors that influence the spread of HIV. A significant part of the U.S. school health education program is an alliance with national organizations interested in education and/or youth health and welfare.

A critical target for AIDS education, but one which is paradoxically the hardest to reach, is the adolescent who has dropped out of school. In some systems, as many as two students out of five fail to graduate from high school. Those teens have been recognized as persons at high-risk of drug abuse, teen pregnancy and sexually transmitted disease; hence, they are also at high-risk of HIV infection. By law or regulation, AIDS education funds must be spent on special efforts to reach these young people, through such broader educational strategies as "schools without walls" and work–study programs. Funding also has been provided to organizations that can work with networks of local organizations that provide youth services to adolescents not in school, to runaways, and to other such target groups of high–risk young people. The Centers for Disease Control funds 51 community–based organizations to provide HIV education and counseling services to youth who are not in school. Many of these service agencies use peer educator or combined peer/professional counselor models as well as group educational sessions to teach out–of–school youth about HIV and to reinforce safe behavior.

Twenty percent of AIDS cases in the United States involve persons aged 20–29. Many young adults in this age group may be reached through college and university health services and health education efforts. Recent serologic surveys suggest that two of every 1 000 college students surveyed are presently infected with HIV. Over the past few years, the American College Health Association has received federal funding to assist colleges and universities in monitoring HIV prevalence and in conducting educational efforts to prevent its spread.

Health promotion innovations in school settings offer exciting potential to reduce behavioral risks. Schools have been providing AIDS education for too short a time, however, for us to evaluate the impact of such programs on HIV–related behaviors. A recent report by the National Academy of Science/National Research Council strongly urges careful and thorough evaluation of school programs. Detailed research strategies for properly evaluating the programs are being designed and initiated.[17]

17 *Ibid.*

Programs Directed Toward Persons Who Engage in High–Risk Behaviors

The patterns of HIV spread in the United States indicate some Americans are at much higher risk of acquiring the infection because of their behavioral practices and current patterns of HIV seroprevalence. These are high–priority populations for AIDS information and education efforts. Americans with highest risk of acquiring or transmitting HIV are those who use illicit injectable drugs and share needles; engage in anal intercourse (especially men who have sex with men); have many sexual partners; practice prostitution; or engage in sex with those who practice those behaviors. Another high–priority population for information and education includes women who can infect offspring (i.e. reproductive–age women who engage in high–risk behaviors or who are already infected with HIV and might become pregnant).

Many different strategies are being used to reach these high–risk groups. In the United States, private AIDS support groups and public health departments maintained by state, city and county governments, with financial and technical assistance from the federal government, have been the main source of information and education for high–risk audiences.

In the first three years of the AIDS epidemic in the United States, many local organizations and some local health departments initiated a substantial amount of educational activity, particularly in the few American cities that first reported large numbers of cases. CDC reviewed the status of AIDS education in nine of these cities in 1985 and discerned a number of lessons.

The most frequent audience for AIDS education in these cities has been gay men, although health workers and the general public also have been targets. Particularly in local organizations, volunteers often contributed greatly, both in terms of the numbers of volunteers and the array of talent that was mobilized to create programs. Early efforts often took the form of information campaigns that focused on using communications channels designed to reach persons at high risk, rather than education designed to create behavioral skills for change. In those early years, program managers frequently cited resource constraints and lack of community support as barriers, whereas community organization efforts, collaboration with other organizations, availability of communication channels such as state–wide task forces, and supportive public stances by political leaders helped to secure educational efforts. Critical local needs included the capacity to train volunteers and to obtain data needed to guide and redirect educational programs and messages.

Today, the national HIV prevention program has several components directed to persons at high risk. All states and several large cities receive funds from the CDC for community–based Health Education and Risk Reduction (HERR) programs. State health departments and organizations funded by the states conduct a variety of community interventions. These include:

- assessing community needs and intervention resources that may be mobilized;
- acquiring base–line and trend data, particularly changes in HIV prevalence and in the knowledge, attitudes and practices of high–risk groups;
- developing street outreach programs that target information to persons who inject drugs or who exchange sex for money or drugs (These have been successful in helping some drug users who are not in treatment to gain access to treatment and stop their risky behaviors.);
- delivering prison education programs as a focused way to reach the high proportion of inmates who use drugs.

Health departments are responsible for developing a comprehensive AIDS prevention plan and for coordinating HIV prevention efforts by community and minority organizations. Obviously an area's education programs should be directed by a needs assessment and by the epidemiologic and behavioral data bases. HIV prevention programs are also made available for persons at increased risk in such settings as sexually transmitted disease (STD) clinics, family planning and perinatal care clinics, tuberculosis (TB) clinics, drug treatment centers and other health care settings.

In the United States, HIV infection is relatively more prevalent among certain racial and ethnic minority populations. African Americans constitute 12% of the U.S. population, but they represent 29% of reported U.S. AIDS cases. Hispanic Americans constitute nine percent of the reported population but 16% of the cases. Among pediatric AIDS cases and cases among women, the overrepresentation of African Americans and Hispanics is even greater. Thus, special prevention efforts directed to racial and ethnic minorities remain a top priority for the national AIDS initiatives. Some HERR and minority grants or cooperative agreements mandate such emphases in all states and cities funded. In addition, the CDC directly funds programs run by community–based organizations that represent a broad cross –section of minority groups in the United States. The CDC funds nearly 340 minority community organizations through its HIV/AIDS prevention/surveillance cooperative agreements. Additionally, 94 local minority community organizations are directly funded by and receive technical assistance from the CDC, as are 32 national and regional minority organizations. The CDC also funds 20 to 25 local minority organizations annually through a cooperative agreement with The United States. Conference of Mayors. These minority organizations develop programs for both communities at large and for persons who engage in high–risk behaviors. Typically such programs offer

culturally sensitive adaptations of messages and community–based educational approaches for minority population subgroups whose sexual or drug
use practices increase their risk of HIV infection. In addition to these
targeted programs, many HERR programs, such as Street'community
outreach, risk eduction, community-level intervention, and HIV *prevention*
case management, are likely to reach minority groups among the risk
groups targeted. Much of the impetus and direction for these programs
emerged from a series of national minority HIV conferences that began in
1987. While they did not necessarily assure consensus, such national
conferences offered a forum for expressing concerns, highlighting common
issues and creating a dialogue with public health officials at the state and
national levels regarding HIV–related issues pertaining to racial and ethnic
minority populations.

Testing for HIV antibody status has been used as a mechanism to inform
and counsel persons who are likely to be practicing high–risk behaviors. By
1991, more than 8 291 public counseling and testing sites were operating in
the United States, performing 1 336 537 test in 1991. In addition, the CDC has
recommended that all patients seen in STD clinics, drug treatment centers
and tuberculosis clinics be counseled—to help patients evaluate their risk
of HIV exposure and to educate them about how to reduce risk. In addition,
clinics are urged to recommend testing for their clients and to provide
access to testing for HIV antibody, counsel patients about both the test and,
once antibody status is known, about risk reduction (i.e. skills to avoid
future exposure if currently seronegative, or steps to avoid further transmission if seropositive). In addition, these sites should have referral
systems for psychological, medical and drug treatment services. Given the
increase in pediatric AIDS cases in the United States, and the preventability
of perinatal transmission, increasing attention is being given to education
and counseling strategies in this area as well. Perinatal spread of HIV can be
prevented by educating reproductive age women to avoid exposure to HIV
or, if infected, to avoid pregnancy. Therefore, at all testing and counseling
sites, seropositive women should be routinely counseled about the potential consequences of pregnancy. In areas with high rates of HIV seroprevalence among women delivering babies and with large numbers of AIDS
cases among women and children, it is recommended that family planning
clinics also offer education, counseling and testing services.

Since 1987 the National Institute on Drug Abuse (NIDA) has conducted
research regarding the efficacy of "street outreach" projects in changing the
risk behavior of the estimated 85% of drug users who are not in drug treatment programs; 40% had never been in treatment. Street outreach involves
repeated face–to–face encounters by street outreach workers with drug
users and their sex partners in neighborhoods with high drug usage. Inter-

vention activities include establishing rapport and trust, individualized risk assessment and risk reduction counseling, referral for drug treatment and other needed prevention services. Outreach workers live in the community and are often recovered drug users. Outreach workers counsel drug users to stop using drugs, start drug treatment, stop or reduce needle sharing, use bleach to clean needles, use condoms, and to seek HIV counseling and testing and tuberculosis prevention. NIDA project researchers have found street outreach projects to be highly successful in increasing the proportion of drug users who seek treatment, who stop or reduce the sharing of needles/works and who use bleach to decontaminate needles if they continue to share them.

Many principles of health education are reaffirmed by the early results of these efforts. Like all types of health education, AIDS education should be targeted to specific, carefully defined risk group populations and should, to the maximum extent possible, be developed with the participation of these groups and, where appropriate, peer educators. HIV prevention crucially requires behavior changes that are lasting; such changes are best achieved by providing consistent messages, using multiple methods and channels and by repeating these methods to reinforce new behaviors. Strategies must be culturally sensitive and use language and concepts understood by the target audience. Educational design must take into account the epidemiologic characterization of the risk groups and the behavioral attributes of the targeted population. Program designs must pay careful attention to factors that encourage or discourage persons from adopting protective behavioral practices. Finally, as the National Academy of Sciences has recommended for AIDS education, appropriate and well-designed evaluation of the educational efforts is essential.[18]

The Importance of Evaluation

Evaluation is critical to the success of any program or intervention. It has become increasingly important for HIV prevention programs to demonstrate and prove their worth, as the U.S. budget deficit has increased cost–consciousness throughout government. In addition, prevention programs face increasing competition for resources from treatment programs as the number of persons with HIV infection and AIDS grows. Thus, it becomes more and more important to evaluate the effectiveness of educational and informational prevention programs. Evaluation of HIV educational interventions is particularly difficult because of the long latency between the

[18] S.L. Coyle, R.F. Boruch, C.F. Turner, *Evaluating AIDS Prevention Programs* (Washington, D.C.: National Academy Press, 1989).

high–risk behavior and development of infection or symptoms and because so many different determinants can affect both behavior and health outcome.

The following types of evaluations should be addressed in all HIV prevention programs. Formative evaluations occur during the planning and design stages of developing an intervention. Examples include early focus group testing to evaluate the effectiveness of the brochure *Understanding AIDS;* story–board testing in the early phases of developing public service announcements; assessing state HIV reporting practices to develop a consensus on standardization of data collection in those states where HIV infection is "notifiable."

Efficacy evaluations test the effectiveness of the interventions in controlled settings under ideal conditions. These studies often produce results that are less generalizable. Two examples follow. An efficacy study involving controlled and confirmed administration of a drug like Azidovudine (formerly azidothym) on a population of otherwise healthy patients with normal gastrointestinal and hematological functions provides the first example. An effectiveness trial would look at the results of prescribing the drug to a broader population with a range of ailments and providing instructions for use. In this effectiveness trial, some patients might not even have their prescriptions filled; others might not take the drug as prescribed. The first trial would assess the drug's efficacy; the second trial would assess its effectiveness. A second example would be an efficacy study of HIV education materials which might examine the knowledge, attitudes and beliefs of a selected group of literate adults in a classroom setting by administering brief examinations before and after they receive the educational materials to read. The efficacy of those materials in this setting must be differentiated from the effectiveness of those same educational materials when mailed to all households.

Process evaluations answer the questions: What was done? To whom? And how? Examples include assessing AIDS case surveillance by using process measures to evaluate completeness, timeliness, accuracy and other aspects of surveillance systems; monitoring health education/risk reduction programs implemented by community–based organizations; monitoring the number of school systems delivering and students receiving HIV education; monitoring the time and frequency of public service announcements being aired by a city and monitoring general audience recall of exposure to the announcements.

Outcome evaluations (or effectiveness evaluations) measure the effects of the intervention as actually delivered, by tracking the outcomes that were observed and determining whether these outcomes were actually attributable to the intervention. Examples include assessing the impact of

CDC's recommendations for universal precautions to prevent transmission of HIV in hospitals in terms of consequent infections (not in terms, for example, of the extent to which precautions are followed, which would be process evaluation); evaluating the effectiveness of laboratory training through ongoing performance evaluation programs; evaluating the effects of couples counseling on condom use and sexual behavior in HIV–discordant relationships; and, evaluating the impact of school–based HIV health education in terms of consequent HIV–related knowledge, beliefs and behaviors.

Cost–effectiveness/cost–benefit evaluations take measures of effectiveness from outcome evaluations and match the effectiveness (or benefits, if the outcomes can be measured in dollar terms) with the cost of the intervention. Examples include comparing the cost–effectiveness of AIDS treatment with the cost–effectiveness of AIDS prevention; estimating the cost–effectiveness of HIV counseling and testing, or partner notification; assessing the costs and benefits of a variety of interventions to prevent and treat HIV infections such as community health center–based case management, T–4 monitoring and prophylactic treatment with Azidovudine or pentamidine.

Strong AIDS education efforts will be necessary in the United States for many years to come. Each new case report and each additional death are sober reminders of the compelling need to maintain a steadfast effort and to improve the effectiveness of our behavioral strategies. This chapter has described ways behavioral science has been applied to HIV prevention and some of the lessons learned in developing education and communications programs at the Centers for Disease Control. The CDC, state and local health departments, a broad array of community organizations, academic health centers, and many other participants in the AIDS prevention effort will continue to work together to apply these lessons and to learn from our experience. Only such a commitment can help eliminate the spread of HIV infection.

The authors wish to thank Jacob Gayle, Wilma Johnson, Deborah Dawson, Ronald Wilson and Robert Kohmescher for their helpful comments and suggestions and Rose Newlin–Clark and Elizabeth Fortenberry for their assistance in the preparation of the manuscript.

The European Response to AIDS

Mukesh Kapila
Maryan J. Pye

THE DIVERSITY OF EUROPE

The thirty–one countries on the continent of Europe represent a great diversity of geography and climate, culture and social organization, economic status and political systems. Europe is not large (about 10.4 million square kilometers, and the smallest continent after Australia) but its 500 million inhabitants manage to speak at least 22 languages amongst themselves. The climate is as varied as its peoples from the Arctic conditions of Iceland and Norway in the north to the warm sunny temperatures of the Mediterranean south in Spain and Greece; from the wet but relatively temperate weather of Ireland and Great Britain in the west to the variable continental conditions of European Russia in the east.

The current political map of the continent reflects the forces of history, particularly turbulent in this century which has seen Europe as the cockpit of two world wars. Postwar Europe has seen the development of two major and deeply polarized political systems. Western Europe has generally democratic forms of government with varying degrees of socialism and mixed market economies contributing to increasingly affluent societies but ones in which inequalities have also grown. In contrast, the Soviet Union and countries of Eastern Europe have pursued a system of centrally planned and controlled economies, and though there is a commitment to equity, standards of living are generally much lower compared to Western

Europe. These political and economic realities have shaped the responses of nations to health and social issues in terms of priorities, resources allocated and organizational arrangements. Not unexpectedly, AIDS prevention and control patterns in Europe reflect these differences.

A few specific points deserve emphasis. For example, unlike their eastern European counterparts, people in Western Europe have traditionally enjoyed unlimited freedom of travel. This is a significant consideration in understanding the initial spread of HIV in Europe.

In this context, it is also pertinent to mention the legacy associated with Western Europe's colonial past—and particularly, the former French, Belgian and British empires. Traditional trade, education, tourism and travel links between these counties and their ex–colonies in the Third World continue and, over time, Europe has seen the emergence of multicultural societies with significant populations of African, Caribbean, Asian and, to some extent, Latin American origin. The extent to which these immigrants have integrated into the mainstream is variable. These "New Europeans" often suffer multiple disadvantages on account of their color, race, religion and economic status. While cultural diversity has enriched Europe as a whole, it has also created difficulties due to differences in values and belief systems. However unjustifiable, it is true that AIDS is popularly seen to have a racial dimension to it. This can stigmatize already disadvantaged people and reduce the effectiveness of education efforts.

Not unexpectedly, Europe displays a range of perspectives on social issues such as AIDS and sexuality, shaped by complex cultural factors. These have been relatively understudied and it is difficult to disentangle reality from popular myths and perceptions of national stereotypes. For example, the Scandinavians are said to have relatively liberal attitudes toward sexuality while so–called traditional values, partly due to Catholicism, are said to be important influences in Spain and Italy. Are these differences between Northern and Southern Europe real? Have they contributed to the different rates of epidemic progression and further, to the style and effectiveness of prevention and control measures in the two regions? Much more comparative research unbiased by the cultural assumptions of the investigators themselves is needed to answer such questions.

THE EPIDEMIC IN EUROPE

It is thought[1] that HIV did not begin to spread extensively in Europe until about 1982; the European epidemic is also considered to be about three years behind that in the U.S., in terms of the magnitude of AIDS cases.

[1] J. Chinn, J. Mann, "Global surveillance and forecasting of AIDS," Bull–WHO 67 (1989): 1-7.

By March 1990, a total of 37 967 reports of people with AIDS had been received from the 32 countries in the European Region by the World Health Organization. Table 10–1 shows the growth of the European epidemic[2] from 47 reported cases up to 1981 to a total of 10 827 reported in 1989.

Table 10–1. *Annual reports of people with AIDS in Europe.*

Year	Annual total of people with AIDS
up to 1981	47
1982	88
1983	287
1984	691
1985	1 740
1986	3 559
1987	6 605
198	9 634
1989	10 827

Source: "Information on AIDS surveillance in Europe," from *The Global Programme on AIDS of the World Health Organization*, Geneva and the WHO collaborating Centre on AIDS at the Institut de Medecine et d'epidemiologie Africaines et tropicales, Hopital Claude Bernard, Paris.

Half of the reported AIDS cases have been in homosexual/bisexual men, and nearly a third in intravenous drug users (table 10–2), while 2.3% of cases have been in children aged under 13 years, mostly due to mother–to–child transmission of the virus. Eighty–seven percent of cases have been in males and 13% in females. The 25 to 34–year–old age group has seen the worst of the epidemic in both men and women.

The AIDS epidemic in Europe (figure 10–1) is characterized in reality by multiple epidemics among at–risk people, and subregional differences can be crudely generalized as follows. Pattern A is predominantly an epidemic among homosexual men with HIV incidence/prevalence that is stable or declining, mostly Northern Europe. Pattern B shows rising HIV prevalence principally from injecting drug use, mostly in the Mediterranean belt countries such as Spain, Italy and Yugoslavia. Pattern C is a mixed pattern with

[2] "Information on AIDS surveillance in Europe," from *The Global Programme on AIDS of the World Health Organization*, Geneva and the WHO collaborating Centre on AIDS at the Institut de Medecine et d'epidemiologie Africaines et tropicales, Paris.

heterosexual and injecting drug use routes increasingly well established, such as in France and Switzerland. Finally, Pattern D shows an emerging picture where the reported epidemic of AIDS is still at an early stage. Significant nosocomial HIV spread has been reported in some countries, such as those of Eastern Europe.

Table 10–2. *Transmission categories of people with AIDS in Europe (cumulative reports for 32 European countries up to March 1990).*

Transmission Category	Adults and Adolescents	Children (<13 yrs)	Total (%)
Homosexual/bisexual	16 166	–	16 166 (46)
Intravenous drug user	10 660	–	10 660 (30)
Homosexual/intravenous drug user	702	–	702 (2)
Recipient of blood/ blood components	2 200	184	2 384 (7)
Heterosexual	2 802	–	2 802 (8)
Mother to child	–	583	583 (2)
Other/Incomplete information	1 618	52	1 670 (5)
Total	34 148	509	34 967 (100)

Source: "Information on AIDS surveillance in Europe," from *The Global Programme on AIDS of the World Health Organization*, Geneva and the WHO collaborating Centre on AIDS at the Institut de Medecine et d'epidemiologie Africaines et tropicales, Hopital Claude Bernard, Paris.

Most countries of Europe now have safe blood supplies and significant numbers of new infection acquired through receipt of infected blood and blood products is not expected. However, sporadic incidents of HIV transmission in health care settings due to use of infected medical equipment such as poorly sterilized needles and syringes continue to be reported in Europe, with particularly catastrophic consequences in some instances. For example, in Spain, transmission of HIV to blood donors through use of infected equipment is said to have caused a crisis of confidence in blood transfusion services and a shortage of volunteer donors. In the Soviet Union and Rumania, poor hospital practices have led to an epidemic of HIV infection in scores of children and adults in a number of cities.

Trend analysis indicates differences across Europe.[3] In the European

[3] *Ibid.*

Figure 10–1. *Cumulative incidence rates of AIDS in Europe (reports for 32 European countries up to March 1990).*

Country	AIDS Cases per Million Population
Albania	0
Austria	54.6
Belgium	65.8
Bulgaria	0.8
Czechoslovakia	1.5
Denmark	112.4
Finland	11.6
France	173.9
Germany, Dem. Rep.	1.1
Germany, Fed. Rep.	75.7
Greece	29.5
Hungary	3.2
Iceland	26.0
Israel	24.2
Ireland	40.6
Italy	105.3
Luxembourg	65.0
Malta	35.0
Monaco	85.5
Netherlands	79.8
Norway	36.4
Poland	0.9
Portugal	39.4
Romania	3.0
San Marino	50.0
Spain	135.1
Sweden	47.8
Switzerland	190.2
Turkey	0.6
United Kingdom	55.1
USSR	0.1
Yugoslavia	5.1

Source: "Information on AIDS surveillance in Europe," from *The Global Programme on AIDS of the World Health Organization*, Geneva and the WHO collaborating Centre on AIDS at the Institut de Medecine et d'epidemiologie Africaines et tropicales, Hopital Claude Bernard, Paris.

Community, which has a population of about 310 million and accounts for 92% of reported AIDS cases in Europe, the overall doubling time was 12.7 months in 1985–88, but was shortest (9.2–10.9 months) in the southern nations of Greece, Italy and Spain, intermediate (12.7 months) in France and longer (15.5–19.3 months) in the northern countries of the Netherlands, Federal Republic of Germany, Denmark and Norway.

This variation is a reflection of the changing face of the European epidemic. In general, the above "northern" countries with the longer doubling times are those in which homosexual transmission is predominant. Homosexual men have made significant behavior changes, reflected in the increase in doubling time of AIDS in homosexuals from 8.8 months in 1983–85 to 20.4 months in 1986–88. In contrast, in "southern" countries such as Spain and Italy, most AIDS cases have so far been reported in intravenous drug users where behavior change has not been as marked and doubling times remain relatively short. For the European Community as a whole, estimated doubling times for AIDS in homosexual/bisexual males was 15.4 months (1985–88) and 9.3 months in intravenous drug users.

Current AIDS reports are a reflection of the pattern of HIV infection acquired several years ago. What projections can be made of the future of the European epidemic? The WHO has estimated that there were 500 000 HIV infected people in Europe, out of an estimated global total of six million in May 1990. By the end of 1991, a cumulative total of 60 000–78 000 AIDS cases are expected in the European countries most affected by the epidemic.

Though the incidence of new infections in homosexual men has declined, they form a large proportion of the population at risk and unless behavior changes are sustained, thousands of additional homosexual men may well get infected over the coming years. But it is the intravenous drug users who are likely to contribute significantly to the overall epidemic in the future. Current information is inadequate to make reliable predictions of the future heterosexual spread of HIV in Europe. However, on the assumption that most intravenous drug users[4] are heterosexual, the potential for a heterosexual epidemic is already established in this region and an increase over the present relatively low numbers is expected. This is already visible in countries such as Italy where a recent rapid increase in AIDS cases attributed to heterosexual transmission is presumed to be due to HIV transmission to partners of intravenous drug users. As a consequence, infection rates in women are expected to rise, which, in turn will contribute to transmission during pregnancy, and a rise in the numbers of children with HIV and AIDS.

As has been noted already, HIV and AIDS affect previously healthy people and the personal and social impact is immense. Apart from the tragic consequences for families from the disease disability and death of their

[4] *Op. cit.* "Information on AIDS surveillance in Europe."

individual members. The cost to national economies is likely to be considerable. For example, it has been estimated that by 1991, the testing, screening and health care costs attributable to HIV disease in the 32 member states of the European region of the WHO may exceed five billion U.S. dollars per annum. Furthermore, there are growing additional costs to society through increasing numbers of years of productive life lost due to premature deaths.

The prevention of HIV infection and AIDS is therefore a major public health priority for the countries of Europe, with information and education the "single most important component of national AIDS programs".[5] The extent to which Europe has been able to respond to this challenge is explored in this chapter.

An Overview of National Prevention Approaches

The extent, scope and style of AIDS prevention programs are an outcome of particular national policies. But the evolving epidemic has highlighted complex social issues, many without precedent, and policy formulation has not necessarily been a systematic process. Some policies have been explicitly stated in legislation and administrative regulations or have emerged as a consequence of precedents established by judicial rulings.

A review[6] of existing AIDS legislation in Europe shows that many countries have taken specific measures on notification and reporting systems, for example, AIDS is classified as a "notifiable disease" in two–thirds of European countries, including 13 states which require HIV seropositivity to be reported in addition to AIDS. Measures have also been taken on follow–up procedures, including contact tracing, counseling of HIV antibody positive people and sanctions against "anti–social behavior" such as willful spread of the disease. Finally, preventive measures have been taken, such as creating information programs for the public, lifting restrictions on condom advertising (for example, in Belgium and France), and encouraging HIV antibody testing in sub–populations such as homosexual men and prostitutes.

However, it is more common for policies not to be explicitly stated but to develop incrementally in response to demands from specialist pressure groups or popular public opinion. Thus, there is now a growing demand

[5] "London Declaration on AIDS Prevention," endorsed by delegates from 148 countries at the World Summit of Ministers of Health on Programmes for AIDS Prevention, jointly organized by the World Health Organization and the United Kingdom Government in London, January 26–28, 1988.
[6] G. Pinet, "Summary of legislative situation and policy on AIDS and HIV infection in Europe" (Copenhagen: WHO Regional Office for Europe, 1988).

for specific measures to protect people with HIV/AIDS from unfair discrimination in schools and work places and to help them in obtaining services such as housing, health insurance and even health care.

A study from the WHO Regional Office for Europe examined national European approaches to AIDS policies and programs to help identify strategic lessons for meeting future needs.[7] The major conclusion was that the presence or absence of explicit policy is not necessarily a critical factor. More important are the mechanisms by which policies and activities are designed and implemented as these strongly influence program effectiveness. For example, national AIDS committees and other state–level coordinating mechanisms that are multidisciplinary, inter–sectorial in representation and include participation of non–governmental organizations appear to achieve greater impact in HIV prevention.

THE SCOPE OF AIDS EDUCATION IN EUROPE

The 1980s have seen a mushrooming of AIDS information, education and communication activities in Europe. Multifaceted strategies have been developed to reach the general population and specific target audiences in appropriate settings through a combination of approaches.

Apart from the general public, specific target audiences include men who have sex with other men, intravenous drug users, prostitutes, patients at sexually transmitted disease (STD) clinics, young people, travelers and tourists, people with HIV/AIDS and their care–givers, minority ethnic people and people with additional communication needs (such as those who are blind or partially sighted, have impaired hearing, are mentally handicapped or have other learning difficulties).

Program delivery has taken place in a variety of settings. These include institutional settings such as schools and colleges, prisons, health care centers and hospitals. Examples of organizational settings have included youth clubs, churches and other religious settings, work places and professional and trade associations. Community–based settings have included clubs and other places of entertainment, neighborhoods and other informally organized groupings.

The intensity with which specific target audiences in particular settings have been addressed in different countries is only partly related to local epidemiology. More significant has been the influence of organized groups representing special interests or lifestyles such as prostitutes in Greece or gay men in Northern Europe. Also important has been the existence of an

---

[7] S. Wayling, "AIDS policies and programmes in the European Region," EURO DOC ICP/ GPA 040. Copenhagen: WHO Regional Office for Europe, 1989.

infrastructure sufficiently adaptable and willing to undertake AIDS education such as the school education system in Scandinavian countries, the prison system in the Netherlands or occupational health arrangements in the work places of some large multinational corporations.

A combination of methods have been deployed in different European programs. Examples include:

- printed material such as leaflets and posters, to create awareness and provide information.
- oral and visual material such as radio and television advertisements, special programs, videos and recorded telephone information to influence public opinion and provide information.
- didactic presentations such as lectures and formal talks to give in–depth information and training to various types of workers.
- small group discussions and interactive workshops to influence group norms, encourage peer group learning and provide support for maintaining changed behaviors.
- person–to–person dialogue such as telephone hotlines or face–to–face contact in individual counseling.

The above approaches represent a hierarchy of communication approaches; some specific examples will be presented later. The choice of methods has depended on the particular audiences that are being addressed, their initial knowledge status, settings employed and specific communication objectives. In part, choices have been dictated by the adequacy, scope and style of existing health education infrastructures. For example, medically dominated systems, such as in Hungary, have taken a more didactic approach to public education while the Dutch were able to develop a national consensus on the main messages to be given to the population, by involving different interest groups in a national coalition right from the beginning.

REACHING THE GENERAL PUBLIC

For most people in Europe, as in other parts of the world, the mass media have been the major source of AIDS information. News coverage and special features started appearing on television and radio and in newspapers and magazines long before officially organized public education efforts got off the ground. Media coverage of AIDS issues has ranged from factual and scientific to inaccurate and sensationalist. In some countries where the press is state controlled, coverage has been restricted and the impression conveyed to citizens that AIDS was a problem for other countries and not for themselves. Major events such as the death from AIDS of public personalities such as Rock Hudson have created intense publicity. Such coverage, often characterizing people with HIV and AIDS as "innocent" (hemophiliacs and children) and "guilty" (homosexuals, promiscuous people) or as "helpless victims" have strongly influenced individual and social perceptions of AIDS and its consequences.

However, the mass media have also made constructive responses. The 1986–87 U.K. campaign was considerably strengthened by impressive and freely provided cooperation which saw extensive T.V. radio and newspaper editorial coverage including an "AIDS radio week" and an "AIDS television week." During the latter at least 35 special programs were screened, during 16 hours of coverage valued at several million dollars. Subsequently some popular soap operas such as "Eastenders," viewed by millions of people each week, have incorporated AIDS into their storylines, generating intense public interest. Other television dramas and documentaries have followed.

Formally organized public education programs have had to operate against this mixed background. Starting from about 1986 onwards, most European programs have had similar concerns, placing more or less emphasis on objectives aimed at:

- providing basic information on HIV transmission and self–protection.
- reassuring anxious people that HIV is not spread through casual contact.
- fostering a supportive social climate to prevent discrimination against people with HIV and AIDS.
- mobilizing public support for AIDS education efforts, including per- suading non–governmental agencies to launch support activities to reinforce official campaigns.
- stimulating personal risk appraisal and, hopefully, behavior change.

For example, the 1986–87 United Kingdom campaign spent about 18 million U.S. dollars on multi–media publicity through national press and youth magazine advertising, street posters in 1500 urban centers, and radio, television and cinema commercials. This was followed, in 1988–89 with a second, more focussed mass media campaign addressing young people, business/holiday travelers and women, with specific messages aimed at each target audience and emphasizing the use of condoms.

In Finland, 9000 posters sprouted along the roadside and on public trans- port throughout 50 major towns and cities in 1986. This was followed in 1987 by radio and television spots and the distribution of a youth magazine and sample condom to each of the 500000 Finns aged 15–24 years.

In The Netherlands, the first public education campaign occurred in

April, 1987 followed by four other mass media campaigns to promote condoms (autumn 1987), alert professionals to safe working practices (spring 1988), encourage safer sex during vacations (summer 1988) and promote AIDS education of young people at home and school (late 1988/ early 1989). Switzerland, France, Belgium, Denmark, Spain and other countries have also made varying use of the mass media.

Campaign styles have shown considerable variation from a neutral factual stance (Switzerland) to the use of fear (U.K.) and humor (Denmark). The Swiss have a well–organized and centrally coordinated program unified by the simple, factual slogan "STOP AIDS" with its memorable campaign logo of a rolled up condom replacing the "O" in "STOP", now familiar in every part of the country. The Spanish T.V. campaign in the winter of 1987 used humorous cartoons and played with the two syllables in SIDA ("SIDA" being the initials for AIDS in Spanish, "SI DA" meaning "does transmit," and the opposite "NO DA" meaning "does not transmit"). The first British campaign exhorted the public "Don't Die of Ignorance" and made use of powerful imagery such as icebergs, tombstones and volcanoes to attract public attention. The second British television campaign had a "softer" style with coy images of a good–looking couple flirting with each other and a message "AIDS, you know the risks, the decision is yours," clearly implying that prudent behavior was a matter for individual responsibility. In contrast, the June 1989 French campaign was aimed at mobilizing a shared social response with its message of "AIDS. It could affect each one of us." In the Netherlands, the first campaign was concerned with persuading people to "Think about it. Stop AIDS." In Denmark, the slogan "Think Twice" brought the positive message to young people that "sex is good and healthy and beautiful, and we want it to stay that way," endorsed by over 200 well–known names such as those of politicians, actors and soccer players appearing on radio and television.

Direct mass media advertising has been supplemented by promotional and publicity activities ranging from the distribution of stickers and postcards to tee shirts, key rings and beer mats. Drawing and song competitions on AIDS themes have been held and results publicized.

Generally directed messages through the mass media have been supported by two major types of activities: large–scale distribution of AIDS information material to households and telephone helplines for use by the public.

Mass Distribution of Information Materials

AIDS leaflets have been systematically distributed to populations in a number of countries. For example, a 16–page booklet was mailed to every Swiss household in March 1986—the first such initiative of this kind, anywhere in the world. The British followed shortly afterwards with a four–page pamphlet to all 23 million U.K. households. Similar initiatives have also been taken in France, Poland and Belgium. In Greece, printed material was enclosed in electricity bills while, at the same time, the main health insurance organization, IKA, distributed educational material to its 3.5 million members. In Sweden, thousands of copies of a brochure were distributed with newspapers. In Spain, 1.5 million copies of simply written leaflets were distributed through pharmacies, primary health care centers, town councils, offices and voluntary organizations.

Evaluations of mass distribution efforts indicate significant impact. For example, 81% of U.K. adults claimed to have seen the leaflet and 58% to have read all or some part of it.[8] Seventy–two percent had seen the leaflet in Belgium with 62% reading at least some of it, with readership related to relative education status.[9] The Swiss report a more comprehensive evaluation[10] with a representative sample of the population approached through two telephone surveys conducted before and two months after distribution of their booklet. Three–quarters of Swiss households received the booklet and 56% of adults read it. Seventy–three percent of parents with children aged over 12 years gave them the booklet to read. Those who read the booklet, compared with those who did not, showed an improvement in knowledge and a better understanding of risk behaviors as well as less fear of becoming infected through casual contact. The evaluators speculate that the booklet "met a more receptive audience because the Swiss are accustomed to receiving official information in this form, and addressed to them personally on various subjects—for example, ballot proposals and information concerning changes of the family code."[11] This importance of social context was also highlighted by the Belgian experience which found that the leaflet style of communication was better received in the Flemish–speaking Flanders region than in the predominantly French–speaking Walloons region.[12]

Telephone Hotlines

Many European countries have found that telephone helplines or hotlines are a cost–effective complement to public education campaigns. A variety of organizational patterns are in existence. For example, some hotlines are

[8] Department of Health and Social Security/The Welsh Office, "AIDS: Monitoring response to the public education campaign, February 1986–February 1987," (London: HMSO, 1987).

[9] "Assessment of AIDS Preventive Strategies," Workshop sponsored by the European Community Working Party on AIDS, Lucerene, Switzerland, November 1988.

[10] P. Lehmann, D. Hausser, B. Somain *et al.*, "Campaign against AIDS in Switzerland: evaluation of a nationwide educational programme," *British Medical Journal* 295 (1987): 1118–20.

[11] *Ibid*.

[12] *Op. cit.* "Assessment of AIDS Preventive Strategies."

directed toward the general public, while others specialize in addressing specific audiences such as people with HIV and AIDS, intravenous drug users, homosexual men and prostitutes. Some hotlines provide a telephone service only, while others offer additional facilities such as "buddying" support and face–to–face counseling. AIDS hotlines also vary in the way they are organized. Some, such as the Italian Telefono Verde AIDS, are highly professional, employing trained physicians and psychologists at the Centro Operativo AIDS inside the National Institute of Health. Others, such as the AIDS–Linien in Denmark, have a core of five staff dependent on 45 volunteers.[13]

Different types of hotlines may coexist in the same country. This can be useful as hotlines can refer clients to each other thus offering them a choice depending on their needs at the moment.

An example is the U.K. National AIDS Helpline, which depends on a pool of 100 trained advisers to staff its battery of telephones which can range from five to sixty lines operating simultaneously, depending on demand. This can vary according to whether or not there are national media campaigns being run, seasonal variations and other externalities such as a major AIDS news story or television documentary. For example, during the 1988 television–based U.K. public education campaign by the Health Education Authority, calls more than doubled to 2 750 per week from their level of 1 250 before the campaign. Each active call lasts about fifteen minutes at a unit cost of about six U.S. dollars. An independent critical scrutiny of the NAH found high levels of customer support for this service with 93% of respondents (selected from a sample of callers) "very satisfied" or "quite satisfied" with the Helpline and over eight out of ten callers expressing an intention, at least, to follow advice given by the Helpline. The NAH number (0800 567 123) is advertised widely through television, radio, press and promotional materials. Its other services include prerecorded messages in a variety of minority ethnic languages such as Bengali, Punjabi, Hindi and Arabic as well as counselors drawn from ethnic minority groups on duty at certain times. The National AIDS Helpline is supplemented by a network of over 100 local AIDS helplines, opening at specific times and days of the week and more specialized helplines such as those of the London Lesbian and Gay Switchboard.

The importance of access to the latest authoritative information, adequate training and support for helplines is important for the quality control of the service. A *National AIDS Manual* has been produced and distributed to helplines accompanied by training in its use and an information updating backup service to ensure that clients get consistent and accurate advice no matter which helpline they call.

[13] First European AIDS Hotline Conference, Amsterdam, April 1989.

The hotline model has also been used very successfully with other types of mass media interventions. For example, in September 1988, BBC Radio One, which has about 17 million young listeners, broadcast a special series of four features on "What's love got to do with it?" AIDS information was presented in the context of sexuality and relationships as part of "growing up" for young people. A national "talkline" received hundreds of calls from young people wanting personal advice on matters of concern generated by the series.

Experience from other helplines[14] such as in Italy, Denmark and France suggests that many callers prefer this channel of communication because it is:

- confidential.
- accessible, whenever and from wherever users may choose to make contact.
- sympathetic and non–judgmental.
- a way of discussing intimate concerns anonymously and is hence less embarrassing than face–to–face contact.
- individually relevant, i.e. advice provided is personalized to the needs of each caller and is therefore more likely to be followed.

In addition, telephone helpline data can be quickly available so as to enable rapid feedback to programmers on how the population is reacting to their efforts. On this basis, timely adjustments can be made to campaign strategies and delivery systems.

As public education efforts have had impact, the nature of the information and advice sought from hotlines has changed.

Callers in the early years (1986–87) were mostly concerned with clarifying basic facts on HIV transmission. More recently (1988–90) as the public have become better informed, they are demanding more complex information relating to the psychosocial consequences of the epidemic, questions relating to employment and insurance, the pros and cons of HIV antibody testing and issues related to discrimination. There is also greater realization that the special needs of minority ethnic people and women have not been adequately addressed so far.

Modern technical developments pose unexpected problems for hotlines. For example, with the introduction of itemized billing, availability of unscrambler devices and central recording of numbers by many telephone companies, there is concern that the anonymity of individual callers could be compromised, thus acting as a disincentive to clients who need to make most use of the service.

14 *Ibid.*

So far programs for the general public making extensive use of the mass media have consumed the lion's share of total resources allocated to information and education work in Europe. Have these programs worked? Are some campaign styles more effective than others?

The evaluations that have been conducted have generally relied upon surveys of samples of the population to track changes in knowledge, attitudes and claimed practices before and after specific campaigns, supported where possible by data on measures of public response such as calls to hotlines and literature ordering services, demand for HIV antibody tests and sales of condoms. The ultimate indicator of successful AIDS education work is a reduction in new infections with HIV. In the absence of adequate baseline and trend data on HIV incidence, and the relatively short time scales over which interventions have been operating, programs have had to rely upon claimed behavioral practices (such as reductions in numbers of partners and greater condom use) and surrogate markers such as reductions in sexually transmitted diseases.

Another complexity relates to the difficulty in linking particular outcomes to specific interventions, as official AIDS education programs do not operate in isolation from the host of other activities and events which influence social opinion.

A convenient and comparative overview of the situation in Western Europe is provided by a public opinion survey of 16 European countries conducted by Gallup between August 1987 and April 1988.[15] About 1000 adults were interviewed in each of seventeen European countries: Austria, Belgium, Denmark, Finland, France, Great Britain, Greece, Iceland, Ireland, Luxembourg, Netherlands, Norway, Portugal, Spain, Sweden, Switzerland and West Germany. The major results are highlighted here:

- The overwhelming majority were aware of AIDS, ranging from 86% in Portugal to 99% in the Netherlands, Austria and Norway.
- AIDS was perceived as a most urgent health problem by nearly two–thirds of respondents in Switzerland and Norway, about 40–50% in Sweden, Great Britain, France and Germany, and a third or less of respondents in Finland, Spain and Greece.
- However, the Swiss, with the highest reported per capita prevalence of AIDS in Europe, exhibited little personal concern of acquiring HIV (10%), compared to 20–25% of Germans, Britons and Danes, while the Greeks expressed the highest levels of concern (45%).
- Generally, populations were well informed on how HIV is transmitted, with eight to nine out of ten people aware that sharing needles and

homosexual intercourse were potential risk factors and seven to eight out of ten people aware that HIV could also be acquired heterosexually.

- At the same time, significant minorities continued to believe that HIV could be acquired through working in close proximity to someone with AIDS (Portugal 20%, Finland 14%), through kissing on the cheek (Spain 12%, Norway 8%), or being coughed or sneezed upon (Portugal 27%, Iceland 24%, France 16%) or from insect bites (Iceland 44%, Sweden 21%, Netherlands 16%).
- Attitudes toward people with AIDS showed mixed sentiments. While most respondents in most countries (93% in France, 70% in Denmark and 57% in Spain) agreed that persons with AIDS should be treated with compassion, a majority (61% in Great Britain, 57% in Finland) also agreed that it was their own fault if they got AIDS, and substantial minorities (Ireland 23%, Austria 22%) would go so far as to refuse to work alongside them.

A number of issues are highlighted by the European experience with general public education programs.

Firstly, though the mass media are very expensive, they can reach very large numbers of people quickly and cost effectively. For example, the 1988 U.K. television campaign cost about six million U.S. dollars, but reached 91% of all adults in the country (population 56 million). Not surprisingly, television is generally the most popular medium compared to radio, cinema, posters, newspapers and magazines.

Publicity through the mass media can motivate people to seek more detailed information. Thus, in Luxembourg, the ten–week period following a campaign saw 35 000 calls to their helpline—a remarkable figure for a population of 350 000.

Mass media campaigns have succeeded in informing the public on the basic facts of HIV transmission and personal protection. For example,[16] U.K. adults' awareness that HIV can be passed on from a mother to her unborn child increased from 62% to 81% following the first public education campaign in 1986–87. Education programs have also helped to reduce unreasonable fears of acquiring HIV from casual contact, and there have been gradual declines in the prevalence of misconceptions. However, certain myths persist despite sustained attempts to root them out. In particular, these relate to uncertainty around whether or not HIV can be transmitted through saliva (as in kissing), from insect bites and in donating blood. The latter concern is heightened from time to time as a consequence of media coverage of incidents such as HIV transmission through use of infected medical equipment to blood donors in Spain and children attend-

[16] *Op. cit.* Department of Health and Social Security/The Welsh Office.

ing hospitals in the Soviet Union. This has led to shortages, usually transient, of blood donations in certain regions.

The persistence of myths is not helped by the confusion caused through the considerable variation in the messages put out by national public education programs.[17] For example, the Dutch advise against anal intercourse, while many other countries do not mention it at all, and rarely still in the heterosexual context. While the British say that "it is safest to stick to one partner," the Dutch advise that "when you have been monogamous with one partner for five years, your sex is always safe." Yugoslavia promotes the view that "good citizens do not have improper sexual relations," while the Norwegians say that "when you have changing sexual contacts, always protect yourself and your partner by using a condom." Iceland and some Eastern European countries give explicit warnings against sex with "foreigners."

The Germans are cautious in stating that HIV transmission through kissing is "exceptional" while the Belgians state confidently that "the virus in not transmitted by kissing and tears." The Swiss regard oro–genital contact as safe but warn "be careful that sperm is not entering the throat" while the British state that "oral sex carries some risk...particularly if you have cuts or sore places in your mouth or sexual parts."

As Europeans make more and more use of the opportunities for travel that are opening up as a consequence of moves towards greater unity, the confusion caused by different campaign messages obtains greater significance. In addition, the communications revolution means that a European country like Belgium or Luxembourg can receive not only its own radio and television, but also mass media transmission from France, West Germany, the Netherlands and the U.K., apart from multiple cable and satellite television stations operated by companies in different countries.

The extent to which information provision through the mass media can lead to behavior change is not clear, but there is some evidence for positive impact. For example, a Finnish campaign between December 1986 and March 1987 to lower the threshold for HIV testing was accompanied by a five–fold increase in the number of people taking the test.[18] In Switzerland, eight months after launching their 1987 general population campaign, the proportion of 17 to 30–year–olds who used condoms all or some of the time had increased from 33% to 62%.[19] In the U.K. a similar, but less marked

[17] H. Moerkerk, "AIDS prevention strategies in European countries," Address to the International Workshop on Prevention of sexual transmission of AIDS and other STDS, The Netherlands, May 1989.

[18] J. Tikkanen, K. Koskela and O. Haikala, "Finnish response to HIV infection," *Hygiene* 7 (1988): 23–31.

[19] D. Hausser, P. Lehmann, F. Dubois–Arber *et al.*, "Evaluation des campagnes de prevention contre le SIDA en Suisse," Cah Rech Doc IUMSP No. 23 (Lausanne: Institut universitaire de medecine sociale et preventive, December 1987).

trend was associated with the 1988 campaign directed at young people where claimed condom use increased from 23% before the campaign to 26–29% during the campaign and 32–33% afterwards. In France, a survey in 1987 showed that 33% of people aged 18 to 49 years who practiced high–risk behavior claimed to have made changes such as a reduction in partner numbers, more careful selection of partners and increased use of condoms. Condom sales from pharmacies increased from 35 million in 1984–85 to 45 million in 1986–87.[20]

Much of the public education work that has been conducted is based on the traditional belief that acquisition of accurate information influences the creation of favorable attitudes and ultimately leads to changes in behavior. This model is considered to have many limitations. It ignores the role of peer group values and social contexts which are particularly important in influencing at–risk behaviors for HIV infection.[21] Indeed, in the long run, the indirect influence of mass media communications is likely to be as significant as any possible direct impact on behavior change. This secondary role of the media is seen as "agenda setting" or influencing the climate of social opinion so as to:

- sustain open discussion and keep AIDS issues high on the list of national priorities for action.
- counter the stigmatization and discrimination experienced by certain groups which can endanger the effectiveness of prevention and control efforts.
- gain the support of the public and key opinion–shapers for essential public health activities.

Thus, the evaluators of the Swiss campaign note that the national program was accompanied by the emergence of "multiplying phenomena," i.e. supportive actions by a range of local organizations which contributed to reinforcing the main message.[22] In France, the November 1988 campaign had the theme "condoms protect you from everything, even from making a fool of yourself" and was aimed at encouraging people to talk about condoms. There followed widespread discussion, with 32–40% of a sample of 18–55 year olds claiming that they had discussed the campaign with friends, family or at work.[23] Initial public education campaigns were launched in haste, often under ad hoc organization arrangements and special funding from national exchequers. While this resulted in an unprecedented mobilization

[20] Personal communication from L'Agence e Lutte contre le SIDA, June 1989.

[21] A.P.M. Coxon, M. Carballo, "Research on AIDS: behavioural perspectives (editorial review)," AIDS 3 (1989): 191–7.

[22] Op. cit. D. Hausser, P. Lehmann, F. Dubois–Arber et al.

[23] Op. cit. Personal communication from L'Agence e Lutte contre le SIDA, June 1989.

of government bureaucracies not usually noted for swift activation, it also created an "emergency mentality" amongst decision–makers and programmers. Essential research such as pretesting messages, materials and modes of communication was often omitted. The lessons have been well learned. For example, the original advertisements put out by the U.K. campaign were only understood by a minority of readers. Modifications followed as the campaign was developed further.

Subsequent programs have benefitted from the evolution of more thoughtful strategies and better organization. One lesson that has been learned is the importance of ensuring that services are in a position to meet demands generated by campaign publicity, especially adequate and accessible facilities for counseling and HIV antibody testing.

The participation of representatives of the target audiences and people with HIV and AIDS in the design and pretesting steps is critical to the appropriateness and acceptability of messages and materials. The success of the Swiss "STOP AIDS" campaign is partly attributable to such involvement.

After the initial information–giving phase, there is growing realization that the "general population" is not a homogeneous mass with uniform needs. With experience, programs are getting more sophisticated in mixing and matching different types of media to reach specific population segments such as young people, women, certain socio–economic groups and so on.

However, considerable work still needs to be done to mitigate the unintended consequences of mass communications. Experience suggests that a not insignificant proportion of patients at counseling centers and callers to hotlines are the "worried well"—people not at any particular risk of HIV infection but pathologically concerned that they may be. These people are extremely difficult to reassure. In many vulnerable individuals, feelings of guilt, fear, despair and confusion have been generated by poorly designed and imperfectly understood messages not helped by ill–informed media coverage. In the U.K., this has lead to the creation of a voluntary code of conduct for journalists and a guiding set of principles governing the work of the Health Education Authority, the national body responsible for official public education efforts. Prevention messages should:

- be as accurate and clear as possible.
- be honest and truthful about uncertainties around HIV and AIDS.
- not be offensive.
- not be alarmist or otherwise generate guilt, fear or despair.
- be relevant and realistic to peoples' needs and personal situations.
- not be victim blaming, anti–sex, stigmatizing or stereotyping.
- help individuals to build confidence and self–esteem, encourage them to care for and respect others, understand factors which influence

their health chances and develop skills which enable them to cope with conflicting and confusing information, so as to make informed choices for themselves.[24]

The need to adhere to such principles poses a challenge to the creativity of those concerned with designing public education approaches. Furthermore, national level, mass media based education efforts need to be linked more effectively with audience–specific and regional/local activities. This requires a genuine commitment to inter–agency work and overcoming the institutional rivalries which are commonly prevalent, particularly between the state and voluntary or private sectors.

Finally we may reflect on the role of governments in public education to prevent AIDS. Government leadership has been critical to achieving public acceptability of national education efforts. For example, after the first U.K. campaign, 90% of British adults sampled considered it right that the government should pay for AIDS advertising.[25] Many European politicians have shown courageous leadership in addressing the sensitive issues around AIDS, sexuality and drug use, bringing them into the public domain and creating conditions which have permitted widespread and open public discussion. However, governments do not always realize when their task is done and when it is more acceptable and effective for other agencies to take over further public education efforts.

REACHING SPECIFIC TARGET AUDIENCES

European AIDS education programs have begun to address the needs of a variety of specific target audiences and this section discusses experiences from working with three types of populations in which there is high prevalence of HIV risk behavior: men who have sex with other men, intravenous drug users and female sex workers.

Reaching Men Who Have Sex with Other Men
As in the U.S., HIV infection was first introduced in Europe into groups of "men who have sex with other men." This title recognizes that some men are sexually involved with other men and practice high–risk behavior but reject specific labels such as "gay" or "homosexual." As has been noted already, these men have also pioneered health education and health promotion responses to the epidemic long before official programs got under way.

[24] Health Education Authority, "AIDS and Sexual Health Programme Draft Strategic Plan 1990–1995." August 1989.
[25] *Op. cit.* Department of Health and Social Security/The Welsh Office.

One of the earliest initiatives was among gay men in Switzerland. Like elsewhere in Northern Europe, most AIDS/HIV reports in Switzerland have come from among homosexual men, estimated to number about 100000 in a country of 6.8 million inhabitants. Early action to prevent HIV transmission in gay men consisted of the distribution of 5000 safer sex booklets containing sample condoms. This was not well received but the experience catalyzed more vigorous efforts at making the condom "familiar and even smart and fashionable" to gay men.[26] Gay men from the advertising profession joined hands with gay educators in a marketing campaign carefully developed through pretesting the product, its name and attendant publicity materials with members of the target audience. Thus the "Hot Rubber Company" was born in November 1985 selling its high quality condoms at the price of one Swiss franc for two. The "Hot Rubbers" were heavily promoted through bars, saunas and other meeting points for gay men. And so, instead of being induced by panic into deserting such places, existing networks and structures which were familiar and trusted by the community were mobilized to bring about changes in peer group norms. It became the done thing to use Hot Rubbers and in certain bars it is now possible to order "a beer with" and be served a beer with two condoms.[27] Some saunas make them available free of charge. To sustain the changes that have been made, there is constant publicity with new posters appearing in bars and saunas each month. These serve to validate the changes that have already been made and provide a topic of conversation among gay men, thus keeping AIDS prevention high on the social agenda. Sales of the "condom for the gay man" increased from nil in November 1985 to 125000 in 1986 and 300000 in 1987. Since then a variety of other manufacturers have begun to offer comparable products—and condoms can now be obtained in supermarkets and many other outlets. A national survey of homosexual behavior in 1987 showed that 85% of respondents claimed to have changed to safer sexual practices by having fewer partners and using condoms in anal intercourse.

The "Hot Rubber Campaign" is part of the Swiss STOP AIDS family of prevention programs and the synergistic links between the general population and targeted efforts are particularly important to the success of both types of activities.

The Swiss experience illustrates the payoff from careful planning and the importance of involving target audiences in the design of prevention messages and approaches. These lessons can be generalized to other target audiences.

[26] R. Staub, "The Hot Rubber Story," in *AIDS prevention and control—Invited presentations and papers from the World Summit of Ministers of Health on Programmes for AIDS prevention* (Geneva: WHO and Oxford: Pergamon Press, 1988).
[27] *Ibid.*

Most prevention activities have been concentrated on visible social networks and communication channels such as gay pubs and clubs and the gay press. These efforts have been successful in reaching the subculture of well–educated white men who openly acknowledge their homosexuality. These men have made substantial changes in their sexual behavior.

However, significant minorities of men continue to practice unsafe sex. The reasons for this are varied. Some are occasional homosexuals (for example, normally heterosexual men in prisons) while others are bisexuals who refuse to acknowledge that they are at risk. Homosexual men from minority ethnic communities and adolescents who are confused about their sexuality may not have access to or associate themselves with the prevention messages that have been put out to gay men. A valuable insight into why gay men continue to practice unsafe sex despite being well informed comes from a study in Norway which found that the "most influential factor in dealing with the AIDS risk effectively is having social resources: being socially integrated, accepting one's sexual identity and leading a stable life with friends and a lover. Those who practiced unsafe sex were often found to be lonely. They had fewer, shorter and looser love relationships and a large number of partners. They also tended to be more 'closeted' and rarely belonged to a gay organization."[28] In this study other reasons for unsafe sex centered around the emotional meaning of certain sexual acts, such as "accepting semen." Therefore safer sex was seen as cold or lacking in devotion and condom use a negative message, implying rejection of one's partner. This understanding provides a basis for new approaches to be developed through strengthening social networks, influencing peer norms and promoting safer sex so that these come to be seen as "new expressions of appreciation and love."[29]

HIV prevention in this target audience is inextricably linked to difficult issues around discrimination against homosexual men. One dilemma is concerned with the extent to which AIDS as an issue should be detached from homosexuality. On one hand this can help to reduce stigma and indicate to the public that AIDS concerns everyone. However, interest in the specific homosexual aspects of AIDS needs to be maintained if this group is to be reached through general campaigns and sufficient resources are to be mobilized to meet the particular additional needs of men who have sex with other men.

Reaching Intravenous Drug Users

HIV has spread rapidly among drug users in Europe, with studies from

---

[28] A. Preuir, A. Andersen, E. Frantzen et al., "Gay men: reasons for continued practice of unsafe sex," *AIDS Health Promotion Exchange* 4 (1988): 10–1.
[29] *Ibid.*

Italy, Scotland and the Netherlands documenting dramatic increases in seroprevalence from 10–20% to 50–60% or even higher within a time scale of two to three years in selected populations. As has been discussed already, HIV infection in intravenous drug users is likely to form the most significant component of the epidemic in Europe in the coming years.

One of the countries most affected is Italy, which has an estimated 200000 people with HIV, at least half of whom are intravenous drug users. Treatment and prevention services, (substitution with methadone, detoxification units, availability of clean needles and syringes) vary considerably across the country. These differences appear to be associated with the range of seropositivity observed in intravenous drug users varying from 7% to 61% in different parts of Italy.[30]

The importance of providing good quality, user friendly services to reach drug users is exemplified by Amsterdam's "methadone–by–bus" project, which started in 1979. Two converted city buses visit different locations around the city dispensing methadone to clients. Needles and syringes can be exchanged and condoms are also available. Counseling and medical help are accessible, but not forced onto clients. Administrative procedures and checks are kept to a minimum. The methadone–by–bus project is supported by a variety of other initiatives designed to help Amsterdam's drug users.[31] In particular this includes syringe exchange schemes which were established in 1984 when 25000 needles were distributed. This expanded rapidly to more than 700000 exchanges in 1987. Some evidence for favorable program impact has come from studies indicating that seroprevalence in Amsterdam's intravenous drug users has remained stable at about 30% between 1986 and 1988.[32]

Despite initial political and moral objections, syringe exchange schemes have been allowed to go ahead in many Western European countries and are an important though controversial component of the services for drug users. An evaluation of their impact has been conducted in England and Scotland[33] where 15 such schemes were examined in 1987–88. Patients at these centers tended to be very well informed on the risks of HIV transmission and to have already made some behavior changes. This self–selected population used syringe exchanges to sustain already low–risk behavior or

[30] G. Rezza, C. Oliva, S. Sasse, "Preventing AIDS among Italian drug addicts—evaluation of treatment programmes and information strategies," Fourth International Conference on AIDS, Stockholm, June 1988.

[31] E.C. Buning, C. Verster, C. Hartgers, *Amsterdam's policy on AIDS and drugs*, (Unpublished), December 1987.

[32] H.J.A. Van Haastrect, J.A.R. Van den Hoek, R.A. Coutinho, "No trend in yearly HIV seroprevalence rates among IVDUs in Amsterdam 1986–88," Fifth International Conference on AIDS, Montreal, June 1989.

[33] Monitoring Research Group, *Injecting Equipment Exchange Schemes Final Report* (London: University of London Goldsmiths College, November 1988).

adopt low–risk behavior through stopping or reducing sharing of equipment. There were also other desirable changes such as a reduction in the range of drugs used and injected and a reduction in the frequency of injection. In contrast, non–patients were shown to continue risk behavior at high levels. Overall, client retention by syringe exchanges was poor, with only 61% arriving at the second visit, 17% at the tenth and only 6% arriving at the twentieth visit. However, some of these had entered treatment regimes for detoxification. The successful syringe exchanges were those that provided more than just an exchange for used equipment. Clients who became regular patients valued the information, counseling and support with re–socialization that was offered.[34]

European experience of education and prevention work with drug users raises a number of issues. There are a variety of drugs that are used and different patterns of drug use. For example, opiates and tranquilizers reduce libido and hence, sexual activity, while crack users are said to have greatly heightened sexual desire. Many drug users work in the sex industry to support their expensive habit, and the sexual transmission of HIV from infected drug users to their partners is potentially a very serious problem, particularly as drug users are less likely to practice safer sex and use condoms. Generally speaking, the sexual behavior of intravenous drug users has received little attention and staff at drug treatment facilities are poorly trained in counseling on this sensitive aspect.

In many places, services like syringe exchanges may only reach the lower–risk drug injectors or those who are better educated or of higher social class. In contrast, most drug users suffer from low self–esteem and find current services inaccessible for a variety of reasons. Therefore, further innovative approaches need to be developed which are geared to the actual lifestyles of drug users. Such approaches must give information and advice, create a climate of trust between marginalized groups and the "official system," use skills training with drug users to re–socialize them into society, encourage peer group involvement in message design and in the reinforcement of positive changes.

The development of effective strategies in many European countries continues to be hindered by professional and philosophical differences. Should control efforts be directed principally at dealing with the "supply side" or the "demand side"? In the former case, the lion's share of national resources is given over to border controls and punitive law enforcement measures, and drugs issues are seen mainly as a responsibility for police and criminal justice services. Such measures have been marginally effective, but are becoming increasingly difficult to maintain with the greater liberal-

34 *Ibid*.

ization of travel within Europe. On the "demand side," experts continue to be sharply divided on the relative merits of abstinence versus substitution maintenance approaches to treatment. Many service providers have strongly held opinions on this subject, often based on personal beliefs rather than scientific logic. In turn, this dictates the pattern of local facilities available to drug users and the latter's health and survival chances.

The complexity and myriad ramifications of drugs and AIDS issues require strategic planning and central leadership at the highest levels in national governments. Multifaceted, comprehensive strategies need to address the problem at different levels directed at:

- those who have not started drug use, encouragingthem to not do so in the future.
- those who use drugs, to encourage them to give up or at least not inject drugs.
- those who can not give up drug injecting, to inject safely.
- those who have given up drugs, to support them in staying off drugs.

However, providing low threshold, user friendly services like the ones in Amsterdam is not easy in other countries where moral, religious and legal objections create a hostile climate unnerving governments who have to take the necessary radical decisions. An example of this is the situation with regard to intravenous drug users in prison. In 1987, the seventeen member countries of the Council of Europe had a total prison population of about 270000, of which an estimated 25–30% were thought to have been regular users of opiate drugs before they came into prison.[35] The seroprevalence of HIV in European prisons was estimated to be in excess of 10% in 1987, ranging from 26% in Spanish institutions to 11–13% in French, Dutch and Swiss and 1–2% in Belgian and Luxembourg prisons. Policies vary considerably from the HIV antibody testing of all prisoners in Portugal (mandatory) and Italy (voluntary) to at–risk groups in Spain (mandatory) and France (voluntary). Dutch and British prisons only permit testing on request. While information and education is provided in prisons in some countries through leaflets and videos, condoms and clean injecting equipment are rarely available. For example, condoms, but not injecting zequipment are available in Swiss prisons. The U.K. has even refused to conduct essential research into the epidemiological and behavioral aspects of drug use and HIV risk behavior in prisons.

35 T.W. Harding, "AIDS in prison," Lancet, ii (1987): 1260–4.

Reaching Female Sex Workers

Female sex workers, or prostitutes as they are usually called, have been blamed for transmitting sexually transmitted diseases for a long time, and in most cultures, they are stigmatized and submitted to official or unofficial sanctions. Nevertheless, prostitution remains a social reality and legislative or punitive attempts at eradication have never succeeded. In Europe, epidemiological studies of female prostitute populations indicate generally very low HIV prevalence except for those women who also have a history of intravenous drug use. At the present time, non–drug using prostitutes in Europe would not appear to have very high risk of HIV transmission as the vast majority of them do work safely and use condoms. However they can be at risk from their non–paying partners with whom they often do not practice safer sex. This is especially significant as there are some data to indicate that there is a higher proportion of drug users in partners of prostitutes, than in the general male population.[36]

There are many reasons, economic and social, as to why women turn to prostitution. Many do so in order to support drug dependence habits in themselves or their partners. For example, 83% of 166 female intravenous drug users studied in Amsterdam worked as prostitutes.[37] They are at high risk of HIV infection from sharing infected needles or acquiring/transmitting HIV sexually as they are less likely to be practicing safer sex.

There is also a range of prostitute lifestyles which may influence chances of HIV transmission. Prostitutes may meet their clients in bars, clubs, saunas and massage parlors, in hotels or private residences, through contact magazines or escort agencies or solicit on the street. Apart from the link with intravenous drug use, work conditions can vary in the quality and privacy of premises, attitudes of local law enforcement agencies, access to health care facilities such as STD clinics and the degree of exploitation from others such as brothel managers. Other characteristics of lifestyles can include voluntary or non–voluntary prostitution (with some of the latter being migrants present illegally), juvenile or adult and independent or organized prostitution. Attitudes toward prostitution can be professional or non–professional, with the former able to differentiate her working life from her home life. All these factors in lifestyles can influence an individual prostitute's health chances.

Two case studies are presented here of different approaches to HIV prevention work with prostitutes—in The Netherlands and Greece, respectively.

[36] S. Biersteker, J. Visser, H. Verbeek, "Prostitutes and their clients," Paper prepared for the International Workshop on Prevention of sexual transmission of AIDS and other STDs, The Netherlands, May 1989.

[37] J.A.R. Van den Hoek *et al.*, "Prevalence and risk factors of HIV infection among drug using prostitutes in Amsterdam," *AIDS* 2 (1988): 55-60.

In The Netherlands, national public education efforts have been supplemented with specific initiatives for the sex industry,[38] including the following activities:

- radio commercials, directed toward clients, broadcast on national and local radio.
- posters for clubs, cafes and sex shops that attempt to eroticize condom use.
- advertisements in pornographic magazines.
- information brochures for prostitutes, available in five languages.
- multilingual condom promotion slogans on cards that prostitutes can present to clients or on towels used during sexual contact.
- some clients have been used to distribute condoms to other potential clients in red light districts ("peer group education").

Public soliciting is illegal in the Netherlands but many local authorities have established *gedoogzones*, which are particular streets where under specified conditions streetwalking is allowed during set hours. In addition, Utrecht has an *afwerkplek*. This is a special car park with parking bays divided by high fencing panels where prostitutes can come to clients' cars and do business without offending local inhabitants. In these facilities, a prostitute can decide freely without being harassed by police whether or not and under what conditions she will go with a client—thus reducing the risk of unsafe working.

Many Dutch towns have also established *huiskamers* (literally "living rooms"), facilities where counseling, care and assistance are easily accessible to prostitutes. One such enterprise is Utrecht's "Huiskamer Aanloop Prostitutes Foundation"[39] operating a mobile caravan parked in the local *gedoogzone* during permitted hours. Prostitutes can come for a rest or take a shower, buy condoms, receive advice and medical care. Every three months a "playful STD/AIDS prevention campaign"[40] is organized in the "living room" during which the streetwalkers receive attractively packaged "fun parcels" containing unusual condoms, safer sex stickers and other materials. In addition, over 40000 condoms, including those for anal use, have been sold in the first 30 months of the project's operation.

The guiding philosophy of the project includes respect for the women, a non–judgmental acceptance of their lifestyles and the creation of an atmo-

[38] M.E.M. Paalman, D.J.M. de Vries, "Condom promotion in the Netherlands: prostitution," Fourth International Conference on AIDS, Stockholm, June 1988.
[39] Information from Huiskamer Aanloop Prostitutes Foundation, Utrecht, The Netherlands, 1988.
[40] *Ibid*.

sphere which enables the prostitutes to take responsibility for their own decisions. Other support services are made as acceptable as possible. Therefore, when a woman is ready to stop drug use or quit prostitution, an individually designed rehabilitation plan is put into effect in association with local social services, police and vice squad, and alcohol and drug abuse treatment clinics.

Greece has a system for registering prostitutes which obliges them to report for twice weekly health checks at special clinics of the Ministry of Health and Welfare. Registered prostitutes are also required to undergo HIV antibody testing every three months. Between March and November 1985, 12 out of 350 prostitutes (3.4%) had tested HIV positive. Subsequently a group of seronegative prostitutes without history of intravenous drug use were followed up with intense personal education consisting of individual counseling supported by distribution of information leaflets. This intervention was highly successful: condom usage increased from 66% in 1985 to 98% in 1987 accompanied by a reduction in syphilis incidence from 17.1% to 3.2% and gonorrhea incidence from 14% to nil in the same period of time. New HIV seroconversions were 0.7% in 1986 (two out of 270 prostitutes) falling to nil in 1987.[41]

Both the Dutch and Greek approaches to HIV prevention in prostitutes is based firmly within their own prevalent cultural situations and political systems dictating how health and social issues are approached. Both are potentially effective and offer elements in their program design which can be commended to other countries seeking to organize effective prevention work. But neither the Dutch or Greek approaches are likely to be totally acceptable or successful outside their own national milieu. This illustrates both the usefulness and the limitations of cross–cultural comparisons when trying to draw out lessons that can be generalized.

However, there is general consensus on a number of issues highlighted from the European experience of health promotion with prostitutes.[42] Firstly, prostitutes can be most effective educators. They have confronted the issues around sexuality as most people have not and are expert in practising and eroticizing safer sex. These skills should be recognized and supported. Prostitutes can be usefully involved at all stages in the design, implementation and evaluation of educational initiatives as well as in essential research into understanding the many factors which relate to prostitute lifestyles. Examples of pioneering action research projects can be found in London and Birmingham, in England.

Prostitution should be decriminalized and legislation–based control

[41] G. Papaevangelou, A. Roumeliotou, Kallinikos et al., "Education in preventing HIV infection in Greek registered prostitutes," Journal of AIDS 1 (1988): 386-9.

[42] Op. cit. S. Biersteker, J. Visser, H. Verbeek.

attempts abandoned. The legal regulation of prostitutes can result in abuses which make it difficult to establish and maintain safer sex practices. For example, in parts of England, the possession of condoms and safer sex literature has been used by police as evidence for prostitution. Immigration laws also increase the vulnerability of prostitutes to exploitation and there are further instances from throughout Europe of the sexual exploitation of prostitutes by corrupt police and judiciary.

Compulsory HIV antibody testing of prostitutes has been used as a component of successful prevention programs, such as in the Greek experience described above. However, this approach also has serious negative impact. Prostitutes who are most vulnerable, such as drug abusing street walkers, are least likely to cooperate with such schemes and hence can be driven "underground," becoming more and more unreachable by prevention and care services. Compulsory testing and certification can also reduce a prostitute's ability to negotiate safer sex with clients. The latter can refuse to use condoms on the grounds that the woman has been certified as un–infected, even though his own status may be unknown.

Health and social services, including those for treating sexually transmitted diseases, contraception, counseling and help with drug and alcohol abuse problems need to be particularly accessible, with staff trained to give friendly, non–moralizing and expert care.

Finally, an exclusive focus on prostitutes is insufficient and only serves to stigmatize them further. The clients and partners (i.e. non–paying sexual contacts) of prostitutes as well as managers in the sex industry (such as hotel, bar and brothel keepers) have an important role in education programs. For example, the latter can decide on house rules and working conditions which can promote or hinder safer sex practice. The non–paying sexual partners of prostitutes do not tend to use condoms and as they are also more likely to have a history of intravenous drug use, reaching them is particularly important. Prostitutes' clients come from a variety of backgrounds and understanding why some of them insist on unsafe sexual contact, despite awareness of the risks, should assist in more effective programming.

COMMUNITY MOBILIZATION FOR AIDS PREVENTION

The earlier sections of this chapter have discussed the issues raised by European experience with general public education and education of specific target audiences such as homosexual men, intravenous drug users and prostitutes. It is now generally accepted that information provision alone is inadequate to initiate changes in individual behaviors which are greatly influenced by family, friends and other peer group pressures.

The case studies from working with gay men in Switzerland and prostitutes in the Netherlands have illustrated the importance of the close involvement of members of target audiences for the acceptance and effectiveness of prevention efforts.

The significance of community mobilization for AIDS prevention is further illustrated by work with young people in Sweden. The county of Stockholm has about a fifth of Sweden's 8.4 million population, but accounts for more than two–thirds of total AIDS and HIV reports. The Youth Project of the Stockholm County Council AIDS Prevention Programme was set up in 1987 with the aim of preventing HIV and other STDS.[43] The magnitude of the task is illustrated by the fact that STDS are very common in Swedish youth with, for example, 25% of those aged 15–25 years having had chlamydia at some time.

The project started from an appreciation of young people's sexuality and their communication and support networks. As in many other countries, Swedish youth get most of their information on sexual matters from their mothers and at school. However, when it comes to actually discussing sexual issues, others such as youth leaders and sports club leaders and friends are most important. From this followed the project's central strategy, which was to train adults who meet teenagers in everyday life in a variety of social and professional contexts to act as informed advisors on issues of sex and relationships, STDS and AIDS. The project has worked with and through existing structures including formally organized institutions such as schools, youth clubs, social services departments and clinics, and informal networks in local municipalities such as voluntary groups, parish priests, and owners of kiosks which sell sweets, cigarettes and pornographic magazines.

Each school in the county, as well as other agencies, was invited to send representatives to carefully designed two–day courses on AIDS, sexuality and youth issues. Each agency or institution also appointed a contact person who was followed up at six months with a more intensive one–day workshop including training on sex education and counseling, sensitization to the links between alcohol, drugs and unsafe sexual activity, and suggestions for local activities. This was complemented by active condom promotion in venues such as discos and soccer clubs where it was shown that teenagers felt more comfortable in getting condoms from people they knew than from pharmacies and shops. The Youth Project operates within a broader AIDS prevention program which includes information provision through leaflets, videos, exhibitions and advertising in local newspapers.

[43] Urwitz V. "A community-oriented approach to AIDS prevention: the Stockholm Youth Project," Research and Policy Papers No. 1 (London: Community Projects Foundation, 1988).

Through using existing infrastructure, massive outreach was possible in a short time. The three staff members of the project, with a budget of less than 175000 U.S. dollars, managed to organize the training of 3500 people in two years, ranging from teachers, nurses and youth leaders to priests, social workers and members of parent–teacher associations. Ninety–eight percent of Stockholm's schools now routinely integrate STD/AIDS information in their sex education curriculum and various youth clubs have developed discussion groups on sex and relationships. More elaborate local activities are being formulated.[44] In due course, the results of impact evaluation in terms of behavior change, condom use and STD incidence are awaited with interest.

The Stockholm Youth Project illustrates a multi–agency, multidisciplinary approach to community mobilization, working through and strengthening existing structures. Identification of local needs and an intimate understanding of formal and informal communication channels together with processes aimed at boosting the confidence of people in seeking locally relevant solutions are other essential characteristics of successful community–based AIDS health promotion interventions.

Voluntary or non–governmental organizations have been among the most powerful forces in mobilizing communities for AIDS prevention. In many Western European countries, these agencies pioneered the first responses to the AIDS crisis long before official efforts got under way. Examples include England's Terrence Higgins Trust, named after the first person to die of AIDS there. Over time, many of the initiatives have grown into large organizations, such as the Deutsch AIDS–Hilfe. Founded in 1983, this West German non–governmental organization has 75 local AIDS–Hilfe groups affiliated to it, along with scores of other organizations and individuals. In 1987, it organized 65 national training events, and produced educational videos and books, as well as ten million leaflets, posters, stickers and other materials. Its work is targeted at homosexual men, intravenous drug users, prostitutes, prison inmates, teachers, health workers and the general public. Local AIDS–Hilfe groups, run mostly by a network of 3000 volunteers, provide thousands of hours of telephone and personal counseling each year as well as "buddying" people with HIV/AIDS and doing social work with drug users and prison inmates.

Numerous other non–governmental organizations now operate in most Western European countries—working with people with HIV/AIDS, prostitutes, homosexual men, minority ethnic communities, young people, drug users, prison and probation services. They have been called the "third force

---

[44] V. Urwitz, T. Juvall, P. Sennerfeldt et al., "AIDS prevention as community intervention-the Stockholm youth intervention project," Fifth International Conference on AIDS, Montreal, June 1989.

in AIDS control"[45] and their experience is illuminating. Non–governmental organizations have demonstrated their ability to work simultaneously with large government bureaucracies and small communities. Their closeness to the communities from which they have often arisen has made them credible and acceptable sources of information. They have been flexible and innovative, and through their ability to form networks they have helped greatly "to close the distance between communities and national programs, and to amplify the voices of those communities."[46]

In some countries, such as the U.K., governments have not felt willing or able to directly provide certain types of prevention messages, for example, explicitly worded literature for gay pubs and clubs. Non–governmental organizations have filled this gap. However, non–governmental organizations also have limitations and experience considerable difficulties in their work. Their enthusiasm and dedication has not always made up for poor organization and inadequate management. To some extent this has been due to insufficient resources as non–governmental organizations have been used by governments to merely fill resource gaps and not enough has been invested to help them build sustainable infrastructures. This has created tensions between official bodies seeking financial accountability from the non–governmental organizations they fund and the latter's distrust of any controls that are perceived to interfere with their much cherished autonomy.

For the most part non–governmental organizations work cooperatively with each other. However, this is not always the case and conflicts between groups representing specific interests undermine their collective contribution to AIDS control. Sometimes this is due to competition for limited resources or disputes over "territoriality," for example, the right to be involved in a particular area such as representing prostitutes in this or that town. This is particularly marked in some areas of low HIV prevalence where many volunteers have been trained and are all "ready to go into the battle against AIDS" but there is not much for them to do. Skillful leadership and direction is needed to make use of this valuable resource for primary prevention purposes.

In contrast, some volunteers have been on the "front line" continuously since the early 1980s—staffing telephone hotlines, counseling people at risk or the "worried well," providing support to people with AIDS, consoling bereaved relatives, giving public lectures, fighting against insensitive official bureaucracies, lobbying for resources and struggling against hostile, prejudiced public opinion. With intense emotional and physical involve-

---

[45] R.N. Grose, "A Third Force: NGOs in AIDS control," *in The Global Impact of AIDS*, eds. A.F. Fleming, M. Carballo, D.W. FitzSimons, M.R. Bailey, J. Mann (New York: Alan R. Liss Inc., 1988).

[46] *Ibid.*

ment in these complex issues over a long period of time, together with poor support and little recognition for their achievements, these workers increasingly experience "burnout" with serious psychological morbidity. This is not helped by increasing friction between the established volunteers and the newly recruited paid workers who have been taken on by many non–governmental organizations as they "professionalize" themselves. Training and support for all HIV workers, voluntary or paid, needs to be strengthened.

TOWARD A UNITED EUROPEAN RESPONSE?

The European scene is not static. Recent years have seen progressive moves toward closer union, political and financial, among the ten member states of the European Community. The latter represents an increasingly powerful global economic force and indeed the area of Europe roughly bounded by Birmingham in the U.K. Frankfurt in West Germany and Paris in France is called the "golden triangle." In Eastern Europe, the pace of political change seems to be accelerating. These changes, leading to more contacts between countries, create complexity for health planners but also present opportunities to enable more effective joint efforts. The latter is particularly crucial in responding to the challenge of AIDS, which knows no international boundaries.

A variety of pan–European institutions are seen to have an involvement in international AIDS issues. The World Health Organization has been mandated by the United Nations General Assembly to lead and coordinate global efforts, from the Geneva based headquarters of its Global Programme on AIDS. The European Regional Office of the WHO, based in Copenhagen, coordinates the regional component of this program on AIDS, facilitating technical collaboration among member states. The European Community (popularly known as the "Common Market") has an Ad Hoc Group on AIDS, established in 1987 by order of the Council of Health Ministers of its member states. This group has a number of task forces. Due to policy differences between governments and the European Community's laborious mechanisms for decision–making, progress is rather slow and contentious issues tend to be avoided. Another body is the Council of Europe which has a wider membership than the European Community and is concerned with social and ethical aspects of AIDS prevention and control. National professional associations such as those for physicians and nurses are also seeking alliances with counterparts in other countries to develop common approaches, such as professional codes of conduct in dealing with persons with HIV and AIDS. In the voluntary sector, the Geneva-based League of Red Cross and Red Crescent

Societies seeks to unite national Red Cross societies. European Red Cross societies have also established an AIDS Task Force. The multiplicity of these international bodies can be confusing and there is a need to clarify their roles with each other and to enhance cooperation.

European governments vary in terms of the priority they give to concerns outside Europe and the levels of development assistance provided to Third World countries. AIDS has provoked a reappraisal of international duties and responsibilities. In January 1988 the government of the United Kingdom organized (jointly with the WHO) a World Summit of Health Ministers to discuss AIDS prevention. One hundred and forty–eight countries representing the vast majority of the world's peoples came together in London in the largest ministerial gathering ever to discuss a specific health issue. Though this was an impressive demonstration of European and international policy resolve, there has been inadequate recognition that AIDS is linked to poverty and underdevelopment and will not be controlled simply by condoms and leaflets. For example, AIDS threatens to wipe out the gains made through child survival initiatives in developing countries. Furthermore, in Africa the potential loss of their most productive men and women in the twenty– to forty–year–old age group is likely to have grave social and economic consequences, and could lead to further political instability. The rich countries of Europe need to individually and collectively consider their policies on development assistance and trade with the Third World. Specifically European issues on which cross–national collaboration would be fruitful include the following.

- Common research protocols including social and behavioral investigations and operational research evaluating the effectiveness of prevention interventions. This would enable useful cross–national comparisons to be made.
- At the same time, ethical standards in AIDS research need to be consistently high across the continent, as variations and laxity hinder collaboration and are potentially exploitative of vulnerable people.
- Universally agreed upon quality control standards for the manufacture of condoms.
- Restrictions on the availability of do–it–yourself HIV antibody test kits, which are just becoming available and which raise considerable concerns on misuse by ill–informed members of the public.
- Development of uniform work place policies, particularly as labor mobility increases. Many corporations have branches in a number of countries, but may have inconsistent approaches such as compulsory pre–employment screening in one factory, but not in its sister enterprise across the border.

- The life and health insurance industry would also benefit from Europe–wide guidelines.
- Consensus on policy toward people who cross international borders as migrants, refugees and tourists. They have important educational needs as well as the need to have their basic human rights protected. For example, an educational project for seafarers is being developed with support from the European Community.
- Finally, basic prevention messages need to be harmonized because, as discussed earlier in this chapter, the public are receiving diverse messages from a variety of sources. This leads to confusion and perpetuates myths which undermine national campaigns.

CONCLUSION

The richness and diversity of the European response to AIDS has been illustrated in this chapter. Much has been achieved in the past seven years from initial fragmented efforts launched in haste but improved through trial and error to the more carefully considered and sustained programs currently under way. The mass media have made a remarkable contribution in creating unprecedented levels of public awareness on a specific health issue, but not without its cost in also creating undue anxiety, perpetuating myths and fostering prejudice. Lethargic institutions and indifferent communities have been mobilized into action. Previously unmentionable human behaviors such as intravenous drug use and anal intercourse are now more openly discussed. Homosexual men have shown what can be done through solidarity and community organization. Prostitutes have demonstrated that they can continue to practice their business, but safely and responsibly. Politicians have had to make tough policy choices. AIDS prevention and control efforts have exposed weaknesses in public health and other societal infrastructures and have provided opportunities for the future. Relationships between individuals and between nations are being re–appraised.

However, in many ways, it is the easy things that have been accomplished. We have much more to do and it will be difficult to maintain momentum in the face of "information overload," complacency and cynicism. The education and health promotion needs of thousands of people living with HIV and AIDS must be addressed. Information and education initiatives also need to take a more vigorous stand against prejudice and bigotry, which threaten individual human rights and undermine public health efforts.

Finally, it needs to be remembered that the European epidemic of HIV and AIDS is still "dynamic and unstable." Prevention and control strategies will need to remain flexible, responding rapidly to changing needs set against a diverse background of rapid social and political changes in Europe.

We are grateful to colleagues in many European countries for sharing their experience with us, and for the privilege to represent their work in this chapter.

IV. STRATEGIES FOR COMMUNICATION AND THE MEDIA

Preface

Harvey Fineberg

We have learned that information is not enough to promote behavior change, but it is an essential ingredient of all AIDS prevention programs and a necessary first step in any successful public health strategy against AIDS. Advertising or reporting can deliver the message, while other education strategies can bring people to the point of actual behavior change. Above all, the mass media have proven to be very effective in promoting positive attitudes toward people with AIDS and in contributing to sustaining behavior modification over time. Therefore, public health departments, schools of public health, non-governmental organizations and communities need to develop strategies for working with the mass media as one aspect of their campaigns against AIDS.

Thomas Netter and Laurie Garrett, seasoned AIDS reporters, tell us in their chapters that although the mass media should not be regarded as partners in AIDS education programs, they can play an important role in helping individuals and institutions to make informed decisions. The two authors clarify how the needs of reporters and of AIDS prevention programs can both be met, and propose that the mass media be used by AIDS professionals to do what they do best: provide information and keep it before the public eye. Netter stresses that AIDS professionals must give the media clear and complete information in order to avoid creating a situation where the media hurt instead of help an AIDS prevention campaign by misinforming the public. Finally, Garrett reminds us that the news media never reach all elements of society and therefore separate educational efforts must specifically target those individuals the news media do not reach.

In their chapter, William DeJong and Jay Winsten present us with two original applications of the broadcast media for AIDS education. On the one hand, entertainment programs can help create a new normative consensus in favor of condom use. On the other hand, public awareness campaigns can supplement community–based educational programs by publicizing them.

Advertising, adapted to AIDS education through social marketing, is limited in much the same way as news media in that it is not interactive. Recognizing this limitation, Milton Gossett and Jeremy Warshaw have developed a social marketing strategy designed to overcome the barriers to AIDS prevention and to reduce denial so people can accept their risk of infection, an important first step on the road to behavior modification.

Another group of authors demonstrates the use of television for the prevention of AIDS. Thomas Goodgame, Jeanne Blake and Gil Schwartz describe how television can give people with AIDS a forum, an important educational strategy based on the idea that people with AIDS are the best educators for AIDS prevention. In addition, such a forum creates compassion for people with AIDS, which can be of help in positively affecting how the public deals with the politics of AIDS.

REFERENCES

G. Friedland, "AIDS and Compassion," Journal of the American Medical Association 259(19) (1988): 2898-9.

WHO "Guide to Planning Health Promotion for AIDS Prevention and Control," WHO AIDS Series 5, Geneva: World health Organization, 1989.

WHO-Norway, MOH 1988.

The Media and AIDS:
A Global Perspective

Thomas W. Netter

At a June 1989 media seminar on AIDS, attended by journalists from both developed and developing countries, the talk turned quickly to the question of journalists as educators. One speaker from an industrialized country, who like the others was covering the Fifth International Conference on AIDS in Montreal, spoke of the difficulty posed for journalists when faced with the challenges of AIDS education: the need to remain objective, the diversity of information, journalists' lack of formal training in education. But for many of those present from developing countries, the idea that journalists should not be expected to educate the public seemed like a heresy, a shock, and prompted looks of disbelief. As soon as the speaker had finished, the hands of many of those in the room shot in to the air and a lively discussion began.

The meeting helped to crystallize a debate that has been raging for some time now among journalists covering AIDS: should they play the role of "educator," carrying a responsibility for bringing education, so vital to the prevention of the AIDS epidemic, to the public at large? Is there a difference between the role of journalists in developed and developing countries, and do the latter have a different role to play? Is there a real distinction between the concept of "information" and "education" in the process of bringing information about AIDS to the broad general public?

The World Health Organization Global Programme on AIDS is strongly committed to working with the mass media to enhance public knowledge about AIDS and to help implement the WHO global strategy against HIV/AIDS.

Our experience has shown that newspapers, magazines, newsletters, television and radio today provide a vital "front line" in the global struggle against AIDS. Although the mass media should not be expected to shoulder the responsibility for educating individuals, the public and governments, it can provide the information necessary for people and institutions to make informed decisions on both an individual and public level. While information is not enough to promote behavior change, it is an essential ingredient in a comprehensive and successful public health strategy against AIDS. Therefore, it is imperative for the WHO, other non–governmental organizations, public health departments and others involved in AIDS prevention to devise precise strategies for working with mass media because many, if not most, people around the world learn much, if not all, of what they know about AIDS from the mass media.

DEFINING THE MEDIA

For this chapter to focus on the mass media and their broad public audience, it is necessary to define precisely what media are being considered. This article will therefore discuss the role of mass media in its most general application—general interest newspapers, magazines, radio and television—rather than advertising, public relations, and sponsored, or specially designed, mass media campaigns. The purpose of this chapter is to discuss the role of journalists and journalism in AIDS prevention strategy, not to review the impact of highly orchestrated, often government or institutionally–sponsored advertising or public relations campaigns.

This is because unlike planned media campaigns, the non–institutional, often independent mass media present a major challenge for public health officials who would try and work with them. These mass media often involve editors and reporters who may or may not have basic scientific knowledge or background about AIDS, and may have criteria for judging the "newsworthiness" of a story that differs radically from public health workers' own views. Journalists may have little access to accurate, timely or relevant information about AIDS or other health issues. In some developing countries, the media may be short of basic resources or staff. Often, there is a consistent state of conflict between the mass media and institutions and organizations involved in public health. Public health professionals often have little understanding or tolerance for the working methods or approaches of the mass media.

Nevertheless, since the AIDS epidemic became a major public issue in the early 1980s, the mass media have played a powerful role in the struggle against AIDS. For the most part, this role has been positive—it is fair to say that the mass media have helped bring much information, in a short time, to a large public. Granted, sometimes the mass media have played a less than positive role, disseminating falsehoods about AIDS, making facile comparisons with the Black Plague, exaggerating the risks for transmission of casual contact, or seeking to attach blame for "starting" the epidemic to a specific region or group. Some expectations for the role the mass media could play in AIDS education have been naive: calling news about AIDS an "information vaccine" may overstate the actual power of the press to change behavior. Even so, the mass media have been a key element in helping public health professionals bring their messages about AIDS to the general public. Few in AIDS–related professions today would contest the idea that information about AIDS in the past decade has contributed to public health efforts that have had some effect in preventing transmission of HIV.

Thus, there is no question of the importance of the media to the WHO and others involved in this global struggle. The AIDS epidemic has developed in an age of unparalleled media development, with information and communication capabilities expanding faster than ever before. Widespread use of video, computer databases and electronic information transfer, search or mailing, were either in fledgling stages of development or unheard of during the WHO campaign against smallpox in the 1960s and 1970s. Technical developments that increase both the volume and the scope of mass media reporting are continuing to accelerate, although to a certain degree the increase in quantity of news has not been accompanied by a parallel increase in depth of coverage of some issues; instead emphasis has often been placed on shorter reports on a greater number of issues. Just as the constantly accelerating development of scientific and medical knowledge and research capabilities has helped speed the process of identifying and studying HIV and AIDS, so has the rapid explosion of media capability and capacity—especially with the advent of television—in the post–World War II era helped expand the role of the mass media in efforts against AIDS.

In addition, the mass media today often play a greater role than previously in reporting on public health policy formation in many countries around the world. In most industrialized countries, the mass media have unquestionably contributed to the public dialogue and policy formation in response to AIDS, more so recently than in the early days of the epidemic, as reporters gain sophistication and understanding of the public policy implications of the AIDS epidemic. In the relatively short history of the AIDS epidemic, the mass media have helped to force both policy makers and the general public to confront the nature of AIDS and all its related ethical and human rights issues. Meanwhile, in many developing countries, AIDS has come at a time when there is a fortunate improvement in information and communications resources, and has actually helped open a dialogue about wider public health issues. In many countries around the world, public perception, knowledge and attitudes toward AIDS have by comparison to previously frightening diseases covered decades in a matter of a few years.

Based on its global experience, it is the perception of the WHO that this mass media focus on AIDS reached its peak of intensity about seven years into the epidemic, or in 1988, roughly in parallel with the expansion of a global consciousness of AIDS. Although there seems to have been a drop in interest in some parts of the world, especially in developed countries, general media interest in AIDS remains high in most of the developing world. Interest in specific scientific, biomedical or social advances regarding AIDS remains important for the developed world, especially in North America and Europe. The fact that AIDS still acts as a powerful magnet for the media was amply illustrated at the Fifth International Conference on AIDS, in Montreal, where over 1,300 accredited correspondents and journalists covered the meeting, or roughly one journalist for every ten participants.

It is clear then that AIDS will continue to remain an important "story." What is less clear, however, is how the media will treat developments in the AIDS epidemic. There may well be a resurgence of interest as the number of persons infected with HIV/AIDS and dying from AIDS continues to increase. The stories of scientific and research activities regarding a number of treatments being tested will also prompt coverage. But it is equally apparent that the intensity of media interest and reaction that marked the early days of the AIDS epidemic is over. A recent survey published in *The Washington Post* based on a study of an electronic data base index in the United States showed an 11–fold increase in articles on AIDS between 1984 and 1987, followed by a plummeting of the number of news stories —by 50 percent— since then.[1] What is clear from this is that the era when any and every story on AIDS could draw a press conference or press attention is over.

The challenges to AIDS professionals in working with the mass media is therefore compounded by the need to develop strategies that will help stimulate the mass media to maintain a focus on AIDS and keep the issue before the public. This raises the question of whether it is possible to regard the mass media as a vital element in AIDS information dissemination when media interest in and attention to the epidemic may be declining. As a result, when formulating a media strategy, public health professionals must not only consider how to bring information to the attention of the mass media and take advantage of its power of news distribution, but also answer the questions of what we can and can not expect from the mass media in the global struggle against AIDS.

[1] *The Washington Post*, Washington, D.C., U.S. 13 June, 1989.

REPORTING ON AIDS: PAST AND PRESENT

Part of the process of devising a media strategy for governments and non–governmental organizations is the analysis of the mass media's approach to AIDS, past and present. There are two key issues that must therefore be considered: the precise role of the mass media, and how this role and reaction to AIDS develops in parallel to the development of AIDS. An important element in understanding the role of the mass media can be found in their reaction to the AIDS epidemic. Based on international experience, reporting on AIDS appears to generally develop in three phases, which could be described roughly as initial reactions of fear and ignorance, followed by development of experience and understanding, with a third phase moving into concentration on precise scientific and policy developments.

The first phase of fear and ignorance appears to occur everywhere that a society first comes into contact with the onset of AIDS cases. Just as misconceptions, misunderstanding, and prejudice often marked early reporting on AIDS in the Pattern I countries of the industrialized world, such problems occur in the early phases of reporting as the disease becomes known in Pattern II countries in Africa, and Pattern III countries in Asia where cases and prevalence are still relatively low. Early articles on AIDS cases and infections with HIV in the United States, for example, often referred to a "gay plague," a phrase that ignored other forms of transmission of HIV such as through blood or blood products, or from mother to fetus or child. In some countries AIDS is still largely characterized as a "gay disease." There is often a large amount of erroneous information on the modes of transmission, especially casual contact. Authorities are often accused of trying to "cover up" information, such as numbers of AIDS cases, or the number of HIV infections. A widespread rejection of AIDS as a problem of "others" occurs, and is fueled by misguided reports comparing AIDS to other illnesses to which it has no parallel, searching for a country or a region to blame as the source bringing in AIDS from outside a country or a culture, and the publication of often spurious stories about modes of transmission that people should fear. The impact of these stories is often fueled by frightening photographic images that in themselves can arise from misunderstandings and prejudices. Pictures of authorities burning the automobile of an accident victim who was infected with HIV, or of police wearing yellow rubber gloves while arresting protesters only serve to endorse public fear and misunderstanding of AIDS.

Numerous examples abound. In the Philippines, the media struggled to find information in the early 1980s, searching for "Filipino victims" to lend "drama" and "impact" to the AIDS story.[2] In Uganda, initial reactions to AIDS

---

[2] Report at WHO Regional Workshop on the Role of the Broadcast Media in the Prevention and Control of HIV Infection and AIDS, Tokyo, Japan, 12–16 June, 1989.

included fear or disbelief as "AIDS was considered a disease of the developed countries," or "a disease of gay people," again stressing the theme of AIDS as an affliction of "others".[3] In Japan, television crews searched out the houses of persons with AIDS (infected through blood transfusions) or filmed hospitals where persons with AIDS had been treated during what was described as an "AIDS panic" over what was commonly referred to in the Japanese media as a "plague of modern times" and an "epidemic of the gay people."[4] In Thailand, reports that a well–known female fashion model was infected prompted a "stake out" in front of the woman's house, forcing her to flee and to issue a public statement a few days later denying the story.[5] Clearly, the initial reactions to AIDS have often been less than responsible, verging on hysteria in some cases and stressing a fearful disease, often associated with "sinful" activities, promiscuity and the unknown, and invariably associated with danger for an unsuspecting public.

In some cases, intense attention to a "newsmaking" aspect of AIDS can have benefits. Public interest and familiarity with AIDS accelerated dramatically, not only in the United States but nearly everywhere in the world, following the July 1985 revelation that the American actor Rock Hudson was ill with AIDS. The desperate search for treatment, followed by the death of the American actor had the effect on some people of actually bringing the realities of AIDS into their lives for the first time.[6] Nevertheless, such images can be used for some of the worst examples of misunderstanding and sensationalism, that can linger in a country or region, even after most of the mass media have matured in their comprehension of AIDS issues. In the so–called "gutter press" in the United Kingdom, for example, the death of Rock Hudson is still making headlines. The Sunday, May 28th, 1989 edition of the London News of the World refers to "The House That Died of Shame", reporting "The specter of AIDS–ravaged film star Rock Hudson is finally being exorcised from the mansion he once used as a gay pleasure palace."[7] Thus, the first phase of unfounded and prejudicial reaction to AIDS can linger long after the media in general in a country have left such judgmental and irresponsible reporting behind, and despite the best efforts of individuals, public institutions and non–governmental organizations to inform and educate the mass media with facts.

The second phase of reporting on AIDS occurs after initial reactions to

[3] Report at the First International Workshop on AIDS for Developing Country Media, Ottawa, Canada, 2–3 June, 1989.

[4] Ibid.

[5] Ann Usher, reporter for The Bangkok Nation, during a conversation with the author in Bangkok, Thailand, March 1989.

[6] "In a sense, it was as if most Americans for the first time lost somebody they knew." Laurie Garrett, The Newsletter of the National Association of Science Writers 35 (1) (March 1987).

[7] The Independent, London, England, 2 August, 1989.

AIDS have been toned down by a combination of efforts to provide accurate information and general acceptance of AIDS as a new health issue for a society to face rather than fear. Bearing in mind the complexity of the subject itself, and the issues involved, such as the right to travel, anti–discrimination, and ethics in testing and screening, reporting on AIDS in many parts of the world has become surprisingly accurate and responsible over a short period of time. Despite the intense burst of mass media interest and the wide range of experience and expertise among reporters covering the International Conference on AIDS in Montreal, few if any reports monitored by the WHO could be described as hysterical, sensationalist or overly slanted or discriminatory against any particular group. It will not be long before the mass media can begin to play a positive role in the struggle against AIDS. Although deliberate attempts at misinformation, such as books and videos recently circulated in the United States, the Federal Republic of Germany and central Africa have proved troublesome and even counter–productive to AIDS prevention efforts, they have not caused new outbreaks of panic in the United States and Europe, while in Uganda, authorities have managed to counteract allegations about AIDS being produced in a laboratory and deliberately spread to the population.

In most cases, the second phase, or advent of responsible reporting, results from good journalists doing their jobs: reporting the news accurately, responsibly and fairly. Sometimes, peer pressure or pressure from news sources has helped stimulate calm reporting. Laurie Garrett, a science reporter for *Long Island Newsday*, Long Island, New York, spoke at the International Conference on AIDS in Children, Adolescents and Heterosexual Adults in Atlanta, Georgia, U.S. in February of 1987, of reporters being "swayed by criticism from the scientific community, the gay community, and the community at large."[8] An Australian paper delivered at a WHO media workshop in Tokyo spoke of the increasing rarity of having a story which is sensationalist in nature, or which is presented in a pejorative manner about, for example, homosexual men or intravenous drug users.

In North America and increasingly in countries in Europe, Latin America, Africa and Asia, the third phase of media reaction is developing, regarding AIDS as a key public issue deserving of serious treatment and policy review. Recent extensive articles about government reactions to the AIDS epidemic report on the ramifications of findings regarding various treatments for AIDS, and other policy issues are receiving greater, more precise attention in the form of serious reporting, often by a reporter assigned to an "AIDS beat," just as others would specialize in such topics as arms control, environmental issues, trade and the economy, etc. With the

8 Laurie Garrett, "Reporting on AIDS: Who is responsible?", *The Newsletter of the National Association of Science Writers* 35 (1) (March 1987).

continuous development of the AIDS epidemic, such focusing on AIDS as a "beat" could be expected to become more prevalent in all three Pattern areas. In addition, while knowledge of the specifics about AIDS may still prove illusive to the non–specialized reporter, with some exceptions, there appears to be a trend toward greater understanding not only of AIDS as an issue, but for those who are HIV–infected or have AIDS. At the same time the ardor that many reporters brought to AIDS reporting in the early days of the epidemic may also be cooling, as reporters grow "tired" of a story without breathtakingly new news developments. "The perception of AIDS has shifted from an uncontrolled epidemic to a chronic problem that will take years to solve," writes Thompson in *The Washington Post* on June 13th, 1989. "The war on AIDS has, in a sense, gone the way of the war on cancer. It is no longer a new crusade."

THE ROLE OF THE MEDIA: INFORMATION OR EDUCATION?

Clearly then, the media have the power to keep the issue of AIDS before the public eye, and to provide the first information to the public about developments in the AIDS pandemic. The mass media can help set both the tone and the agenda of AIDS prevention activities in some countries. But because of the varying levels of media understanding and commitment to accuracy in reporting on AIDS in all parts of the world, the role of the press in the struggle against AIDS should not, and must not, be taken for granted. This brings us to the second element of strategy planning: the question of the role of journalists in the mass media as educators. There are strong arguments for and against this role.

There are a number of reasons for arguing that journalists and the media should not be expected to play the role of educators. The first is that journalists—even science writers who specialize in the field—are not trained as educators. Education, many reporters argue, is for educators, while the journalist's role is to inform, to cover AIDS as a medical, scientific, social and public policy issue, and to reach for the most "newsworthy" aspects of a development. Education through the media, the argument goes, is imprecise, relying on a distracted reader, or incomplete understanding. There is no classroom or controlled setting, no teacher to provide answers to questions or to immediately correct misunderstandings. Journalism is thus an inefficient means of education, and should not be relied on.

Another argument centers on the role of journalists: it states that their mandate is clearly that of information, rather than education. The argument stresses that journalists must maintain their independence and not become a partner of any government or any non–governmental organization for fear of sacrificing their objectivity or compromising their independence of judgment. The mass media play the role of "asking the tough questions" in the words of Garrett of *Long Island Newsday*, rather than "joining the team."[9]

There is also a strong tendency to cite other attempts at behavioral change in response to a public health issue, such as smoking, or wearing seat belts while driving. Garrett stated that "if the mass media were an excellent source of public education, nobody in the United States would smoke cigarettes. Nobody would misuse pesticides. Nobody would be eating cholesterol–rich foods as a steady part of their diets. And probably nobody would inject heroin or smoke crack. If all it took was to hear something was dangerous, behavior would change [with media coverage]. No medical news report has received the volume of press coverage that AIDS has, and by and large that press coverage has stressed the most crucial points the public needs to know to decide if they personally need to be afraid or change their sexual or drug–abuse patterns. The press is very good at raising the level of fear and concern. But it takes more than fear and concern to move people to take rational, pragmatic action."

Garrett and others argue that the very nature of some forms of AIDS transmission, the fact that AIDS is a sexually transmitted disease, has compounded the difficulty faced by reporters, even if they seek to educate. Garrett speaks of being prevented for three years from using the words "rectum" and "rectal intercourse" in her reports for National Public Radio in the United States. In an October 1987 article in the U.S. magazine *Mother Jones*, reporter Marlene Cimons of the *Los Angeles Times* spoke of language still being a difficult issue, of discussions with editors over the use of the word "epidemic" instead of "outbreak," or of articles with phrases such as "anal intercourse," "swallowing semen," "fisting" and "rimming" being edited out, eliminating information that might have helped some avoid the spread of AIDS. "Words don't kill," Cimons wrote, "but they could have saved lives. And I wonder how many lives were lost in our failure to print them."

Other problems include the prospects of some journalists "getting it wrong," as described in an article by Eleanor Randolph of *The Washington Post* on June 5th, 1987 when "someone in the news media [doesn't get] it quite right—a moment when months of excellent coverage... are lost to a less careful reporter confused about the medical issue of the moment." Filipino journalists spoke in Tokyo of the lack of information about AIDS, which made it difficult if not impossible for them to portray the AIDS situation in their country accurately. A Manila television reporter described how

---

[9] "Skepticism is really the key to good journalism... Joining the team is not our job. Our job is to stand back and take a hard look at what you are doing." Laurie Garrett, *The Newsletter of the National Association of Science Writers* 35 (1) (March 1987).

she received conflicting answers to questions about transmission, resulting in a situation where "journalists reporting on AIDS don't know what to believe, and only end up aiding the confusion." It is worth bearing in mind that for most reporters, the subject is difficult. Randolph in *The Washington Post* reports interviewing many journalists who regarded the AIDS story as "one of the most difficult they have covered."[10] This applies, of course, to journalists who want to "get it right." As all experienced members of the media must know, there is little if anything that one can do to prevent a journalist or any other interviewer from ultimately making an error if the writer comes to the subject with an agenda that is either preconceived to make a point counter to the facts, or prejudiced in one way or another.

THE CHALLENGE FOR AIDS PROFESSIONALS

If these arguments are valid for not relying on the media to educate, then what is the sense of working with the mass media, other than to merely answer questions and try and avoid misunderstandings? While all the arguments cited above are valid, and the problems of erroneous or squeamish reporting have occurred and will continue to occur, we firmly believe that the mass media remain a vital conduit for providing information that is educational to the public. While the mass media should not automatically be regarded as a "partner in prevention," public health workers at all levels in the struggle against AIDS must continue to regard the mass media as vital to the prevention of HIV transmission and the understanding of the AIDS issue. This is true because the speed of developments in the epidemic and its constantly changing elements make definition and explanation in official or formal documents slow; however, these rapid developments are of immediate relevance to many in the general public.

Just as we should not regard the mass media as partners in preventing HIV, nor should we assume that the mass media have an obligation to report on AIDS, although many reporters will themselves see their work as such an obligation. AIDS professionals should not regard the media as partners, since to see the press as a partner is to be seen as wanting to control or manipulate the media. They should not regard the media as a substitute for any form of education, which can and must continue in its proper setting. But for any form of education to have the widest possible impact, and for public health to realize the potential of the media as an educative tool, we must find ways of merging the concepts of health education with efforts to work with the media.

10 E. Randolph, "AIDS Reporters Challenge: To Educate, Not Panic, the Public," *The Washington Post* 5 June, 1987.

The importance of this is underscored by numerous surveys. A Roper poll in the United States stated that most U.S. residents "get information about AIDS from television. Newspapers came in second; the medical profession was third."[11] In New Zealand, a nationwide survey on the impact of HIV/AIDS in 1987 found that the most common way people heard about HIV was on the television news, followed by newspapers and subsequent television programs, radio programs, magazine articles, television advertising and finally word of mouth.[12] In Uganda the media play a vital role in promoting or hindering the work of the national AIDS programs.[13] In other countries, the patterns may vary according to public accessibility of print or broadcast media, but the principle remains the same.

Mass media stimulation of interest in AIDS functions not only as a form of AIDS education, but also can help public health implement its strategies. "As long as the media kept AIDS in the forefront of society's consciousness, it was easier for public health professionals to get across the message of prevention through safe sex and avoidance of drug abuse," writes Thompson in *The Washington Post*, June 13th, 1989. Reporters are often committed to reporting graphically on AIDS and how HIV is transmitted because of a belief that by providing the most detailed information, at least some readers or listeners will change behavior or ask their medical practitioner for advice. In Australia, "the potential for radio and television to address issues related to HIV infection, such as fear, prejudice and discrimination... is significant. Television has helped develop far more sensitive and informed community attitudes towards people with HIV/AIDS."[14]

In countries around the world, AIDS reporting has also led to increased media coverage of other health issues, such as a resurgence of tuberculosis in some cities in the developed world as well as in developing countries; the interrelationship of various illnesses and diseases in the developing countries, and what impact they have on public health systems and policies; and social issues such as human sexuality, prostitution, and illegal drug use, with positive results.

What then are the challenges for the media, and for public health professionals? At the WHO Media Workshop in Tokyo, reporters from Asia identified three objectives: to increase public awareness of HIV/AIDS in order to promote positive attitudes and behavior; to prevent stigmatization of people infected with AIDS; and to support and monitor government and

[11] *USA Today*, 14 April 1987.

[12] *Op. cit.* Report at WHO Regional Workshop on the Role of the Broadcast Media in the Prevention and Control of HIV Infection and AIDS, Tokyo, Japan.

[13] Report by Dr. Kamasomero, Media Specialist, Radio Uganda, to the WHO Media Workshop in Ottawa, Canada, June 1989.

[14] *Op. cit.* Report at WHO Regional Workshop on the Role of the Broadcast Media in the Prevention and Control of HIV Infection and AIDS, Tokyo, Japan.

community efforts in the achievement of the above objectives. These three basic objectives can be expanded into more specific recommendations.

- Reporting the news about AIDS accurately, objectively and without prejudice.
- Avoiding the sensational aspects of the AIDS story and realizing that solid, informed reporting on AIDS can help facilitate public health work against AIDS without compromising a news organization's independence or objectivity.
- Applying the same degree of skepticism and professionalism to all aspects of reporting on AIDS as would be applied to any other story of global importance.
- Reporting on people with AIDS with the same understanding and compassion that would be provided to those suffering from any other disease, including the avoidance of any form of judgment or prejudice.
- Being as well–informed as possible, in part by making AIDS a "beat" so that the best and most accurate information about any aspect of the AIDS epidemic is made available to the public.

The challenges to the international health care community and national public health sectors are broader, and apply to all organizations involved in campaigns against AIDS. Bearing in mind that the mass media should not and can not be co–opted into the process as partners in the public health or health education process, it is essential to find a balance between the requirements of the press for a story and the AIDS professional's need to get accurate and timely information to the public. While the press will cover AIDS as an important social, medical and ethical issue for our time, public health and AIDS professionals have an obligation to provide the media with the best information available to help make the reporting informative and accurate, while maintaining the reporters' interest in the subject. In order to gain maximum advantage from the power of the media, the AIDS professional must be informative when questioned by the media, and provide the most complete information, or a reasonable explanation of why this is impossible; they must be timely, bearing in mind that for the reporter, newsworthiness is synonymous with timeliness; and AIDS professionals must be patient, realizing that unless a reporter is a bona fide specialist in the field, only a willingness to explain the issues carefully and clearly can help the reporter to understand.

AIDS professionals and all those working against AIDS must seek ways to combine health education with public information. They must find ways to add substance and focus to messages given to the mass media, and they need to help maintain both the quality of reporting and interest in the subject. To this end, some organizations, including the WHO, have under-taken a series of media workshops that will continue to educate reporters around the world in the basic issues of AIDS and to forge contacts that can improve not only the quality of reporting, but access to accurate informa-tion. Public health workers should draw attention to erroneous, misleading or damaging reports, not only to educate reporters, but also editors, instill-ing a sense of responsibility among the members of the media, and a super-vising function for themselves. Many AIDS reporters will agree that educa-tion is important not only to them, but also to their editors, who must often be swayed to provide them with the mandate to concentrate on AIDS, the space to print their reports in newspapers or include them in newscasts and help them make the judgments necessary to maintain high–quality reporting.

In addition, ministries of health and information can contribute to the effectiveness of the mass media's role in the AIDS epidemic by working openly with the mass media, providing accurate, up–to–date information on cases, legislative and governmental activities, and policy development. Non–governmental organizations must aggressively work with the media, providing the best information possible on their specific areas of interest.

The discussion on whether the media should be expected to play the role of educator will continue. But the goal of any media strategy must ulti-mately be getting as much accurate information as possible to the public. Although we cannot hope to reach everyone, or know precisely if working with the mass media is prompting behavior change in much of the world, the information presented by the mass media can and will save lives. Help-ing to promote good reporting on AIDS will contribute to the development of a public consciousness and awareness, help to overcome fear and igno-rance, and provide the basis for understanding and development of further knowledge about AIDS. For public health professionals amid a continuously worsening epidemic who have access to a rapidly developing mass media there is no other acceptable alternative.

The Strategic Use of the Broadcast Media for AIDS Prevention: Current Limits and Future Directions

William DeJong
Jay A. Winsten

Since World War II, public communication campaigns designed to effect behavior change have been a mainstay of health promotion and education efforts in the United States.[1] Public health advocates have often vacillated in their enthusiasm for such campaigns, with naive and unrealistic expectations alternating with a hard–boiled skepticism about the strategic use of mass media for health promotion. During the 1980s, however, there has been a growing clarity that mass media campaigns can indeed play an important role in changing health–related behaviors and lifestyles, when they are designed and executed according to certain principles, and when they are in operation for several years.[2]

Thus, confronted this decade by the growing menace of the AIDS epidemic, and with a cure or vaccine a distant hope, U.S. public health officials have turned to the mass media as a means of quickly educating the American general public about the disease and the changes in behavior that are required to stem its spread. The broadcast media have emerged as one of the principal vehicles for conveying these anti–AIDS messages because of their capacity for transmitting artful and potent messages and their efficiency in reaching vast audiences.[3]

[1] R.E. Rice and C.K. Atkin, *Public Communication Campaigns*, 2nd ed. (Newbury Park, CA: Sage, 1989).

[2] W. DeJong and J.A. Winsten, "Recommendations for Future Mass Media Campaigns to Prevent Preteen and Adolescent Substance Abuse," *Health Affairs* 9 (1990): 30-46.

[3] K. Warner, "Television and Health Education," *American Journal of Public Health* 77 (1987) 140-2.

Resulting from a combination of television and radio public awareness campaigns, news media coverage, print advertising for condoms and television entertainment programming, most American adolescents and adults now know a great deal about the AIDS threat, modes of transmission and available prevention measures. Unfortunately, these gains in factual knowledge do not often enough lead to health–protective changes in sexual behavior. Of special concern is condom use, for aside from sexual abstinence or a stable, mutually faithful relationship with another uninfected person, using condoms is widely acknowledged to be the best protection against sexually transmitted AIDS.[4] Other changes in sexual behavior could be stressed, such as reducing the number of one's sexual partners, using other "safer sex" practices, or, for adolescents, delaying initiation of sexual activity. But we concur in the belief that the greatest progress in preventing AIDS transmission can be made at this time by promoting greater condom use.

The successful promotion of condoms requires moving beyond basic factual information about AIDS and prophylaxis to motivating messages that address in specific ways the various psychological barriers that impede their use—specifically, widespread concerns about condoms interfering with sexual pleasure and the difficulties often faced in negotiating condom use with one's sexual partners.[5] Targeted messages are needed for homosexual, bisexual and heterosexual audiences. However, because the U.S. broadcast media seek to avoid alienating large segments of their mass audience and the political or economic pressures that would ensue, they cannot be readily mobilized to communicate the specific information that is necessary for motivating condom use, even among heterosexuals.

To establish a context for examining the strategic use of the broadcast media for delivering AIDS prevention messages, we begin this chapter by providing a brief overview of what can be accomplished in health promotion through the mass media. We then describe what the nation's anti–AIDS public service campaigns have actually achieved to date, noting that news media coverage has both helped and hurt the health community's efforts to inform the American public. Next, we examine what is required to motivate greater condom use—namely, addressing the public's specific concerns about using condoms.

We next describe how the standards enforced by the national broadcast media have thus far made it impossible to deliver these motivating messages

[4] L. Liskin and R. Blackburn, "AIDS: A Public Health Crisis," *Population Reports L6* (Baltimore: Population Information Program, Johns Hopkins University, 1986).

[5] M.Z. Solomon and W. DeJong, "Recent Sexually Transmitted Disease Prevention Efforts and Their Implications for AIDS Health Education," *Health Education Quarterly* 13 (1986): 301–16; and M.Z. Solomon and W. DeJong, "Preventing AIDS and Other STDs Through Condom Promotion: A Patient Education Intervention," *American Journal of Public Health* 79 (1989): 453–8.

through paid or public service advertising. While television entertainment programming offers greater leeway for bringing these messages to the American public, they cannot be incorporated into programming often enough to make a critical difference. News programming is similarly limiting as a vehicle for providing motivating messages on condom use.

With the reality of these current restrictions in view, we urge that current public awareness campaigns be supplemented by an expansion of community–based educational programs that focus on condom promotion and can be assisted in various ways by local mass media. New and expanded programs that focus on adolescent and young adult heterosexuals who are at risk of AIDS, similar to model community–based programs that target homosexuals or IV–drug users and their partners, are especially necessary.

WHAT MASS MEDIA CAMPAIGNS CAN ACCOMPLISH IN HEALTH PROMOTION

During the past 15 years, several studies have established that long–term mass media campaigns can have a meaningful impact on health–related behaviors and lifestyles. There are two keys to designing and executing a successful campaign: 1) adoption of the "consumer" orientation typical of commercial marketing, and 2) a full understanding of how behavior change occurs and how a mass media campaign can facilitate each step of that process.[6]

Specifically, communications researchers have pointed to the following elements of successful mass media campaigns: 1) the specification of well–defined target audiences, differentiated according to geographic, demographic, psychological and other relevant characteristics; 2) extensive use of formative research (e.g., focus groups, in–depth interviews) to understand the target audience and to pretest campaign materials; 3) messages that build from the audience's current levels of knowledge and skill; 4) messages that satisfy the audience's pre–existing needs and motives, especially those that are not related to health per se and can be gratified within a short time; 5) a media plan guaranteeing that the target audience is exposed to the campaign; and 6) procedures for evaluating progress.

Often, the behaviors that public health advocates seek to change are ingrained habits or have accrued a cultural meaning or personal significance that makes them resistant to change.[7] This is especially true in the case of AIDS prevention, with both sexual behavior and addictive drug use

[6] *Op. cit.* W. DeJong and J.A. Winsten.
[7] T. Robertson and L. Wortzel, "Consumer Behavior and Health Care Change: The Role of the Mass Media," *Advances in Consumer Research* 5 (1977): 524-7.

at issue. As a result, short–term public communication campaigns should not be expected to produce sweeping changes in behavior. Commitment to a long–term effort is usually necessary.[8]

Rather than focusing on immediate behavior change, it is often more realistic and appropriate for a campaign to concentrate on achieving objectives that set the stage for behavior change in the long term. In this regard, mass media campaigns can accomplish the following:

1) increase awareness of a health problem and establish it as a priority concern;
2) increase knowledge and change beliefs that impede the adoption of health–promoting attitudes and behavior;
3) stimulate additional information–seeking through hotlines or other mechanisms;
4) motivate change by demonstrating the personal and social benefits that the desired behavior can bring;
5) teach new behavioral skills;
6) link the performance of newly acquired behaviors to cues in the physical and social environment;
7) demonstrate how various barriers to behavior change can be overcome;
8) teach self–management techniques for sustaining changes in behavior;
9) provide supports for maintaining the behavior, both directly and by stimulating interpersonal communication and the support of opinion leaders, spouses or peers.[9]

Mass media campaigns can also support school– or community–based programs in a variety of ways: by publicizing important changes in public policy; recruiting new program participants and volunteers; supporting fund–raising and coalition building; announcing the availability of self–help materials and program activities; and reinforcing the face–to–face instruction provided by these programs.

As described more fully below, AIDS prevention campaigns have contributed significantly to the American public's relatively high degree of knowledge about AIDS, both directly and through the promotion of information hotlines. These campaigns have also helped maintain the AIDS crisis at the top of the nation's health agenda. Unfortunately, what they have been unable to do is address the psychological barriers that impede the

---

[8] D. Roberts and N. Maccoby, "Effects of Mass Communication," in *Handbook of Social Psychology: Special Fields and Applications* (Vol. 2), eds. G. Lindzey and E. Aronson (New York: Random House, 1985).

[9] *Ibid*; and *op. cit.* W. DeJong and J.A. Winsten.

greater use of condoms, demonstrate the immediate personal benefits that condom use might bring, or teach the interpersonal skills necessary to introduce their use in a sexual relationship.

NATIONAL U.S. PUBLIC INFORMATION CAMPAIGNS ON AIDS

To date, national U.S. AIDS campaigns by the American Red Cross and the Centers for Disease Control have rightfully focused on increasing awareness of the AIDS threat, modes of disease transmission, and available prevention measures and on addressing common misconceptions about HIV. To avoid the political consequences that might follow more explicit information being presented on–air, the radio and television spots for both campaigns have provided telephone numbers through which the public can seek additional information. Neither campaign has focused specifically on homosexuals or bisexuals, but rather on the general (and presumably heterosexual) public.

American Red Cross: "Rumors Are Spreading Faster Than AIDS"
Assisted by the Advertising Council, the American Red Cross launched a multi–year campaign in 1987 to provide accurate information on AIDS transmission, with a focus on stopping rumors about transmission through casual contact or blood donation. Community outreach is the pillar of the Red Cross campaign, with brochures, films, videotapes and other educational materials disseminated to individuals, schools, churches and other civic organizations through AIDS coordinators working in over 600 local Red Cross chapters. Under the slogan "Rumors Are Spreading Faster Than AIDS," the campaign also provides several radio and television spots both to the networks and to local affiliate stations for their use during unsold commercial time. Each spot features a Hollywood celebrity who speaks directly to the audience. Both English– and Spanish–language spots are available. Media campaign materials also include "live announcer" copy for radio spots, print advertisements suitable for both the business and consumer press and posters. Importantly, all of the campaign materials encourage the public to call the Red Cross as a source of additional information.

Centers for Disease Control: "America Responds to AIDS"
Also launched in 1987, this national campaign sponsored by the U.S. Centers for Disease Control (CDC) began with a focus on providing the general public with basic factual information about AIDS, encouraging public discussion of the epidemic, and introducing the National AIDS Hotline as a source of more detailed information. First, in June 1987, under the leadership of U.S.. Surgeon General Koop, a brochure entitled, *Understanding AIDS*

was mailed to every U.S. household.[10] Three months later, the media campaign began. Campaign materials serving this general information function have also been developed in subsequent phases of the campaign.

The CDC's 1988 campaign targeted sexually active, heterosexual adults, especially those with multiple partners, and women at risk because of a sex partner's intravenous (IV) drug use. A mix of radio and television public service announcements, print advertisements, transit cards and posters presented information on the role of IV drug use in spreading AIDS to women and unborn children, advice to women to leave a man who refuses drug treatment, and pointed admonishments to avoid extramarital sex.

During this second phase, a large number of print advertisements were developed to promote condom use. One series ("What Have You Got Against a Condom?") merely informed readers that properly using a condom could be lifesaving. A second series, designed to encourage women to discuss condom use with their sex partners, depicted a woman who says, "If he doesn't have a condom, you just have to take a deep breath and tell him to go get one." Unfortunately, guidance regarding how that discussion might proceed was not provided. Only one print advertisement was bold enough to use sexual innuendo: Under a large black box, meant to be suggestive of a darkened bedroom, the headline reads, "If you want him to use a condom, this is all you have to say." Above, superimposed on the box, is a white–lettered caption: "Let me help you." During this campaign phase, only one Spanish–language television spot but no radio spots mentioned condoms explicitly.

CDC's 1989 campaign was designed to raise awareness of young people's vulnerability to AIDS and to encourage and enable parents and other adults to talk with young people about AIDS. *An AIDS Prevention Guide* —available through the national hotline and promoted through public service announcements—provides facts about HIV infection and AIDS, suggests techniques for delivering those facts effectively, and provides age-appropriate educational materials for adults to give to children and teenagers. Additional print advertisements promoting condoms were developed for this campaign phase; one English–language radio spot but no television spots mention condoms explicitly.

While the CDC was recently authorized to buy media time, the campaign previously relied solely on donated time by the networks and local affiliates. According to campaign reports, an estimated $18 million in air time was donated from October 1987 through June 1988, which resulted in reaching an estimated 80% of all U.S. households. By February 1989, the campaign had received more than $28 million in donated air time. A 1989

[10] Centers for Disease Control, "Understanding AIDS," HHS Publication No. (CDC) HHS–88–8404. (Rockville, MD: U.S. Public Health Service, Centers for Disease Control, 1987).

survey showed that 22% of U.S. adults recalled seeing or hearing during the previous month a public service announcement with the slogan "America Responds to AIDS."[11]

THE ROLE OF NEWS MEDIA COVERAGE

Both local and national news media have also played a major role in educating the American public about the AIDS crisis. Despite its overall positive contribution to increasing public understanding, U.S. news coverage has been frequently criticized by the public health community for undermining its efforts to eliminate misinformation about the routes of AIDS transmission. This criticism was especially vocal in the early 1980s, as the nation first became aware of the AIDS crisis.

Initially, when the disease was not perceived to be a major threat to the public at large, the news media did not cover AIDS extensively. Then, once it was learned that blood transfusion recipients and the sexual partners of intravenous drug users were also at substantial risk, the amount of press coverage soared. With public interest aroused, the competitive pressures on news reporters frequently resulted in incomplete investigative reporting and the sensationalist treatment of tentative scientific findings, both of which contributed to public confusion and panic.[12]

In one especially important case, a study reported in a 1983 issue of the *Journal of the American Medical Association* hinted that "routine contact" among household members might be sufficient for AIDS transmission to occur. Although subsequent studies showed that the disease was not spread through casual transmission, and although these studies were covered in turn by the news media, the initial news stories nevertheless had a residual effect.[13] This residual effect was sustained in the mid–1980s by extensive coverage of public hysteria about AIDS, as manifested in the boycotts of schools attended by AIDS victims, public arrests of AIDS patients by police wearing protective gloves, and so forth.

Critics of AIDS news coverage have also asserted that public confusion about casual transmission of AIDS is in part due to the vague terminology typically used by news reporters during the early days of the epidemic to describe AIDS–risk behavior (e.g. "sexual contact," "bodily fluids").[14]

[11] D.A. Dawson, "AIDS Knowledge and Attitudes for January–March 1989: Provisional Data from the National Health Interview Survey," Advance Data for Vital and Health Statistics, Public Health Service, 1989.

[12] J.A. Winsten, "Fighting Panic on AIDS," *The New York Times*, July 26, 1983.

[13] J.R. Milavsky, "AIDS and the Media," Paper presented at the Annual Meeting of the American Psychological Association, Atlanta, 1988.

[14] *Ibid*; and R. Shilts, *And the Band Played On: Politics, People, and the AIDS Epidemic* (New York: St. Martin's, 1987).

Although motivated by the existing standards of good taste, this initial reluctance to use explicit and clear language helped perpetuate several myths about AIDS transmission among sizable numbers of Americans.

Coverage in recent years has used more direct language, largely because news reporters are more appreciative of the need for absolute clarity, but also because such directness is more permissible now. Responding to the forthrightness of Surgeon General Koop's public statements about AIDS, the American public over time has become desensitized to and more accepting of explicit prevention messages about AIDS and other sexually transmitted diseases, a process that continues to the present day.

THE CURRENT STATE OF AMERICANS' KNOWLEDGE ABOUT AIDS

The National Health Interview Survey (NHIS), a periodic household interview survey of U.S. adults by the National Center for Health Statistics, has conducted a supplemental survey on AIDS since the last half of 1987. These surveys have shown consistently that an overwhelming majority of Americans are knowledgeable about the cause, transmission and prevention of AIDS. As noted by Louis Harris and Associates in describing the results of their own poll, "In general, Americans are highly knowledgeable about AIDS in areas which have been the center of media attention."[15]

As public information campaigns and news coverage on the transmission of AIDS have continued, increasingly fewer American adults perceive themselves to be at risk of getting AIDS. In late 1987, 60% of adults polled for the NHIS said there was no chance of their getting the AIDS virus.[16] By 1989, this figure had increased to 78%.[17]

Although fewer Americans now believe that AIDS can be transmitted through casual contact, unfortunately those who remain misinformed or confused on this point still represent a sizable group. A 1987 Harris poll, for example, showed that 23% of U.S. adults believed that AIDS was more contagious than the common cold.[18] According to NHIS statistics, in late 1987, only 53% stated correctly that it is either "very unlikely" or "definitely not possible" for a person to become infected by working near some-

---

[15] Louis Harris & Associates, Inc., *The National AIDS Awareness Test: Summary Report* (New York: Harris, 1987a).

[16] "HIV Epidemic and AIDS: Trends in Knowledge—United States, 1987 and 1988," *Morbidity and Mortality Weekly Report* 38 (May 26, 1989): 353–8.

[17] *Op. cit.* D.A. Dawson; and A.H. Hardy, "AIDS Knowledge and Attitudes for April–June 1989: Provisional Data from the National Health Interview Survey," Advance Data for Vital and Health Statistics, No. 179 (Hyattsville, MD: National Center for Health Statistics, Public Health Service, 1989).

[18] *Op. cit.* Louis Harris & Associates, Inc. 1987a.

one with AIDS.[19] By 1989, 71% stated this to be the case.[20] This represents a significant improvement over the earlier figures, but still leaves 29% of U.S. adults who remain to be thoroughly convinced that working near someone with AIDS is not a risk factor. Of great concern, a 1986 study of Massachusetts adolescents showed that 61% believed that giving blood puts one at risk of AIDS.[21] By 1988, this figure was still distressingly large, at 51%.[22]

Awareness of condoms as an effective means of reducing AIDS risk has been consistently high since the NHIS was first administered. In late 1987, 82% of adults polled said that condoms were "very" or "somewhat" effective in preventing AIDS transmission.[23] By 1989, 85% said this was the case.[24] Still, not all the facts about condom use are known. A 1987 poll of U.S. adults showed that, when asked to select from a list which barrier method would be the best protection against AIDS, 48% selected the correct response, latex condoms, but 28% selected natural–skin condoms, 6% selected the diaphragm, and 17% did not know. Moreover, 23% incorrectly identified as true the statement, "Condoms need only to be worn during anal sex."[25]

This relatively high degree of knowledge about AIDS is not necessarily translated into greater condom use, however. One study of sexually active black women college students showed that, while 94% knew that condoms reduce the risk of AIDS, 17% reported never using condoms, and 48% said they used them only rarely.[26] Similarly, a 1988 study of Massachusetts adolescents aged 16 to 19 showed that, of those who reported having sexual intercourse or other sexual contact during the past year, only 19% had adopted condom use because of AIDS. Among these sexually active adolescents, 63% said they had used condoms during the past year, but half of these respondents had failed to use them all the time.[27]

Another recent study provided more hopeful results: in a 1988 survey of never–married young men aged 15–19, 57% of those who were sexually active indicated in an in–person interview that they used a condom the last time they had intercourse. Among men aged 17–19 living in metropolitan areas, reported condom usage at last intercourse had more than doubled

[19] Op. cit. "HIV Epidemic and AIDS: Trends in Knowledge—United States, 1987 and 1988."

[20] Op. cit. D.A. Dawson; and op. cit. A.H. Hardy

[21] L. Strunin and R. Hingson, "Acquired Immunodeficiency Syndrome and Adolescents: Knowledge, Beliefs, Attitudes, and Behaviors," Pediatrics 79 (1987): 825–8.

[22] R. Hingson, L. Strunin and B. Berlin, "AIDS Transmission: Changes in Knowledge and Behaviors Among Adolescents: Massachusetts Statewide Surveys, 1986–1988," Pediatrics (In press).

[23] Op. cit. "HIV Epidemic and AIDS: Trends in Knowledge—United States, 1987 and 1988."

[24] Op. cit. D.A. Dawson; and op. cit. A.H.. Hardy.

[25] Op. cit. Louis Harris & Associates, Inc. 1987a.

[26] V.M. Mays and S.D. Cochran, "Issues in the Perception of AIDS Risk and Risk Reduction Activities by Black and Hispanic/Latina Women," American Psychologist 43 (1988): 949–57.

[27] Op. cit. R. Hingson, L. Strunin and B. Berlin.

since a similar 1979 survey.[28] While heartening, these figures still point to the need for continuing education efforts.

National public awareness campaigns and continuing news coverage have made a critical difference in educating the American public about AIDS and keeping this health problem at the top of the nation's health agenda. Although a shrinking minority, there are large numbers of people who remain ignorant of the basic facts about AIDS, making the continuation of these public awareness campaigns a clear necessity. At the same time, there is also a strong need to move beyond current information campaigns to motivate the wider and more frequent use of condoms.

THE LIMITED POTENTIAL OF THE U.S. BROADCAST MEDIA FOR MOTIVATING CONDOM USE: THE CONDOM'S NEGATIVE IMAGE

Despite their effectiveness, relatively low cost, and convenience, condoms are much maligned in the United States. The chief objection to condoms is their supposed impact on the pleasure of sexual intercourse— by reducing physical sensation, by interfering with the "naturalness" of the sexual act and by reducing spontaneity.[29] Furthermore, because they are associated in the public mind with "illicit" sex and venereal disease, condoms have a notoriety that makes their introduction an unwelcome commentary on the sexual act.[30]

Another objection to condoms is that suggesting their use can raise issues of interpersonal trust or can be personally embarrassing.[31] Some people fear their partner would be insulted or angered. Others simply do not know how to bring up the subject with their partners or what counter–arguments to give if objections are raised. For couples in what is purported to be a monogamous relationship, the sudden desire by one of the partners to use condoms can be especially troublesome.[32]

In short, condoms are seen as an imposition, an unwanted intrusion on the sexual act.

[28] F.L. Sonenstein, J.H. Pleck and L.C. Ku, "Sexual Activity, Condom Use and AIDS Awareness Among Adolescent Males," *Family Planning Perspectives* 21 (1989): 152–8.

[29] "Condoms," *Consumer Reports*, October 1979: 583–9; and W.W. Darrow, "Attitudes Toward Condom Use and the Acceptance of Venereal Disease Prophylactics," in *The Condom: Increasing Utilization in the United States*, eds. M.H. Redford, G.W. Duncan and D.J. Prager (San Francisco: San Francisco Press, 1974).

[30] N.J. Fiumara, "Ineffectiveness of Condoms in Preventing Venereal Disease," *Medical Aspects of Human Sexuality* 6 (1972): 146–50.

[31] *Op. cit.* M.Z. Solomon and W. DeJong, 1989.

[32] D.C. DesJarlais and S.R. Friedman, "The Psychology of Preventing AIDS Among Intravenous Drug Users: A Social Learning Conceptualization," *American Psychologist* 43 (1988): 865–70.

Recent commercial condom advertising has served to reinforce the public's negative image of the condom. Largely restricted to print ads, much of this advertising has exploited public fears of sexually transmitted diseases, and of AIDS in particular.[33] This advertising has also emphasized the specific features of the condom itself that enhance its performance as a protective device (e.g., Nonoxynol–9 spermicide, lubricants, adhesive seals). Such advertising does serve to enhance awareness of the AIDS threat and to inform the public that using condoms could reduce the risk of HIV transmission. Indeed, because of the AIDS threat, condom sales soared during the mid–1980s.

But with a focus on disease prevention and the technical aspects of product quality, this advertising also inadvertently portrays the condom as a device to be tolerated. By failing to suggest how the product can be enjoyed or how to introduce its use to one's partner, the advertising fails to address many consumers' primary concerns. As a result, the growth in condom sales has leveled off since 1988, falling far short of manufacturers' expectations.[34] In consequence, U.S. condom manufacturers are now largely abandoning AIDS—inspired scare tactics in favor of humor appeals and other traditional strategies used for packaged goods promotions, such as price–reduction coupons.[35]

REQUIREMENTS FOR SUCCESSFUL CONDOM PROMOTION

With a "consumer" orientation in view, what must be done to promote greater condom use is immediately evident. First, the image of the condom user has to be changed by associating condom use with other personal

[33] Although fear appeals of this sort have strong intuitive appeal, such campaigns are difficult to execute effectively and rarely succeed (C.K. Atkin, "Mass Media Information Campaign Effectiveness," in *Public Communication Campaigns*, eds. R. Rice and W. Paisley (Beverly Hills, CA: Sage, 1981); F. Boster and P. Mongeau, "Fear–arousing Persuasive Messages," in *Communication Yearbook* (Volume 8), ed. R Bostrom (Beverly Hills, CA: Sage, 1984); R.F.S. Job, "Effective and Ineffective Use of Fear in Health Promotion Campaigns," *American Journal of Public Health* 78 (1988): 163–7.). In limited circumstances, a recommended action might be adequate to remove a threat that is highly probable and immediate, making a fear appeal viable. More often, however, there is the real risk that a fear appeal will backfire and inadvertently make the problem behavior even more resistant to change (R. Rogers and C. Mewborn, "Fear Appeals and Attitude Change: Effect of a Threat's Noxiousness, Probability of Occurrence, and the Efficacy of Coping Responses," *Journal of Personality and Social Psychology* 34 (1976): 54–61). There is an additional problem with using fear appeals. While realistic fears may temporarily inspire condom use, such fears can dissipate or can be rationalized away in a moment of passion (or intoxication), when the risks of pregnancy or disease are reassessed against the potential disruptiveness of using condoms and the possibility of a sexual partner's strong negative reaction to their suggested use (M.Z. Solomon and W. DeJong, "Recent Sexually Transmitted Disease Prevention Efforts and Their Implications for AIDS Health Education," *Health Education Quarterly* 13 (1986): 301–16).

[34] M. Gladwell, "Condom Consciousness: Unexpected Slowdown in Sales Worries Health Officials," *Washington Post Health*, February 21, 1989, p. 6; and R. Rothenberg, "Condom Makers Change Approach," *The New York Times*, August 8, 1988, p. D1, D6.

[35] *Op. cit.* R. Rothenberg.

qualities that are considered desirable such as power, status, popularity and intelligence. In particular, condom use should be more strongly associated with a modern masculine image. In Jamaica, for example, condoms were introduced under the Panther brand name, a name chosen after thorough marketing research for its "macho" connotations.[36]

Second, promotion efforts should demonstrate that there is a new normative consensus in favor of condom use. Peers are a major influence on normative expectations concerning all aspects of sexuality, especially among adolescents and young adults.[37] This suggests that if adolescents and young adults can see, through advertising and other promotions, that condoms have widespread acceptance among both men and women, they will be more likely themselves to begin using the product.

Third, the condom should be positioned as a product that couples rather than individuals use. Accordingly, these promotions should model how a sexual partner might be persuaded, through a mix of logical argumentation and sexual innuendo, to use condoms.[38] It should be cautioned that this may be an especially difficult message for certain target audiences to act on. In particular, Hispanic women, who are traditionally expected to be sexually modest, run the risk of stigmatization and rejection if they raise the subject or supply condoms for their sexual partners.[39]

Most important, promotion efforts should suggest that condoms need not interfere with sexual pleasure and might even enhance it if their use is approached in a sexually appealing way.[40] This does not require graphic depictions of sexual acts, but does necessitate a frank presentation of how condom use can be mutually satisfying to both partners.

Past and current U.S. marketing efforts have tried to accomplish this objective by emphasizing the condom's thinness and by devising evocative brand names (e.g. "Sensitol")[41] and advertising slogans (e.g. "Trojans: For That Certain Feeling").[42] On the other hand, past U.S. advertising has rarely suggested the possibilities of sexual pleasure directly. One exception is Schmid's Fiesta™ brand: "Fiesta: A Little Color Can Add a Lot More Fun to Your Sex Life."[43] More recently, American manufacturers have offered

[36] W. DeJong, "Condom Promotion: The Need for a Social Marketing Program in America's Inner Cities," *American Journal of Health Promotion* 3 (1989): 5–10, 16.

[37] C.S. Chilman, "Adolescent Sexuality in a Changing American Society: Social and Psychological Perspectives," (Washington, D.C.: U.S. Government Printing Office, 1980).

[38] *Op. cit.* M.Z. Solomon and W. DeJong, 1986; and *op. cit.* M.Z. Solomon and W. DeJong, 1989.

[39] *Op. cit.* V.M. Mays and S.D. Cochran.

[40] *Op. cit.* M.Z. Solomon and W. DeJong, 1989.

[41] S.A. Baker, "Advertising Male Contraceptives," in *The Condom: Increasing Utilization in the United States*, eds. M.H. Redford, G.W. Duncan and D.J. Prager (San Francisco: San Francisco Press, 1974).

[42] L.R. Brenner, "Condommunications," in *The Condom: Increasing Utilization in the United States*, eds. M.H. Redford, G.W. Duncan and D.J. Prager (San Francisco: San Francisco Press, 1974).

[43] *Op. cit.* S.A. Baker.

condoms in a wider variety of shapes, colors, textures and scents, and while condoms themselves are not effective in sexual stimulation, the use of color and rough surfaces can help make them seem so.[44]

Not surprisingly, condom promotion in other countries has been more adventurous. For example, a Swedish campaign aimed at adolescents was much more open about the pleasures of condom use. A new condom was developed for the campaign and introduced with a randy tagline asserting that the condom "just grows and grows." In describing this campaign, Ajax writes: "It should be fun to use the condom if the product is made attractive to the consumer. This is the only way to reach those who are not highly motivated to use contraceptives."[45]

A research–tested videotape developed in the U.S. for inner-city blacks provides a good example of how the use of condoms can be "eroticized" while still adhering to mainstream standards of propriety.[46] Through presentation of a dramatic "soap opera" entitled "Let's Do Something Different," the videotape acknowledges the widely perceived disadvantages of condom use, but emphasizes the ways in which condoms can actually enhance sexual pleasure by reinforcing a modern masculine image for the male partner, by prolonging intercourse,[47] and by giving both partners peace of mind.[48] Most important, the videotape presents the idea that putting the condom on can be imaginatively integrated into foreplay. In the final scene, the lead character, Diane, playfully suggests to her reluctant boyfriend that, when they next make love, she be the one to put a condom in place. Coupled with her factual arguments, this sexually appealing promise finally wins him over.

RESTRICTIONS ON CONDOM PROMOTION THROUGH THE BROADCAST MEDIA

The use of condoms is morally unacceptable to large numbers of people because of their opposition to contraception. Because the U.S. broadcast media seek to avoid alienating large segments of their mass audience and the political or economic pressures that would ensue,[49] they cannot be readily utilized to communicate the specific information that is necessary for motivating condom use.

[44] Y.S. Matsumoto, A. Koizumi and T. Nohara, "Condom Use in Japan," *Studies in Family Planning* 3 (1972): 251–5.

[45] L. Ajax, "How to Market a Nonmedical Contraceptive: A Case Study from Sweden," in *The Condom: Increasing Utilization in the United States*, eds. M.H. Redford, G.W. Duncan and D.J. Prager (San Francisco: San Francisco Press, 1974).

[46] *Op. cit.* M.Z. Solomon and W. DeJong, 1989.

[47] R.A. Hatcher, "Reasons to Recommend the Condom," *Medical Aspects of Human Sexuality* 12 (1978): 91.

[48] *Op. cit.* "Condoms."

[49] K.C. Montgomery, *Target: Prime Time* (New York: Oxford University Press, 1989).

While some local affiliates do accept commercial condom advertising, the major U.S. television networks do not. A 1987 poll showed that 60% of U.S. adults were in favor of contraceptive advertising on television, versus 37% who were not.[50] When reminded that Surgeon General Koop and others have called for increased condom use to stem the AIDS epidemic, support for contraceptive advertising increased to 74% of those polled. While such statistics embolden critics of the television industry to pressure the networks to air contraceptive advertising, the fact remains that the minority opposed to this is still a sizable and highly vocal group.

The concerns of national broadcasters have decidedly influenced the way in which AIDS prevention public service campaigns have dealt with the issue of condom use. As recently as 1988, this meant that condom use could not be mentioned in television or radio public service announcements as an AIDS preventive. Consider the contrast between print and broadcast advertising developed for the CDC's "America Responds to AIDS" campaign in 1988, its second year. A print advertisement from that year showed a young black woman who describes how she and her baby both contracted AIDS because a man she was involved with was "shooting up" drugs and sharing needles. The advertising copy depicted her saying, "Had I know better, I would have made him use condoms... In contrast, a similar radio spot, entitled "Baby," did not mention condoms but instead referred vaguely to the need for "protection." A corresponding television spot did **not** even include that reference, but merely ended with the plea, "Please, **don't** let this happen to you." As noted before, the only CDC television spot that has mentioned condoms explicitly was in Spanish, "Sandra y Luis," also developed in 1988.[51] A single radio spot developed in 1989 also mentions condoms.

In 1989, with Surgeon General Koop's continuing outspokenness on the need to promote condom use and with the public's evolving tolerance of direct AIDS prevention messages, a new public service campaign has focused more narrowly on motivating condom use. This campaign, developed by the American Foundation for AIDS Research (AmFAR), the National AIDS Network (NAN), and the Advertising Council, introduces condoms as an AIDS preventive with the slogan, "Help stop AIDS. Use a condom." The campaign's general acceptance by television "gatekeepers" was considered a major breakthrough by the Advertising Council. Consistent with current

[50] Louis Harris & Associates, Inc., *Attitudes About Television, Sex and Contraception* (New York: Harris, 1987b).

[51] The CDC campaign did test the limits of the network rules by developing its famous "Socks" spot, in which condom use is alluded to but not cited explicitly. As a young man puts on a crew sock, he says: "If I told you I could save my life just by putting on my socks, you wouldn't take me seriously. Because life is never that simple. But watch... Okay. You're right. That wouldn't really save my life. But there's something just as simple that could." Network reaction to the spot was mixed. ABC accepted the spot for late–night airing, but CBS rejected it outright.

network policies, which prescribe that condoms be mentioned as a small part of larger health–related messages, the television spots developed for this campaign take a straightforward, factual approach, emphasizing the frightful consequences of the disease and the impossibility of knowing who might be carrying the AIDS virus.[52] Unfortunately, like its predecessors, this campaign also fails to address the key psychological barriers to condom use.

THE POTENTIAL ROLE OF TELEVISION ENTERTAINMENT PROGRAMMING

Television entertainment programming provides an additional opportunity for presenting AIDS prevention messages to the American general public. For many people, and for children and adolescents especially, such programming is an important source of information about how the world works and how one should behave in that world.[53] As summarized by one researcher, "…people are as likely to acquire attitudes, emotional responses, and new styles of conduct from filmed and televised models as from live models. The basic modeling process is the same."[54]

In recent years, a number of weekly entertainment programs have periodically dealt with the subject of condoms, with treatments ranging from joke punchlines to entire episodes that explore issues related to responsible sexuality.[55] During one week in early 1989, for example, three situation comedies—"Golden Girls," "Head of the Class," and "Hooperman"—all included scenes in which a main character goes to a pharmacy to purchase condoms. During the previous television season, an episode of "The Hogan Family" showed the oldest teenage boy declining to have sex with an attractive girl because he had no condoms.

In judging the suitability of such treatments, network executives responsible for reviewing program content do not apply hard and fast rules but general guidelines. For example, condoms can be introduced in a program if doing so is "dramatically relevant" and if the treatment is "tasteful." And, in general, discussions of condoms must be balanced against discus-

52 A spot entitled "Vilma" is typical. On camera, we see a young black woman holding her baby. She says, tearfully, "I have AIDS. And my baby has AIDS. My husband may have it, but he won't go to the doctor. In the beginning, he wouldn't even talk about it. My mother helps us, but sometimes I think she's afraid. Every night I kneel by my baby's crib and pray to be strong for him. Every night I pray that my baby won't die." The announcer then intones: "Protect people you love. Use a condom."

53 C.K. Atkin, "Television Socialization and Risky Driving by Teenagers," *Alcohol, Drugs and Driving* 5 (1989): 1–11.

54 D.F. Roberts, "The Impact of Media Portrayals of Risky Driving on Adolescents: Some Speculations," *Alcohol, Drugs and Driving* 5 (1989): 13–20.

55 B. Mondello, "From Broadway to Hollywood: The Imprint of AIDS on Modern Drama," *Washington Post Health*, December 29, 1987, pp. 10–14.

sions of sexual abstinence, especially when adolescents are involved. Importantly, what is allowed by the networks also depends on the time of day the show airs and the audience's expectations of the show and its characters. Thus, network executives have no in-principle objections to dramatic portrayals that address the psychological barriers to condom use. Each treatment is reviewed carefully, its acceptability depending entirely on the specific execution and its context.

Still, even with this greater leeway, it remains doubtful that entertainment programming can by itself make a critical difference in overcoming the psychological barriers to condom use. As already demonstrated by past programming, entertainment programs can easily and routinely portray a new normative consensus in favor of condom use and can associate product use with a modern masculine image. On the other hand, addressing public concerns about the condom's supposed interference with sexual pleasure or suggesting how condom use can be successfully negotiated with a sex partner requires fuller treatments, and there are practical limitations on the frequency with which such scenes could be introduced. An additional difficulty is that, given current broadcast practices, such entertainment programming would stand alone, unsupported by paid or public service advertising providing the same message.

THE POTENTIAL ROLE OF BROADCAST NEWS COVERAGE

Broadcast news programming also provides limited opportunities for providing clear and consistent messages to promote condom use. This fact was amply demonstrated by press coverage of New York City's announcement of its 1987 AIDS campaign aimed at promoting condom use among heterosexuals (see Gossett and Warshaw, this volume). Several television reports aired the campaign's spots as part of their news coverage, thereby furthering the objectives of the campaign. On the other hand, these reports also featured interviews with a clerical spokesman for the Catholic Archdiocese of New York, who objected strongly to the "graphic" portrayals in the campaign's television spots and their implicit endorsement of "promiscuity." In further support of his attack on the campaign, this spokesman asserted that the condom's high failure rate made it a poor choice in AIDS prevention efforts. This claim, which failed to account for consumers' sometimes improper or inconsistent use of condoms, was not challenged in any of the news reports.[56]

[56] J.D. Sherris, D. Lewison and G. Fox, "Update on Condoms: Products, Protection, Promotion," *Population Reports H6* (Baltimore: Population Information Program, Johns Hopkins University, 1982).

A NEED FOR EXPANDED COMMUNITY–BASED EDUCATION PROGRAMS

Because current restrictions in the broadcast media are unlikely to change radically in the near future, we urge that current public awareness campaigns be supplemented by an expansion of community–based educational programs that stress condom promotion. Such programs targeted at male homosexuals, IV drug users, prostitutes and runaway youth are already in place or being developed in many communities and will continue to be implemented elsewhere.[57] These programs need to be expanded. In addition, new programs are needed that target sexually active adolescent and young adult heterosexuals, especially in well–defined neighborhoods where AIDS is more prevalent. These new programs should rely on direct "selling" approaches, with outreach through school–based health clinics, family planning services, drug rehabilitation centers, churches, and community/neighborhood organizations or even through door–to–door sales.

For certain inner–city neighborhoods, community–based social marketing campaigns similar to successful programs that the U.S. government and others have helped create in Third World countries should be developed.[58] Going beyond education, social marketing programs can be designed to promote, distribute and sell condoms and other forms of contraception or prophylaxis through existing retail outlets at a relatively low, subsidized price, thereby reaching markets not normally reached through profit––driven commercial efforts.[59] Even in countries where all direct advertising of condoms is expressly forbidden, and where initial public acceptance is limited due to religious or political dictates, such programs have been adapted and eventually succeeded in generating increased condom use.

While time–intensive and expensive, programs that emphasize person–to–person and social marketing approaches, with the opportunity for dialogue they present, are currently our best hope of motivating people to use condoms. Importantly, such community—based programs could be supported in the local broadcast media in two important ways. First, daily news coverage, editorials, documentaries and station–developed public service announcements could publicize these programs along with local information hotlines, thereby helping to recruit new program participants and volunteers and to build financial support. Second, local affiliates could

[57] U.S. Conference of Mayors, "Local Responses to Acquired Immunodeficiency Syndrome (AIDS): A Report of 55. Cities" (Washington, D.C.: U.S. Conference of Mayors, 1984); and U.S. General Accounting Office, "AIDS Education: Reaching Populations at Higher Risk" (Washington, D.C.: U.S. General Accounting Office, 1988).

[58] *Op. cit.* W. DeJong.

[59] D. Altmann, P. Piotrow, "Social Marketing: Does It Work?" *Population Reports J21* (Baltimore: Population Information Program, Johns Hopkins University, 1984); and *op. cit.* J.D. Sherris, D. Lewison and G. Fox.

substantially increase their commitment of air time for spots developed for the AMFAR/NAN campaign ("Help stop AIDS. Use a condom.") and any new campaigns that might emerge. Depending on local public sentiment, individual television and radio stations could choose to air paid condom advertising or to produce and air their own public service announcements that explicitly address the psychological barriers to condom use.

Preparation of this chapter was supported by grants to the Center for Health Communication of the Harvard School of Public Health, from the Exxon Corporation, the Esther A. and Joseph Klingenstein Fund, the Pew Charitable Trusts, and the Helena Rubinstein Foundation.

AIDS, Government and the Press

In the best of circumstances, the relationship between the press and the AIDS public health community constitutes an uneasy, sometimes tense, alliance forged by a shared bottom-line desire to disseminate accurate information about the epidemic.

In the worst of circumstances, the two institutions are either in a state of outright animosity coupled with distrust or, at the opposite extreme, the public health establishment directly dictates the content and tone of all press reports on the subject.

As the AIDS epidemic has expanded both in volume and geographic distribution many health officials and well–meaning scientists have spoken of "using the media to educate people about AIDS" in order to promote behavior changes, discount improper fears, even forward political agendas.

For their part, some reporters wedded to "the AIDS beat" have adopted the AIDS battle as their own, joining the physicians in the trenches without maintaining sufficient distance to judge how well the battle is being fought. Both cases represent a failure to serve the needs of the public.

There are two terms that are often used interchangeably: the media and journalism. This confusion of terms underscores a larger and troubling misunderstanding of the role of the Fourth Estate.

The media, which occasionally include some semblance of journalism, in fact, comprise a set of technologies including movies, television, radio, wire services, facsimile transmitters, photocopiers, computer information services and offset press machines. The media can be bent to any purpose, from artistic expression to advertising and propaganda.

Journalism is a profession, which, under ideal circumstances, operates under a very specific set of ethical rules. Journalists use a set of technologies to relay their information to the public. When a journalist is in top form, he or she often is ready to attack other uses of the media–certainly to question their accuracy, ethics and efficacy.

Appreciation of the distinction between the media and journalism is central to understanding why the media can be used effectively to educate people about AIDS; journalism cannot, and should not, ever be "used" to that end.

It would be monumentally tragic if well–meaning public health officials were to use techniques to control the pandemic which ultimately undermine the distinction between the media and journalism. Unfortunately, it appears that throughout the world this is already occurring, and the press has by and large acquiesced.

AIDS in the Pattern I Nations

The World Health Organization has identified three classic AIDS epidemic patterns, with Pattern I being that seen primarily in industrialized Western nations. For these countries, AIDS is already a comparatively old story, receiving less press attention as the populace adjusts to the idea that the disease is, at least for the present generation, a permanent, albeit loathsome, feature on the public health landscape.

At the present time the key problems in Pattern I AIDS press coverage are complacency, homophobia, increasing need for reporter specialization, sophisticated manipulation of the press, and what, for lack of a better term, might be called "the despair factor."

It is perhaps ironic that a problem which shows no sign of subsiding and which eludes solution should cease to constitute news in some quarters, but AIDS rarely grabs the front page or top of a newscast any more, and many reporters complain that it is increasingly difficult to convince their editors and producers that there is a need for continued coverage.

In the United States and some European nations there are indications, according to the WHO and the U.S. Centers for Disease Control (CDC), that the numbers of newly diagnosed cases of the disease are at a plateau, perhaps even declining, among gay and bisexual men. Some observers assert a decline can also be seen among intravenous drug users in some cities. Several major publications and broadcasters have concluded, therefore, that urgency, and a concomitant mandate for strong levels of journalistic commitment to the story are no longer required. It is commonly said that "the AIDS story is over," and many top reporters in Europe and the U.S. have, in the last year, switched off the AIDS beat. For example, one of Sweden's top T.V. reporters had to fight for air time to broadcast reports from the Fourth International Conference on AIDS, which was held in Stockholm.

It should be noted that when many say "the AIDS story is over" they are, in fact, sighing with relief that "the general population isn't affected." In 1987 and 1988 a great number of news column inches were devoted to discussion of whether or not the epidemic would soon spread into the middle class heterosexual community. As "alarmists,"such as William Masters and Virginia Johnson, were silenced, the press rooms of North America and Europe turned away from the story.

The epidemic, however, continued to expand, affecting, according to recent CDC and WHO estimates, upwards of 50% of the urban homosexual populations in such cities as Geneva, New York and San Francisco and an alarming 60–80% of the intravenous drug users of New York and New Jersey. Lack of attention from the press to this toll reflects the racial, cultural and social attitudes of those in the news rooms of the industrialized world.

Complacency has set in, as the death toll mounts: by 1993, one U.S. resident will be diagnosed HIV positive every 36 seconds, but in the eyes of those who make command decisions for the press it is the color, class and sexual preferences of these unfortunates, not their numbers, which dictate their relative news value.

In Pattern I nations there is a press room term for riveting stories: "sexy news." The story needn't be about sex to fulfill the necessary criteria for "hot" headline–grabbing news. In press room thinking AIDS was a "sexy story" when American movie star Rock Hudson died, when parents surrounded a New Jersey schoolboy with AIDS to prevent him from entering a classroom, when the human immunodeficiency virus was discovered and a Franco–American rivalry—better yet, scandal—developed, and when famed anti–Communist Roy Cohn succumbed to the disease.

In the future AIDS will be "sexy news" when other famous people die from the disease, and if either a vaccine or cure is found. Barring such events, the epidemic will, realistically, continue to fall victim to news room boredom, and coverage will depend greatly upon the dedication of individual journalists, editors and producers.

Faced with such nonchalance, many members of the AIDS community have turned to manipulative tactics to inject a new sense of urgency into the journalistic community. Reporters are now commonly given exclusive leaks on stories involving policy confrontations between AIDS activists and government figures. In some cases, scientific and policy meetings are held with "selected press" access, a bald attempt to control which reporters and institutions can observe unfolding events. Most top scientists, policy makers, pharmaceutical companies, hospitals and AIDS activists now have public relations officers; many have hired Madison Avenue–style promotions firms to screen out press calls and "leak" information when desired.

Journalists have all too often succumbed to such manipulation, savoring their special relationships with top government and scientific sources and failing to ask themselves why people who are allegedly leading the war against AIDS have the time and inclination to selectively feed information to members of the press. Writing in the March 1989 issue of the American magazine Esquire, San Francisco journalist Randy Shilts expressed dismay over what he described as a rather cozy relationship between the U.S. press and government officials: "AIDS had spread because indolent news organizations shunned their responsibility to provide tough, adversarial reporting, instead of basing stories largely on the Official Truth of government press releases."

In short, as AIDS becomes more institutionalized its players take on all the propaganda and press tactics used by other multi–billion dollar efforts, such as national defense, foreign policy and environmental disputes.

Meanwhile, the seasoned AIDS reporters are burning out. Some cite increasing difficulties in both researching a story and getting it past editorial roadblocks. Others are simply overwhelmed by the despair of AIDS, particularly when coupled with the economic and political obstacles to equal care for all the planet's HIV targets.

Pattern II: The Information Gap

In Pattern II nations, where the epidemic is predominantly heterosexually and perinatally transmitted, the power of the press is limited by a combination of political, economic and social factors.

Per capita income of Pattern II nations is far below that of Pattern I (see table 13-1), as is per capita health spending.

Illiteracy rates in some Pattern II nations are strikingly high, illustrating the shortcomings of reliance on newspapers and the printed word.

In addition, many languages have no words for such things as viruses and cells; fewer can describe immunology or virology without resorting to European languages. For example, one Swahili term for HIV is *vinidogodogo*, which is best translated as very tiny germ. It is accurate, yet fails to convey the rather special threat viruses pose to human beings compared to other microorganisms. This may affect attitudes about transmission risks and self–protection.

Table 13-1. *Per capita income, literacy and percent of urban population in relation to the three patterns of the AIDS epidemic.*

Pattern/ Country	Per capita income 1985	Education & literacy spending 1985 as % of GNP	% of literate adults M	% of literate adults F	% of urban population in 1987
Pattern I					
United States	16 240	6.7	>95	>95	74
France	8 932	6.1	>95	>95	74
United Kingdom	7 882	5.2	>95	>95	92
Pattern II					
Kenya	291	6.7	49	70	22
Mozambique	156	(NA)	12.2	44	23
Nigeria	1 155	1.8	31	54	33
Tanzania	250	4.3	88	93	28
Uganda	300	2.7	45	70	10
Zaire	150	3.4	45	79	38
Pattern III					
Brazil	1 527	3.3	72.8	76.3	75
China (PRC)	342	2.3	51.1	79.2	21
Hungary	7 331	5.7	99.3	98.5	58
Japan	10 920	5.1	>95	>95	77
Philippines	520	1.7	82.8	83.9	41
Soviet Union	7 635	7.0	>95	>95	66
Saudi Arabia	6 950	10.6	>95	>95	75
Mexico	2 139	2.1	88	92	71

Colleagues from several African nations tell me the language constraints, alone, force less precise, often simplistic coverage of AIDS. It is not uncommon, for example, to hear the same story covered by a given reporter in five languages on East African radio, with all but the English language version confined to very basic concepts of the disease.

This implies that the well–educated European language speaking population has better access to AIDS information.

In addition to language, class and literacy, there are other limits to press information. Radio is by far the most powerful medium in most of the Pattern II nations; it is also state–owned and operated. Where television exists, it, too, is often under state control. State control does not by definition mean direct state intervention and censorship are common, but it does ease the way for such government interference. One need not envision a dictatorship to illustrate the point; the current United Kingdom government has censored several major BBC reports in the last two years.

Public health officials might mistakenly take comfort in this, thinking their AIDS efforts will proceed more smoothly without the scrutiny of a critical press. Similarly, these officials may be loathe to waste their time with foreign journalists whose training dictates that they ask tough questions and maintain a skeptical distance from the answers.

However, each country, and the global community as a whole, are best served by a press which is able to question health authorities. It is well documented that the belated U.S. government response to the epidemic was the final result of a combination of press pressure and unrelenting political activism from the gay community.

When foreign journalists first turned their attention to Africa's AIDS epidemic in 1985–86, there were two unfortunate outcomes: health officials recoiled from questions that placed the origin of AIDS in Africa and attacked Western racism, and the foreign reporters felt restricted in their access to information, crying "cover up." In the years that followed, tensions between the two groups eased as each gained a greater appreciation of the professional, cultural and political needs of the other. Nevertheless, the two forces continued to view one another with shared suspicion, much of which transcends the orientations of their respective professions. Racism, cultural misunderstandings, anti–Western sentiments, and understandable government (and individual) reluctance to release information which puts its country in a bad light all continue to impede the flow of accurate nformation.

There are two reasons why it is in the interest of national public health officials to improve this situation: foreign aid and global understanding. If foreign scientific and financial assistance is needed for a given nation to combat its epidemic, foreign press coverage should logically be encouraged; it may draw attention to a nation's plight and point out specific areas of concern. But opening the visa offices to Western reporters, in particular, is not without risks. These journalists are aggressive, competitive, trained to smell scandal and ask tough questions. Rather than take offense, officials would be advised to anticipate such behavior. For their part, foreign correspondents should consider whether or not the standards to which they hold officials in a developing country exceed those they would apply to officials at home.

From a global perspective the flow of information is vital to understanding and controlling the pandemic; anything which impedes that flow should be discouraged. Journalists would do well to remember their historical role as chroniclers of the epidemic and avoid sensationalism for the sake of short-term headline glory.

Finally, the ever–shrinking "global village" should consider the implication of two facts: at the International AIDS Conference in Stockholm one out of 800 registered journalists was African, and a handful came from other developing countries; the 1988 Montreal meeting was attended by over 40 journalists from developing countries. There was a staggering improvement in both the volume and quality of reporting from Montreal to developing countries. The reason was economic.

What made the difference between Stockholm and Montreal was a program of journalist sponsorship, funded by the WHO, Canada's IRDC and the Ford Foundation. In the coming years the International AIDS Conference is scheduled to take place in expensive cities in the Northern Hemisphere such as San Francisco, Florence and Boston. These meetings, and smaller AIDS gatherings, should consider the lesson of Montreal and seek ethically sound ways to underwrite the travel, communications, and per diem costs of journalists from developing countries. Lacking such support, a journalist from, for example, Zambia can't possibly travel to Florence in 1991 to attend the international meeting. In their absence, the AIDS information gap will persist, perhaps even expand.

PATTERN III NATIONS: THE MIX

Because the epidemic is relatively new in a typical Pattern III nation the predominant modes of transmission may not be clear. Health officials have not always identified educational target groups and AIDS campaigns, where they are under way, tend to be fairly generalized.

The character and structure of the press in Pattern III nations also defies definition: it runs the gamut from free–wheeling privately owned competitive journalism to uniformly state–run tightly controlled press. All the press issues raised in the discussions of Pattern I and II nations may be applicable in Pattern III (see table 13-1).

Pattern III nations do have one golden opportunity which was not available to those of Pattern I and II; that of learning from history. Their epidemics are just beginning. Unfortunately, the short history of AIDS shows lessons are rarely learned.

The key lessons I might venture to pass on, as a journalist who has been covering the epidemic since it was known merely as an unusual incidence of Pneumocystis carinii and Kaposi's sarcoma among gay California men, include the following three general policy suggestions in relation to the media and AIDS.

First, prejudicial attitudes journalists and health officials may harbor towards members of high-risk groups should be confronted immediately. When honesty prevails, every reporter or scientist who dealt with AIDS in the early years of the epidemic, from 1981 to 1984 in the U.S. and Europe, made statements they would like, today, to retract, statements which reflected their homophobia, or, if they are gay, their defensiveness. All scientists and reporters mirror the culture in which they work, and there are times, as in the era of AIDS, in which the general biases of society as a whole must be overcome by the individual to allow truly professional performance.

Such biases are not limited to homophobia: AIDS has highlighted such attitudes as racism, ethnic rivalries, nationalism, hatred of or disdain for drug addicts, economic class attitudes and the exaggerated personal fears of disease held by many reporters. For accuracy's sake, as well as that of human compassion, all involved in the early stages of the epidemic need to constantly consider the social filters through which they are viewing the epidemic and those it attacks.

Second, officials should never delude themselves with the belief that the press reaches all elements of society. Indeed, in both the U.S. and Europe, it is obvious that many of the individuals at highest risk for AIDS are alienated from mainstream press sources by a combination of language difficulties, illiteracy and cultural differences. The bulk of the press in Western nations reflects the language and cultural perspectives of the majority populations. If, however, foreign immigrant workers, unemployed drug users, semi–literate homeless women and recent immigrants are at risk of infection by HIV, educational efforts must be specifically targeted at these individuals, through methods other than the use of the mainstream media. Furthermore, where the majority of the population relies upon electronic media as the primary source of news information, as is the case in the U.S., health officials should note the peculiar limitations of such outlets. Television and radio cannot be considered reliable AIDS information outlets if they are not permitted to discuss anal intercourse or condoms.

Finally, public health officials should never rely solely upon the press to disseminate such vital information as modes of transmission, methods of protection and reasons not to fear particular social groups. In countries such as the U.S., in which the government allowed the epidemic to unfold without federally sponsored education efforts, the results have been catastrophic. The press did its job in the U.S. for six years, pointing out debates and controversies that no government institution or final authority ever stepped in to resolve. While some heads–of–state in Africa and Europe embraced AIDS patients publicly to allay public hysteria, no such action was taken in the U.S. until 1987. The public was deluged with conflicting press information about AIDS which was not addressed at a top federal level until the spring of 1988, when U.S. Surgeon General C. Everett Koop mailed an AIDS pamphlet to every American household.

As a result, polls show the American public continues to harbor dangerous misunderstandings about AIDS. While the term "AIDS" is more familiar to U.S. citizens than the name of the nation's President, a 1988 survey by the U.S. National Center for Health Statistics found that a quarter of the population felt they "knew very little about AIDS." Over one–third were unaware that the disease was caused by a virus, and 40 percent thought one could get AIDS from a toilet seat.

A *New York Times*/CBS poll released in October 1988 found that three–quarters of the American people said they had "no sympathy" for homosexual and intravenous drug using people with AIDS. A startling 19% said they had "no sympathy for people with AIDS regardless of how they got the disease."

AIDS is directly related to the two subjects people, regardless of their culture, are least likely to discuss openly and honestly: sex and death. Worse yet, AIDS means sex can equal death, pleasure can be hell, life–giving may be life–taking. It should, therefore, not be surprising to anybody that the press, public health leaders and the public throughout our planet have difficulty accepting the reality of AIDS for what it is: a disease, caused by a virus, which spreads through very specific means and theoretically endangers the lives of anybody who practices activities which put them at risk. Nothing more, nothing less.

SUGGESTED READING

Committee to Protect Journalists. *Attacks on the Press*. New York, 1989.

Kirp, David L. *Learning by Heart: AIDS and Schoolchildren in America's Communities*. Rutgers Press, 1989.

Moore, Mike. *Health Risks and the Press: Perspectives on Media Coverage of Risk Assessment and Health*. The Media Institute, American Medical Association, 1989.

Panos Institute. *AIDS and the Third World*. New Society Publishers, Philadelphia, 1988.

The New York City Campaign

Milton Gossett
Jeremy Warshaw

In the fall of 1986, Saatchi & Saatchi, the world's largest advertising company, and New York City, America's largest city government, became partners in a marketing communications program. The objective was to acquaint the heterosexual community in New York City with the dangers of AIDS. This partnership resulted in the first comprehensive paid media program on the subject of AIDS and turned out to be a pioneering effort that taught both sides some interesting lessons in dealing with social concerns in a political environment. It also revealed the difficulties of dealing with public and religious mores as well as often ambivalent attitudes of the media world in relation to AIDS.

Saatchi & Saatchi Advertising has a heritage of a merger between two major advertising agencies—Dancer Fitzgerald Sample and Compton Advertising —and of a long history of public service advertising. One of its more famous campaigns, McGruff the Crime Dog ("Take A Bite Out Of Crime"), has become a part of the American scene. The agency, and particularly its creative people, have always looked forward to public service campaigns because they allow a freedom of expression and opportunity for recognition over and above that offered by packaged goods and service industry advertising.

On October 15, 1986, Jeremy Warshaw, a vice president of Saatchi & Saatchi Advertising Inc., called Deputy Mayor Herb Rickman and volunteered the services of the agency to the City of New York. Jeremy Warshaw had in mind involvement in some sort of civic campaign similar to the famous "I Love New York" campaign. His offer was quickly accepted and he was asked if Saatchi & Saatchi would work with New York City in developing a campaign aimed at communicating the dangers of AIDS to the heterosexual population. Jeremy Warshaw, at that time, like most of New York's population, had only a sketchy idea what AIDS was and how it was transmitted. To be absolutely candid, he and his partner—Creative Director Charlie Abrams—were interested in putting together a brilliant advertising campaign on any public service subject and not necessarily in helping to solve the problems associated with the modern epidemic of AIDS. That was before they were educated themselves about AIDS and became heavily involved in AIDS education along with others in the agency.

Once Warshaw and Abrams received agency management approval to become involved, a briefing meeting took place at the agency in November, 1986. There, Deputy Mayor Herb Rickman, Public Health Commissioner Dr. Stephen Joseph and Assistant Health Commissioner Peggy Clarke outlined for them the health care project the City had in mind. Their outline went as follows: The statistics on the spread of AIDS were alarming, and continued to rise. At the time there were thought to be four hundred thousand people with the AIDS virus. There were thousands more people with AIDS-related diseases, and ten thousand people diagnosed with AIDS.

Mayor Koch and the city commissioners had been alerted to the present and potential dangers of the spread of the AIDS virus. It was recognized that the groups most at risk were the gay community and intravenous (IV) drug users. However, the Mayor and the Health Commissioner felt that there was a pressing need to alert and inform the heterosexual population of the nature and danger of AIDS as well. Heterosexuals were either ignorant of the danger of AIDS or considered themselves at low risk. The City did not agree. In the words of Dr. Stephen Joseph:

"We knew the virus was being transmitted primarily through the high–risk behaviors of sharing needles with HIV–infected drug partners, and sharing high–risk sexual activity with HIV–infected partners of either sex. We felt it was important to launch the first of a series of advertising campaigns targeting specific audiences by delivering the AIDS prevention message to sexually active women who might not realize their own danger of infection. Our great concern was that the large numbers of infected and infectious men in the city presented a potentially deadly pool of infection for the women who were their sex partners—and, of course, for any children they might have together. We had the chance to reduce the inroads the AIDS virus could make in the heterosexual population, and we wanted to make the best use of that chance."

At that first meeting, it was decided that a clearly written marketing plan, including a marketing objective and copy strategy, had to be prepared before work could begin. This was the classic first step in a communication process that is as necessary for developing a health care campaign against AIDS as it is for selling a major consumer brand.

Those on the agency side began work on the project. They had some basic information but needed a better understanding of the attitude of the individuals and the groups at which the advertising should be aimed. A city/agency team was formed headed on the client's side by Peggy Clarke and on the agency side by Jeremy Warshaw. As information began coming in and was analyzed, a working marketing plan and strategy was agreed on with the aim of sharpening the focus of the message.

It is a commonly accepted belief at Saatchi & Saatchi that the best and most relevant advertising comes out of a mutually agreed upon strategy aimed at consumer benefit. When the creative team is asked to accommodate too many "selling" points in the advertising or when the briefing has not been discussed and agreed on by both advertiser and agency, the result can lead to blandness or irrelevancy. It is vital that discussion take place regarding advertising's role, objectives, central message and tonality before the creative department applies their problem-solving skills to the task at hand.

AIDS ADVERTISING AND MARKETING STRATEGY

The strategy that the agency in fact used read as follows:

Marketing Objective
- To help stem the spread of the AIDS virus within the heterosexual community.

Advertising Objectives
- To communicate that the AIDS virus can be transmitted heterosexually.
- To provide education and practical information as to the best means of avoiding transmission.

Accepted Consumer Belief
- "I'm not a homosexual so I can't get AIDS." Target Audience
- Primary: Sexually active heterosexual adults 18–34.
- Secondary: All sexually active heterosexual adults.

Proposition
- You can catch the AIDS virus from anyone unless you take preventive action.

Rationale
- The AIDS virus can be transmitted heterosexually. It is not confined to homosexuals or IV drug users.

- The person you have sex with may not even know they are infected so you must protect yourself. You cannot rely on claims that your partner is not a carrier.
- Abstinence is the only sure way to avoid the virus but use of a condom will radically reduce the risk.

Tonality
- Frank, explicit, direct, informative.

Requirements for Execution
- New York City hot line number always to be featured. It should be pointed out here that pre–agreements were made between the City and the agency before the assignment was actually undertaken.
- The City of New York placed no creative or strategic restrictions on us except in the words of Mayor Koch, "Do not talk only to minorities—it is everyone's problem."
- The agency insisted that assuming the creative work was consistent with the agreed upon strategy, it should be accepted without further consideration. The principle at stake was that if it ever came to a question of one person's taste versus another then the agency believed it should prevail over the city government.

Once the strategy had been agreed on by both parties the creative director, Abrams, felt it would be appropriate to offer the challenge to any team within the agency willing to participate. Because of the nature and importance of the project the work was approached in a myriad of ways. The campaign included advertising whose purpose was to shock the viewer into accepting the central premise, i.e. that we are all at risk. Advertising that used a more cerebral and rational approach was also developed. Abrams applied his best judgment and knowledge of the known facts to push his teams to dig further, be more provocative, and avoid the easy option.

Charlie Abrams' first step was to identify the character or tonality of the advertising. "At the time the language of AIDS in newspapers and on television seemed to adopt a kind of "scientist speak." For instance, you'd read 'Exchange of bodily fluids. Well, what did that mean? If it meant semen, vaginal secretions and saliva, we should say so and not pussy–foot around in an effort to avoid upsetting delicate sensibilities. I figured we needed to break out of this conspiracy of gentility and tell it like it is."

"AIDS—If you don't think you can get it you're dead wrong." This was the theme line that came about as ideas and phrases were lobbied about. When the actual line was put forth it sounded right to everyone present. Although it was "creative" it came about as a result of hard work and a tighter and tighter focus on the essence of the message.

Now at last a character for the advertising was beginning to take shape.

What had been happening at the same time was the realization that one or two ads would not be sufficient to do the job. First of all, the agency knew that because of the likely reaction of the media, they would have to prepare a range of print and T.V. advertising from fairly frank to very explicit. The menu of ads thus created would increase the likelihood of at least one of the executions being adopted by every publication that was approached.

In addition, it was decided a number of print ads, posters and T.V. commercials were required because of the comprehensive nature of the problem. The campaign had to be a multi–media effort which addressed the multiplicity of issues such as the role of parental responsibility, bisexuality, condom usage, sex outside a long–standing monogamous relationship, abstinence and so forth. All these issues could be tackled under the theme line umbrella, "AIDS. If you think you can't get it you're dead wrong!"

At a formal meeting held in January, 1987 the creative work was presented after being approved within the agency. It was not an easy decision to go forward with the boldest, most explicit advertising the agency had ever presented. Ads, posters and commercials like those included here were the first of their nature ever recommended to be put before the public. It represented a startling departure from any other advertising campaign heretofore developed, and everyone in the social marketing world who viewed them realized what a battle it was going to be to get them produced and then placed in the media.

The first to view the samples were Dr. Joseph, Peggy Clarke and Mayor Koch and his advisers. To the surprise and gratification of the agency, the advertising was unanimously approved. There were comments and suggestions, but they were all manageable. Now that the advertising had been approved in layout and storyboard form, the next steps in the communications program were put into action.

Press production, type, photographic and T.V. production companies were asked to give their best price for the production elements, and to do so in consideration that this was a pro bono or voluntary effort of the City of New York. They were also informed that the advertising agency was only covering its expenses. The list of companies and individuals who gave their best talents at low or no cost is shown at the end of this chapter. This generosity is not exceptional in the communications business when it comes to good causes.

While the ads and television commercials were being prepared, another form of communications was being involved, i.e. publicity/public relations. The press was an important element in getting the AIDS message across to the public. Therefore the press had to be educated as to what we were doing and why we were doing it. A comprehensive and fairly dramatic press kit was designed. It included a tape of the television commercials, reprints of all the ads, an explanation of the intent of the campaign, and finally the inclusion of a packaged condom.

The storyboards and layout copy had to have legal approval and also go through the clearance procedures of the press and the networks.

Meantime, Milt Gossett, co–chairman of Saatchi & Saatchi Advertising Worldwide, proposed to the City that he and the agency make an attempt to get private funding for this campaign so that it need not depend on the space and time slots donated by the media (these are often after midnight or Sunday morning). If the advertising space and time could be purchased, it could also be scheduled. One of the handicaps of pro bono advertising is that there is no way to know in advance when the advertising will run, how often it will run or where it will run.

Milt Gossett had an "ideal" media program put together encompassing radio, T.V., bus and subway posters, newspapers and magazines to show what a campaign covering all the right target markets at the right advertising levels would look like. The cost for a full year came to six million U.S. dollars. It was proposed that it be broken into quarters and that 1.5 million U.S. dollars be the first target.

A further benefit of a financed campaign was that its effects could be monitored and measured by properly utilized research. Yankelovich, Clancy, Schulman, a well known social research company agreed, to contribute a research program at cost.

The agency then went to outside sources for advice and counsel on sources of money to finance the campaign. The first stop was Jim Burke, at the time chairman and CEO of Johnson and Johnson. He and some of his management were shown the campaign. Mr. Burke told us what we already suspected, that this campaign in its candid, no–holds–barred approach was the only way to tackle the problem. But, at the same time, he felt our approach was going to give us all kinds of political, religious and censorship problems. His advice was sought on sources of finance. He advised us to look to the insurance industry. The potential impact of AIDS was clearly apparent to the insurance companies, and they might be very receptive to supporting a communications program that could help to fight the spread of AIDS.

Another source of information and expertise was Dr. Mathilde Krim, founding chairman of the American Foundation for AIDS Research. She was invited to a presentation of the campaign to the New York Life Insurance Company, a client of Saatchi & Saatchi. Taking Jim Burke's advice, Milt Gossett had asked for an audience with Don Ross, the chairman.

Mr. Ross called his executive committee together and they viewed the campaign as presented by Jeremy Warshaw and Charlie Abrams of Saatchi & Saatchi. As a group they were highly approving. Don Ross asked what was wanted of New York Life—and was told of our hopes, that we wanted to have a funded campaign at 1.5 million U.S. dollars a quarter. Would New York Life supply us with the money to initiate a campaign which would be measured and quantified over a period of time? Three days later Don Ross called Milt Gossett to say that New York Life would underwrite the introduction of the campaign to the sum of one million U.S. dollars if Milt Gossett and the agency would make every effort to enlist the aid of other companies in defraying the first quarter cost of the campaign. We agreed with alacrity. Even as we spoke the advertising was being prepared and a press launch was scheduled for mid–May, 1987. New York Life scheduled a meeting for Gossett, Warshaw and Abrams with the American Association of Insurance Agencies, led by former Pennsylvania Senator Richard Schweiker. The work was presented in Washington to Schweiker and his group of insurance representatives. Comments and suggestions were made and general approval was received. However, the organization volunteered no financial help. The agency also made a presentation to the Metropolitan Life Insurance Company. This company was in the midst of its own plans for combating the AIDS threat. New York City's efforts were welcomed and Metropolitan pledged $100 000 to offset some of New York Life's costs.

The campaign now had funding, a plan for testing its effectiveness, a media schedule and a date for announcing the City's plans to the press and to the public. On May 11th the Mayor called a press conference at City Hall. It was attended by all of the New York press and T.V. and radio stations. For the first time the press saw blow–ups of print ads, posters. and car cards and were shown the television commercials via T.V. monitors. The impact was tremendous. The media reporters had a field day questioning an advertising campaign that spoke plainly and dramatically about AIDS, sex and the use of condoms. Such was the controversy at the press conference, that Dr. Joseph had to remind all those present that he was "in charge of public health and not public morality."

The press kits were swiftly picked up. The fact that they included a condom was news in itself. The agency and the City did not have long to wait for the impact of the press announcement. That night's news and the next day's press showed clearly that the campaign was the most controversial and talked about ever announced by the City. Some columnists praised it for its courageous tactics and others bitterly criticized its approach.

John Woolsey, spokesman for John Cardinal O'Connor:
   "The ads explicitly endorse sexual promiscuity and mislead people into thinking that there is such a thing as safe sex."

Ray Kerrison, New York Post (May 14, 1987):
"From the same people who gave us a sex ed course with books so damaging in their misinformation they had to be withdrawn for review, comes the latest contribution to the well–being of New York: A condom advertising campaign so utterly lacking in taste and propriety that even the T.V. stations are declining to run them...What next will they dredge up to trample on our sensitivities and flout the tenets of decency which have served this nation so well for so long?"

Gerald McKelvey, the father of a four–year–old girl, wrote a Newsday editorial, "Prevention is not the disease," (May 15, 1987). Distressed at the "head–in–the–sand attitude taken by the city's three commercial television stations, women's groups and the Roman Catholic hierarchy" over the City's AIDS awareness campaign, he wrote:

"The ads are punchy, no doubt of that, and they get the message across...Yes I cringe when I read the word 'rubbers,' recalling the word my classmates and I whispered in junior high school 30 years ago in furtive conversations about sex. But the time for furtiveness has ended...Disease like sin flourishes in ignorance. Whatever the reasons to hesitate, we can't afford knowingly to tolerate ignorance of AIDS."

Newsday (May 13, 1987):
"The shocking tone of the ad campaign is to some degree unavoidable. As bold as the catchy graphics and blunt dialogue may be, they're overshadowed by the looming reality of an unchecked AIDS pandemic...For a lot of people, ads that cannot be ignored may be the only way to pound home the lesson of one way to help guard against AIDS: 'The use of condoms'."

U.S. News and World Report (May 25, 1987):
"The commercials in Denmark and Sweden make ours seem soporific. The British, not noted for their licentiousness, have set an example with a vigorous drive to publicize risks and precautions...The stations should take the ads—and, for good measure, they should devote one percent of the profits from doing so to AIDS research."

The campaign was off and running. The Yankelovich research people had started their survey shortly before the press announcement. Meantime, the agency media people were running into a stone wall with some of the television stations and press. As the attached T.V. clearance chart shows, only WOR, some of the cable stations and WNYC showed all three commercials produced. Stations WXTV and WNJL (an Hispanic station) also showed all three commercials. As for the local networks, affiliates WNBC and WCBS only cleared one ad providing it was not aired before 11 p.m. The agency argued that this was probably the hour that the target audience was engaged in the risky sexual behavior the advertising was intended to influence, but to no avail. WABC, on the other hand, would not even clear this commercial as their station policy banned the display of a condom.

The New York Daily News refused to run any of the ads (see T.V. and print clearance charts). *The New York Times* ran two of the ads and the rest of the newspapers varied. Of the magazines, only *Rolling Stone* and *Night Life* showed all of the advertisements, although other magazines ran at least one ad. On the other hand, there were no problems with the subway posters. It is ironic to note that a Lou Harris Poll commissioned by the Planned Parenthood Federation of America on "Sexual Material on American Network T.V. During the 1987–88 Season" showed a preponderance of sexual/promiscuous behavior on America's television stations with over four thousand references to intercourse and over four thousand references to deviant or discouraged sexual practices. It also showed that there were hardly any references to sex education on sexually transmitted diseases, birth control or abortion to counterbalance the sexual content on T.V.

EVALUATION OF CAMPAIGN EFFECTIVENESS

The purpose of the research by Yankelovich Clancy Schulman, was to gauge the impact of the anti–AIDS communications campaign on the key target group—single New Yorkers between the ages of 18 and 34. A pre–campaign survey was carried out in May, 1987 just before the advertising campaign was launched.

Table 14-1. *Method of Study.*

The survey was conducted by telephone September 30 to October 8 with 400 single New Yorkers between the ages of 18 and 34.

The sample consisted of:

193 Whites/Asians	201 Women
98 Blacks	199 Men
109 Hispanics	

The results were weighted to their true proportions in the population (based on U.S. Census data) according to race/ethnicity and age.

Table 14-2. *Recall of AIDS advertising.*

Have you seen or heard any advertising in the past month about how to prevent getting AIDS?	Oct. 1987 %	May 1987 %
Yes	86	70
No	14	30

Table 14-3. *Slogans recalled from AIDS advertisements.*

Do you recall seeing or hearing any advertising about AIDS that:	Oct. 1987 %	May 1987 %
Has the slogan: "If you think you can't get AIDS, you're dead wrong."	89	60
Shows a black mother telling her child to use a condom to prevent getting AIDS.	66	8
Suggests that parents talk with their children about AIDS: "Before it hits home."	53	32
Has the slogan: "Don't die of embarrassment"— when having sex, say no unless a condom is used.	51	20
Has the slogan: "Don't go out without your rubbers."	41	20
Has the slogan: "Bang, you're dead."	23	11

Table 14-4. *Messages recalled from AIDS advertisements.*

Do you recall whether any of these AIDS advertisements made the point that:	Oct. 1987 %	May 1987 %
Using condoms helps prevent AIDS.	90	85
Sexually active people should carry condoms with them.	90	76
People should always use condoms when having sex with someone they do not know well.	89	88
Women should tell their partner to use a condom.	86	68
Anyone who is sexually active runs a risk of getting AIDS.	84	78

The sample consisted of 193 Whites/Asians; 98 Blacks and 109 Hispanics. Of this total, 201 were women and 199 were men. The results were weighted to their true proportions in the population based on U.S. Census data according to race, ethnicity and age.

The second study was conducted in October, 1987. These surveys examined the changes that have occurred in young singles' attitudes and behavior following their exposure to the anti–AIDS advertising. It should be noted that the May percentage figures were probably higher than they normally would be because of the great publicity generated by the press at the announcement of the campaign. Following is a compendium of the results.

The campaign ran from May, 1987 until January of 1988. Because of discounts from the media, the originally proposed 1.5 million U.S. dollars went much further than originally envisaged. The greatest impact of the campaign was in the first several months. The longest running component was the series of subway posters that ran throughout the year.

Table 14-5. *Feelings about AIDS advertising.*

Is there anything you disliked about this AIDS advertising?	Oct. 1987 %	May 1987 %
Yes	15	16
No	85	84

What is that? (asked of those who disliked AIDS advertising)		
Too explicit/too frank.	3	7
Hear too much about AIDS/see ads everywhere.	1	2
Promotes sex, promiscuity.	1	1
Exaggerates the dangers/ tries to scare people.	2	1
Other (answers receiving single mentions).	8	5
Not applicable (nothing in advertising that was disliked)	85	84

Table 14-6. *Attitudes toward using condoms.*

Do you agree, somewhat agree or disagree with the following statements?	Oct. 1987 %	May 1987 %
People should always use condoms when having sex with someone they do not know well.	95	84
Women should tell their sex partner to use a condom.	88	78
Sexually active people should carry condoms with them.	84	76

Table 14-7. *Reactions from AIDS advertising.*

Do you agree or disagree that seeing or hearing these AIDS advertisements:	Total %	Age 18-21 %	22-28 %	29-34 %
Made you more aware that condoms help prevent AIDS.	85	90	85	77
Made you more careful in choosing who you will have sexual intercourse with.	80	88	79	72
Made you discuss more often with your sexual partner how to prevent AIDS.	71	74	72	66
Made you use condoms more often when you have sexual intercourse.	70	78	69	62
Made you more worried that you might catch AIDS.	52	55	54	43

SUMMARY

In the words of Mayor Koch, the campaign was a useful communications effort to fight the AIDS epidemic.

"This hard–hitting campaign is very direct. It may offend some people. But being direct and being provocative is worth it if people are reminded that they need to protect themselves and their loved ones against the risk of AIDS transmission. The more openly, honestly and directly we talk about AIDS and how to prevent its transmission, the less likely it is people will suffer its tragic consequences."

The City is now in the process of looking for effective ways of communicating to the IV drug user. This will necessitate a new marketing and creative strategy. Whether or not it will utilize advertising in the usual sense of the word remains to be seen.

The City has also commissioned a campaign aimed at homosexuals. So far, the advertising has not been aired on T.V. except as shown in news programs on the subject.

There are lessons to be learned from the New York City advertising campaign on AIDS that might apply to others planning a communication program. Advice for other cities, communities or groups considering advertising as an educational force against AIDS:

- Do not expect miracles from advertising where the ultimate aim is behavior change. Be realistic and expect advertising to deliver the message. It will take a variety of forces over time to drive it home and result in change.
- Although it will not be easy, do not sugar coat the message no matter how fierce the opposition or formidable the outcry. The AIDS issue is too critical to skirt.
- Do not expect a lot of support from politicians once your program gets real heat. Realistically, AIDS polarizes religious, educational and community groups. Politicians will find it tough to stay the course in the face of resistance from these groups.
- Once you have a soundly organized campaign, seek help from the business community. Business has much to gain by helping to fight the AIDS virus. Companies can be valuable allies in terms of funding and moral support.
- Avoid re–inventing the wheel. Federal Agencies, states, cities and community organizations have created communications programs and have experience in AIDS education. Before you start your own, check on what has already been done.

Television's Response to the AIDS Crisis: One Company's Experience

Tom Goodgame
Jeanne Blake
Gil Schwartz

It is a blistering hot July afternoon in the heart of the Bronx, the northern-most borough of the city of New York. The air is heavy and stagnant; heat is radiating from the brick of the tenements and the cracked concrete side-walks. Young children scream with delight as they run through cool water spraying from an open fire hydrant. Rhythmic music blares from cars cruising by. Store owners stand in their doorways hoping for a cool breeze, nodding to passersby. "Got us another hot one here." These are the sounds of summer in the ghetto.

Medical Reporter Jeanne Blake of Boston station WBZ-TV is on the street too, with a production crew, working on a story about AIDS. An excruciat-ingly thin black woman stumbles by, wearing giant sunglasses and a short, cotton, sleeveless dress. Her face, arms and legs are covered with ulcers and large, purple lesions. "Kaposi's sarcoma," Blake explains to an awe–struck production assistant, who wonders aloud, "How can her skinny legs hold up her body?" Clearly, the woman is near death. She has emerged from a boarded–up brownstone around the corner, which Blake is told is a "shooting gallery," a place where addicts buy and inject drugs.

Business is hopping in the "drugstore." A steady stream of men, women and youngsters moves up and down the stairs, into the house. A commu-nity outreach social worker accompanying Blake's team gestures down the street. "Imagine," he says, "five years from now, a hundred people on each block here in the Bronx will be dead. So little is being done to address the AIDS problem. There is no education here." Blake's eyes drift to the third floor of a building across the street. The window is open and filled with little faces. The social worker asks, "Who will take care of the children?"

A television camera crew always attracts a crowd. A young, well–dressed man approaches Blake. "Whachu guys doin'?" he asks. "A story about AIDS." Blake tells him. "Oh," he responds immediately. "I know 'bout AIDS." "Really?" Blake asks hopefully. Perhaps, she thinks, the warnings are being heard. The man continues, proud of himself and his knowledge. "Yeah," he says. "I know you can't get AIDS through casual contact, right?" "That's right," says Blake, wrapping her arm around his broad shoulders and pulling him close. "If you had AIDS and I gave you a hug like this, you couldn't infect me. If I had AIDS and hugged you, you couldn't get it from me." The man nods. "Right!" he says cheerfully. "So, that means I can have sex with a lady just once, 'cause that's casual, right?"

"I stared at the man for what seemed like two minutes, feeling dizzy," Blake now says. "Then I realized how stunned I was by his words. 'My God,' I thought. 'the task ahead is so great. Not only do we have to hope people hear the message, we have to say it in a way they will really under-stand. One word can skew the whole meaning of the message.' From that moment on, I never underestimated the enormous challenge we, as communicators, faced. We had to attempt to break through denial, sensitiv-ities about sexual issues and a deep resistance to change. And we had to be explicit. Explaining the basics was going to be more difficult than I ever dreamed. And I had a tremendous sense of sadness that the epidemic would be with us for a very long time."

We in the media have a statement that sometimes comforts us when story we have to tell our audience is bad. "We don't make the news," we tell each other. "We just report it." On the other hand, there are times when the media have a chance to affect the way people lead their lives. Along with this power comes a huge responsibility: the responsibility to use our influence for the good, to make a positive impact on a problem, perhaps even to help in solving it.

Nowhere has this power and responsibility been more evident than in the AIDS crisis, where public information was, and continues to be, one of the only weapons against the illness. Early on—and by that we mean in the early 1980s—it became quite clear to those on the front lines of reporting that something massive and terrible was happening in the communities we serve. And yet the story, as it unfolded, presented challenges, particularly to the broadcasting media.

The questions posed by the epidemic were immediate and many: How were we to convey critical, life–saving information to the public—within the boundaries of "taste" and "propriety" that people had come to expect from television news? What if the public didn't want to know? What if a large segment of our audience didn't care to hear much of anything about a disease that always seemed to happen to "them," to other people of whom, perhaps, a majority did not approve?

Westinghouse Broadcasting faced these problems early on, and, we believe, went about meeting the challenge more aggressively than any other broadcast organization in the United States. In the following pages, we'd like to relate the story of how our television station group reacted to the AIDS crisis, first in one community, then in two, then in an effort that spanned the United States, reaching more than 60% of American viewers. It is a story of journalists and their managers making a decision to take on an unpopular subject and communicate it to a public that was squeamish and uninformed—and essentially satisfied to remain that way.

It is the story of an organization that saw a need, and moved to meet it head-on, with all the resources it could muster.

This story is part history, but it must also be told in the voices of some of those who covered it, because there —on the front lines of AIDS coverage— is where important lessons were learned. Finally, we will take a brief look at what still remains to be done, for the tasks that lie ahead are in some ways even more significant than those which came before.

EARLY DAYS

In 1983, KPIX-TV presented its first comprehensive report on AIDS. The four–part series concentrated on debunking myths that were causing fear and panic across the country. What KPIX began to understand was that the statistics and the dire predictions for the future were frightening enough, without being augmented by the force of ignorance and prejudice that went along with them.

Without a treatment or a cure, information was the key to stopping the AIDS epidemic from spreading. Covering the stories and reporting new information was not enough. Within two years, KPIX became the first local television station in the country to make a complete commitment. The station gave it a name: AIDS LIFELINE; and a goal, to educate and inform the public in a comprehensive way never before attempted by the electronic media.

Instrumental in the development of this first ongoing, complete AIDS coverage effort was KPIX reporter Jim Bunn. Bunn joined KPIX EYEWITNESS NEWS as a general assignment reporter in June, 1983, bringing with him almost ten years of experience as an investigative and general assignment reporter. Shortly after his arrival, Bunn's responsibilities were expanded to include the tracking of the AIDS epidemic in the Bay Area and around the world. To accomplish that task, Bunn traveled extensively, seeking out and reporting on every aspect of the disease and its prevention. In 1987, Group W loaned Mr. Bunn to the World Health Organization, to assist in that group's establishment of a worldwide information office. By that time, he had reported nearly 500 news stories on AIDS for KPIX.

Bunn was among the first to face some of the critical problems in reporting the story that would later be encountered by reporters nationwide.

Jim Bunn, Journalist:

"It was within the first few months as a reporter at KPIX, in September of 1983, that I was assigned to a three–part series on the disease. But it had become very obvious that it couldn't just be San Francisco story. I went to people running the newsroom at the time and said 'I think, one, it needs to be bigger than a San Francisco story, and two, it needs to be five parts, and three, I think we need to do a considerable amount of travelling." So in the space of a week, I went to Atlanta, to Washington and to New York. The important thing for me was that from a professional standpoint, they were willing to take a chance.

"They gave me the roll of the dice... and that commitment to covering the issue never really let up. It would be easy to look at KPIX and say, "Well, of course, it was San Francisco." The fact of the matter was, that television station was like every other T.V. station in the U.S. in that at a given point in time this was a story that didn't seem to affect a great number of people in its viewing audience. Nevertheless, management of that newsroom and the television station responded in a way that transcended a 'normal' response. The only person doing anything at the time was Randy Shilts. As a result he was the bell-wether I measured my reporting against.

"One of the things we did early on was report on people with AIDS, and the various things they were going through—whether it dealt with housing, financing, discrimination or whatever. We didn't get into how they got the disease or what their sexual preference was. The editors were quite comfortable with that and our viewing audience as well as the editors saw that you could do a story that would be of interest to the mass audience. We did stories about people who were sick and dying. It wasn't that we were soft pedaling the truth of the epidemic. It showed that people who have the disease are human beings."

Early on, however, Bunn knew the public's questions on how the disease was transmitted had to be answered. New ways of transmitting essential information had to be found, and they would challenge the notion of what was acceptable on local television. In the first AIDS LIFELINE special, Bunn interviewed Dr. Connie Wofsey on AIDS, and how its transmission could be contained. During that show, Dr. Wofsey produced a condom and placed it over a syringe to demonstrate its proper use. Bunn explains how the decision was made to employ this graphic illustration on broadcast television:

"Connie had been at a press conference in February of 1987 in Atlanta, about AIDS and adolescent children. She pulled out this condom and stretched it over her hands. I just sat there and watched the reporters. They were collectively aghast. You could have driven a truck through the collective space that their mouths created. I saw that it had tremendous impact.

"The fact of the matter here was Connie Wofsey was one of the preeminent clinicians in the world, a highly respected AIDS researcher... also a woman, who cut a very dignified figure visually for someone who didn't know her credentials. It didn't seem staged, it didn't seem intrusive, it didn't even seem mildly offensive. So having seen that in the press conference, when we got to the point of planning the program I asked Dr. Wofsey if she could bring some of her 'stuff.'The reason for doing it was much less the 'wow factor.' It was to move the issue to a place where it had never been before on television and it was so apparent to me that for all the little checks we look for in T.V., it worked for T.V.

"When Dr. Wofsey put the condom on the syringe we did not get one negative call. We did get calls from people who said 'thanks for doing that.'"

Bunn knew that general descriptions would not serve when public education was at stake. He had learned this lesson through first–hand reporting of the AIDS epidemic:

"I did an interview in a the Lower East Side health clinic. I was talking to a health care worker who had dealt with outreach education for women. I said that I felt the need to educate people about how to use condom was overblown. 'This is not brain surgery we are talking about here,' I told her. 'There aren't any gears or strings to pull; you just open the package and it should be obvious.'

"So she said, let me tell you a story. She proceeded to tell me how they have one woman who came in for sex education and birth control education and they had gotten out a package of condoms and opened it and said, here is how you put it on, only they reached into the closet pulled out broom and slid the condom down over the broom handle, and said now, this is how it fits and when you are done you take it off tie it in a knot and throw it away. So, six month later she comes back three months pregnant and they asked her what happened. She said I did what you showed me, I made love with my husband, I put the condom on the broom and...

"The health care worker insisted she wasn't joking. And what she basically was saying was, we have to show them. You can't assume anything. I got the message that if you are going to talk about things—don't mess around! Show it!

"That was a passage for me because it armed me with fodder to convince people in the newsroom, and they didn't need much convincing, that we needed to be frank and blunt and clear, and that we needed to educate, and that we couldn't make assumptions when we used terms. It was a turning point for me in that I had to reevaluate the degree of education I needed to put into my stories."

Based on Bunn's reporting and the station–wide perception that a full effort was required to face the growing health crisis, the AIDS LIFELINE total station campaign was created in 1985. The campaign was designed to use the resources available in every department of the television station, and was built along the lines of previous Group W public affairs and programming campaigns. In the 1980s alone, Group W had programmed and syndicated "Second Chance" (which explored the need for organ donation), "Whispering Hope" (which reported on the plight of those suffering from Alzheimer's disease) and "For Kids' Sake" (an ongoing campaign exploring issues pertaining to children). Each of these total station campaigns was successful in its local markets, and eventually went into syndication, reaching a national audience. In syndication, they served non–Group W television stations that did not have the resources to mount such a local effort themselves, with programming, public service announcements and a wide variety of special reports and printed material.

The full AIDS LIFELINE effort brought documentaries, special programs and news response with the latest information about AIDS to the San Francisco community. Public service announcements and an information pamphlet helped reinforce the campaign's basic message: that the facts must be known, because AIDS is preventable.

In preparing the programming material for public viewing, KPIX drew on concerned individuals and organizations from within the community that were only too happy to help in this essential effort.

Holly Smith, Media Director, Shanti Project, San Francisco, California:

"[KPIX AIDS coverage] legitimized the topic. It helped focus the public on the fact that we were talking about people. Remember that in 1983, '84 and '85 there was great confusion and misperception about contagion and transmission, partially because we were still discovering what AIDS was all about.

"KPIX and Westinghouse didn't allow it to be a sensational topic, and continuously looked at its various elements through the eyes of people, looking at its medical issues, family values, education issues, the human toll that was being taken... as well as all the political, research, economic stuff. It helped the Bay Area get a solid jump start on preventing the spread of the virus and diminish the homophobia and AIDS phobia inherent in this topic. KPIX treatment of it gave it that legitimacy where people paid attention, where they didn't just see it as a gay issue, or issue of drug using, but constantly people were being told that AIDS was an equal opportunity claimer, that anyone could potentially be exposed based on risk activity, not groups.

"In those days I was creating a media relations program at the San Francisco AIDS Foundation, and Jim Bunn and I had lunch and we created the program. As we started out that first documentary, it was clear that they were willing to work with us, and we with them. And we said, 'Let's create a situation so it doesn't stop when this documentary airs, let's make sure there is a brochure people can call and ask for, that it's tied into the hotline, so people know there is a place they can call and get nonjudgmental information.

"KPIX's and Group W's coverage of AIDS goes against the grain of the industry standard. Because to do this work right, people had to care, ultimately. And as much as people talk about being objective analysts, everyone who has made this effort work successfully has gone beyond that point to say 'I care about these people, these people have an impact on me even though I am just reporting about them.' It wasn't just a new reporter coming in every week to do a story on the political scene or whatever. And I don't believe that's the norm in a T.V. newsroom."

The first one–hour documentary for the AIDS LIFELINE campaign, "Our Worst Fears: The AIDS Epidemic," drew an unprecedented response, not only in the San Francisco Bay area, but across the country. It was the highest–rated public affairs show in the history of the television station. The San Francisco AIDS Foundation's AIDS Hotline recorded the highest number of calls since the organization began. The program was rebroadcast because of the enormous viewer response. In all, more than one million people viewed it locally. The special also was broadcast in all Group W markets and was syndicated across the country in New York, Cincinnati, Miami and Honolulu. Requests came from around the world to use the documentary as a teaching tool—from Canada to Guam to Australia, and from more than 100 organizations including school systems, colleges, hospitals and major corporations. With the cooperation and expertise of the San Francisco AIDS Foundation, a basic information pamphlet was designed and distributed to the general public. The AIDS LIFELINE pamphlet soon became the most widely available in the country, with more than half a million distributed in several different languages.

With the total campaign now gathering momentum, in September of 1986 KPIX (in association with Chen Sam Associates) produced an AIDS public service announcement campaign. More than 45 celebrities, including Bob Hope, Joe Namath and Dionne Warwick contributed to the more than 60 spots. The public service announcements were distributed to television stations across the country. The effort was at that time the largest single public service announcement campaign ever produced for any single cause.

The heart of San Francisco's AIDS LIFELINE campaign came from the KPIX news department. Over a four–year period, more than 1000 news reports on AIDS were presented. News crews traveled around the country, and around the world, to bring the AIDS story home and to put it in perspective. In addition to the California coverage, stories were filed from Australia, Paris, Brussels, Geneva, Washington, D.C., New York City, Phoenix and Indiana among other locations. In addition, talk shows, documentaries and community call–in programs continued to answer viewer questions and keep people informed.

Although honors were not the motivation behind the campaign, KPIX received unprecedented recognition for its local AIDS LIFELINE efforts. The station was honored with a Presidential Citation, a regional Emmy, a Peabody and the National Emmy For Community Service. More importantly, viewer response and the ongoing need for information compelled KPIX—and Group W as a national organization—to continue AIDS LIFELINE, and expand its efforts.

In Boston

While San Francisco was gearing up its total station campaign, its sister station, Group W's WBZ–TV in Boston, was moving in its own way to meet the growing AIDS crisis in that city.

In the fall of 1985, six weeks after the world was shocked by news that Rock Hudson was dying of AIDS, WBZ–TV aired its first AIDS information program. It was "Our Worst Fears: The AIDS Epidemic." Programming elements had been picked up from KPIX in San Francisco, but the station made the effort to customize the show for its local audience. The live, two–hour program was broadcast during prime–time on a Sunday night in September. As host, WBZ–TV's medical reporter Jeanne Blake invited viewers to "join us in search of answers to some of the questions surrounding the AIDS epidemic."

Because the broadcast involved remote interviews from Atlanta, San Francisco and Boston, the entire technical staff of WBZ–TV was involved. In Boston, Blake interviewed a young, gay man with AIDS, Paul Cronan. Cronan was an employee of New England Telephone and was claiming that his supervisor at work had breached his confidentiality by disclosing his diagnosis.

What the viewers didn't see behind the scenes was that WBZ–TV, a leading force for AIDS education in the community, was having its own struggle over the issue. Group W management was aware that television stations around the country had encountered a reluctance among staff members to work with AIDS patients. To ward off difficulties, executives held an AIDS educational seminar at the station the week prior to the AIDS special. Dr. David Witt, an infectious disease specialist from Boston City Hospital, was on hand to answer questions. The meeting was well attended, and it eased concerns for many employees. But not for all. The issues surrounding this first shoot were emblematic of similar deep–seated problems and fears that beset the broadcasting industry across the nation.

Producers of the special intended to shoot pictures of Paul Cronan in his home on Saturday, the day before the program. The videotape would be used in a special, follow–up series, later that week. That Saturday morning, four photographers refused the assignment. They admitted they were afraid of people with AIDS. Finally, photographer Jim Frances, reached at home the next morning, accepted the assignment.

> "I was fascinated by AIDS," he now says. "I had shot video of people with AIDS before. I welcomed the opportunity. I actually felt I could learn a lot from them. I knew from reading news reports and covering AIDS stories that it wasn't contagious in the sense that I could get it through casual contact."

Later that day, technicians arrived at Paul Cronan's house to set up for the live interview. That meant running cables, establishing a microwave signal from a van parked in front of his house, and setting up the camera and the lights. Packed in their gear was a new microphone.

A technician from WBZ–TV recalls, "There were photographers and technicians that were reluctant to do a live shot with Paul Cronan. But they were persuaded to do it when the operations manager said he would purchase a cheap microphone that would be used in the interview, then thrown away. And they were promised they could keep their distance from Paul." Monday morning, the Cronan live remote was the talk of the newsroom. There were stories about how the technicians determined who worked outside in the microwave truck, who ran the camera, and who drew the "short straw," and had to pin the microphone on Cronan. Also, there was plenty of talk about the cheap microphone and what happened to it after the program. One technician, not assigned to the shoot recalls:

> "The mike probably cost $30 and they must have figured, 'Why throw it away?' But they wouldn't pack it away in the truck. The story goes, they taped it to the bumper. Can you imagine? They had to have realized at some point, 'This is crazy!' But they carried that mike back to the station on the bumper. For months, it sat in the maintenance shop, where it was referred to as the 'AIDS mike' and no one would touch it."

In the following months, others refused to work around people with AIDS. One cameraman remained committed to his policy of not entering a room where there was AIDS virus, whether it was in a person or in a test tube. One afternoon he was the only available cameraman when an AIDS–related story broke. It was explained to him the assignment included shooting an interview with a doctor and pictures of his laboratory. He asked, "Will there be any AIDS virus in the room?" Blake told him, "I imagine in the laboratory, but it won't be flying around the room." He couldn't be persuaded.

He agreed to shoot only the interview, explaining "You never know, 10 years down the road, we might find out you can get infected that way."

Another technician gave a particularly unique excuse for not working on an AIDS–related story: 'My wife won't let me," he said. There was proof, however, that education can help. Within a few weeks of the station–sponsored seminar, a cameraman who had previously refused AIDS–related assignments agreed to shoot an interview with a woman who had AIDS. As the news van pulled away from the television station, Blake turned to him and inquired, "How come you're doing this?" "I read some stuff," the man responded. "I went to the seminar and I got comfortable." "Good for you." Blake said. The subject was dropped, and they got on with their work.

Blake, who has reported on the epidemic for five years, describes how she learned, early on, the value of education in overcoming the fear of AIDS:

"John and I met through friends of his who had AIDS. John had AIDS, too. I never interviewed him for television, but we were friends. I called him occasionally to check on him. He called me to talk. Those conversations proved educational. They taught me about the gay lifestyle, about the struggle and desperation of living with AIDS, and the agony one suffers when rejected by family. He called one day sobbing. 'My sister told me a week ago she was coming to Boston to see me. She promised. That was a week ago. She hasn't shown up. I am so angry.' John's family had never accepted his homosexuality. And now, his unspoken words said 'They can't even put that aside when I am almost dead.'

"Not long after that conversation, a mutual friend called to say John was in the hospital desperately ill. As I walked into his room I found him in the midst of a coughing jag. He lifted a silver bedpan to his mouth and spit a mouthful of blood into it. Leaning back he moaned, 'Oh God.' Only the look in his eyes acknowledged my presence. Then, the coughing began again. I sat down in the orange, vinyl chair a few feet from his bed. When he coughed I pushed back in the chair. I wondered to myself, 'Is he spraying the AIDS virus all over me every time he coughs? Am I getting infected just sitting here?' It was obvious to me that John needed help supporting his body. But I was paralyzed by fear. I wanted to run from the room.

"Finally a nurse came into the room. She wiped the blood from his mouth and propped up pillows behind his back. Turning to me she said 'I think you ought to leave. He needs to concentrate on clearing his chest.' I felt so ashamed. I knew they both saw that I was afraid. As I jumped from my chair, I leaned over to John, took his thin, damp hands in mine and kissed them. Then I walked out of the room, and ducked into the ladies room next door. I turned on the hot water and lathered up my hands with disinfectant from a soap box on the wall. I splashed water over my face and the part of my lips that had touched his hands.

"When I got home, a half hour later, I peeled off my jeans and tee shirt and jumped into the shower. The room was so hot. I could feel the virus in the air. I must have gotten infected! I kissed his hands right after he coughed! My husband, who had followed me into the room, stood watching me, dumb struck.

'I cannot believe what you're saying,' he said. 'You know you cannot get infected that way.' That night I slept poorly, waking several times drenched with perspiration. 'Night sweats. I am positive it's night sweats.' My mind turned to my sexual past. 'What if I am infected. What if I suffer like John has suffered. Who will take care of me?' The next morning I called an AIDS researcher whom I had interviewed. After I relayed the events of the night before, he said, 'I understand your fear. I have gone through my own fears. I have been spit upon, phlegm has gotten in my eye, and on my mouth when patients coughed around me. But I am not infected and you didn't get infected last night either.'

"I persisted. 'But the air in the room was so conducive to germs and bacteria growing.' Calmly he reassured me, 'That's not warm enough to keep the virus alive. The air would kill it.' I had more questions. 'I shouldn't have kissed his hand. What if I had a crack in my lip.' I said, running my fingers across my lips to check for breaks in the skin. 'Jeanne. The virus wouldn't live on his hand. You didn't get infected.' I was quiet. 'Do you have any more questions?' He asked. 'No. I believe you. I really do believe you. Thanks.'

"There were important lessons for me in that experience. I learned that irrational fear of AIDS is real. Emotions, by nature, are not logical. If the doctor had told me to 'stop being afraid' it wouldn't have helped. I needed to talk through the fear, turn it inside out, approach it from every possible angle. Only then could I let it go. It helped me be more tolerant of the public's fear of AIDS in the initial stages of the epidemic. A short time later, we aired our first program to help people get the facts about AIDS. We formatted the program so people could follow up on their questions. That, in a sense, was their opportunity to 'approach their fear from every angle.' It's a crucial element in successful education. The experience also taught me the importance and necessity of repetition. It takes a while to break through fear."

Two days after "Our Worst Fears" aired, Blake contacted Cronan to thank him for his participation, and, at the suggestion of WBZ Special Projects Producer Barry Ahrendt, asked Cronan to consider another request. Blake explained that she wanted to follow Cronan with their cameras for an indefinite period of time, and chronicle his life with AIDS.

When Cronan said he would consider it, photographer/editor Jim Frances spent a few hours with him, describing the project. "I explained the way I wanted to shoot it," Frances recalls, "that it would be relaxed and laid back. I also told him I hoped he would get as much out of it as we would, that I hoped it would be therapeutic for him, going over issues he wanted to talk about. I told him I had done that before with other people who had serious diseases. Actually, I had done that with my father and a very close friend who had cancer before they died, so I said that with confidence."

"We all realized the nature of our request," Blake says. "We were asking a young man in a vulnerable position to expose the most intimate aspects of his life before hundreds of thousands of people. But we had worked with AIDS, measured the public's reaction to the disease and realized that for too many people, AIDS was a disease of statistics."

Producer Ahrendt recounts, "As we learned with Rock Hudson, people weren't interested in paying attention to the disease until it had a human face. Paul seemed to be the perfect person because he was articulate, he had a rare talent for storytelling, and he was willing to talk about the most intimate details of his private and emotional life."

Several months passed with no word from Cronan. Finally, he called Blake on Christmas Day 1985. "I have decided it would be OK if you filmed me," Cronan told Blake. "I think it could be good. There is so much ignorance about AIDS. Maybe it would help people understand."

Producer Ahrendt carved out a shooting schedule. He knew what he wanted on tape. "What we were hoping to show was the day–to–day reality of living with AIDS," he says. "Most of the stories that were in the news were medical stories or about people dying from the disease. We wanted to show what it was like for people to wake up to the reality of AIDS every morning, and wrestle with it as they tried to get to sleep at night."

Frances would videotape milestones in Cronan's life, including doctor's visits, his birthday and the annual trip to his parents' grave site. Periodically, he would let the camera roll as Paul recounted his fears and frustrations. Frances, Ahrendt and Blake spent many night and weekend hours at Cronan's Dorchester, Massachusetts, home. For sixteen months the three experienced the pain, tenderness and exhilaration of Cronan's life. "We shared his emotional highs and lows as he passed through stages of anger, denial and acceptance," Blake recalls.

"It was incredibly invigorating." said Frances. "He would call me at home to tell me about something that had happened, just to chat. That showed he was comfortable with the process and that what we were doing was not just good for us, but that he was getting something out of it. That's when I knew it was ultimately going to be a successful program."

One hundred and fifty video cassettes later, WBZ-TV aired the powerful documentary "The Paul Cronan Story: Living with AIDS." The program was broadcast in prime–time on a Friday night in January of 1987. It aired without commercials, because, in those early years of AIDS coverage, the WBZ Sales Department was unable to find a sponsor—and the station was determined to put it on the air anyway. Skeptics predicted that conservative Boston viewers weren't ready for an hour–long story about a gay man who was Catholic and had AIDS. "For a week leading up to the program, I prayed for a blizzard," Blake says. "Bad weather increases viewership. In Boston, the night of the program, half a foot of snow was whipped around by 30 mile–per–hour winds. 'The Paul Cronan Story' ran a hair behind the time slot's top–rated show. Station executives were ecstatic. But for those of us who worked on the program, testimony to its success came in different forms."

Research assistant Anne Burke volunteered to take calls during and after the program. Into the early hours of Saturday morning, she talked with grandmothers and teens, mothers and fathers, gay men and nuns about the impact of the documentary. She logged more than a hundred calls that night. In the weeks following the broadcast, the WBZ-TV mail room was inundated with letters and postcards. Many said that Cronan's story had enlightened them. A man from Peabody, Massachusetts wrote:

> "It helped change my attitude. I always felt that if someone contracted AIDS then it was too bad, that they knew the risk and they accepted it. After watching, I have to tell you I'm ashamed of that attitude. I have to admire the way Paul is trying to help other victims of AIDS by letting his story be told. It takes guts to do that."

News Director Stan Hopkins received a letter commending him for "a brave and caring program." It read:

> "Most local stations are retreating from any risky topics such as AIDS. Your presentation was not only well done and intelligent, it dared to attack sensitive issues and opinions that make people cringe in fear. I was further impressed that you aired this material in a prime–time slot."

Several hundred letters made a similar point. WBZ-TV received requests and made available copies of the documentary to many schools, corporations, church groups and politicians, including Senator Edward Kennedy, Governor Michael Dukakis and Boston Mayor Ray Flynn. Harvard Business School requested a copy for "classroom teaching for MBA candidates to illustrate the effect of AIDS in the work place." Harvard Medical School wanted a copy to "help educate medical students about the way AIDS is experienced by a young adult, and to help illustrate the psychological and social difficulties that emerge in these cases, alongside the biomedical ones."

The publicity of the Cronan case and the hour–long program proved to be an embarrassment to New England Telephone Company, Paul's employer. As one New England Telephone employee said of the ordeal, "We were definitely flying by the seat of our pants." Executives moved quickly to restore the company's public image. Two months after the program was broadcast, a vice president from the telephone company called a meeting of representatives of eight other Boston corporations. Andrea Dudley, staff director of Human Resources at New England Telephone recalls, "We wanted to say, 'This is what we did, this is what we did wrong. This is what we learned. What are you doing? What can we all learn together?'"

Andrea Dudley, Staff Director, Human Resources, New England Telephone Company:

> "The public nature of the Paul Cronan case had an impact, definitely, on us, and brought to realization that we had not thought in much detail about doing AIDS education for employees. While we had done some thinking about AIDS policy, we hadn't done enough to make that policy a reality, or think about what would happen when an employee with AIDS was assimilated back into the work force. In that sense, I would say that the case was a major factor in our decision to pursue AIDS education."

As a direct response to the Paul Cronan story, New England Telephone led in the organization of the New England AIDS Consortium, a group of nine area businesses dedicated to creating a meaningful industry response to the AIDS crisis. The group's mission was to provide leadership and advocacy in the business community on issues surrounding the HIV epidemic in the work place, including education, policy, legal and medical considerations, community relations and corporate philanthropy. Dudley explains how this group was formed:

> "One of its prime movers was Peter Berchman, who was vice president of human resources for New England Telephone. He realized that there must be other businesses around that shared common concerns around AIDS. He thought it would be a good idea to get together some of those business leaders to talk about what was being done what could be done. This initial discussion took place in the spring of 1987. No one thought two years ago that as much could come out of it as has. Just in our own companies, there are 500 000 employees who have received information and education about AIDS.
>
> "Having nine major companies together speak out on the issue almost validates it for other businesses to be concerned and to realize they should do something too. And I think that is the prime impact the consortium can have now."

Paul Ross, manager of the AIDS Program Office of Digital Equipment Corporation, one of the corporations in the consortium, adds:

> "If you accept the premise that education is the best ally, then you set an environment where people can feel safe in the work place. People don't have to be afraid in the work place of contracting AIDS and most important, those people with AIDS, if they choose to disclose, can find a supportive work force.
>
> "Paul Cronan's story clearly motivated people to say 'this could have been us on the front pages.' So we look at education as an investment, in helping us all

respond to and manage on an independent and collective basis the fact that the epidemic isn't going away."

Ross also notes that, even at this late date, less than 10% of the companies in the United States are doing anything systematic on the problem of AIDS in the work place.

In August of 1988, Paul Cronan died from complications of AIDS. In the final months of his life, Cronan accepted his diagnosis and impending death. But he was also angered to the end by reminders of discrimination against people with AIDS, and the injustice he suffered.

With the Consortium's efforts in full gear, its brochures and videotapes now reach some 500 000 employees worldwide. Blake believes that Paul Cronan would be encouraged at how much has changed since that September night in 1987 when the technician feared he would be infected pinning a microphone on his black velour bathrobe.

David Casey, Cronan's attorney in his lawsuit, agrees:

"I think the lawsuit and coverage of the law suit in general would have effectively reached the relevant legal community, which is to say lawyers for management and employees, and standing alone, the law suit and the legal–issue –related coverage would have been sufficient to educate that group of people to the issues. But I think the effect of the television program was to reach and inform and make more sensitive to the legal and human issues, a much wider audience. I think what the hour–long documentary did was really drive home the issue in all its complexities.

"My sense of the impact of "The Paul Cronan Story" is that it made people more aware of the discrimination in general that gay people feel. I think it gave the disease AIDS a human face. And it made the disease AIDS which had previously been shrouded with mystery and shrouded with fear and resentment another disease in which a person experienced the same kind of suffering people suffer with terminal cancer. So I think people from all walks of life, from different generations with different political perspectives, saw a young man they otherwise would have rejected, they had the time to see his personality, his character and his confrontation with death unfold in a way that made the disease and lifestyle understandable to them.

"I think that it let the corporate world know they had to think about addressing AIDS in the work place before it happened in their shop. They saw that New England Telephone got hurt legally, financially and with the public. They learned they had to think about this problem before it happened to them and to think about creating management structures that would address the problem. That means doing two things: sensitizing their managerial force to be very careful to maintain confidences on the one hand, and second, to alert them to the fact that they had to accommodate people with AIDS in the work place. We established the principal in Massachusetts, anyway, that AIDS is a handicap, that it requires reasonable accommodations. And so the corporate community learned they had to be aware that they had to maintain the confidentiality of persons with AIDS and at the same time accommodate their handicap. That is no small feat.

"In the aftermath of Cronan, there was much more sympathy and much greater public understanding of the disease and a much greater willingness to accommodate people, and so in a broader sense the corporate community realized they had to take this problem seriously because public opinion had moved in the direction of those suffering with the disease."

The "Paul Cronan Story" was the cornerstone of WBZ–TV's AIDS education effort, which they, too, called AIDS LIFELINE. The station dedicated itself to its own total station campaign, which included numerous specials, news reports and public service announcements. Lois Roach, public service director at the station, was instrumental in development of WBZ's public service campaign.

Lois Roach, Public Service Director, WBZ–TV:

"Basically our challenge was to come up with ways to create awareness around the issue of AIDS. We went out into the community. I spoke with people involved with the development of training materials, volunteers, social service folks, I talked to people who ran AIDS hotlines, people whose clients were IV drug users.

"There was always the concern that people with AIDS were the gay, the IV drug users and the people of color who might not be appealing to the 'mainstream' audience. And among the people who were IV drug users, there was the feeling, 'Hey, we aren't worth anything so we aren't worth saving.' In some of the spots we did we tried to counter that feeling they might have. We produced a series of spots geared toward that person. One featured a recovering addict who had turned his life around completely and was working at one of the agencies as an outreach worker. He went from a life of shooting–up to being out on the streets to tell people how to get off the stuff.

"There was a spot done with a really creative outlook that was a different approach, that was geared toward the IV drug community. It was dealing with a harsh and unpleasant subject and at the same time it would give the contrast of the beauty that life without some of these conditions has to offer. For example, the main characters were male and a female, it was done on film, very soft lighting, smooth dissolves... smooth dance. The goal was to create a dream life effect of a man and a woman. If you just looked at the shot you would say, 'Oh, isn't this pretty, isn't this dreamlike,' but if you listened to the words you realized it was something very serious.

"One of the workers at AIDS Action Committee made a couple of comments to me about how her clients who had seen the spot had felt this was a spot that talked to them, or was directed to them. Basically she said it was the first time they felt that someone reached out and talked to them... and the committee knew that the woman who walked in off the street did so because she felt cared about for the first time."

THE NATIONAL CAMPAIGN

In the summer of 1987, KPIX approached Group W management in New York City with a proposal to create a national version of AIDS LIFELINE, one that would run on all five Group W Television stations and be syndicated nationwide through the Television Group's distribution arm, Group W Television Sales.

At that time, there was significant discussion among the TV Group's stations and New York management as to whether there would be a national audience for such programming. Many markets were sure to feel, it was said, that because AIDS had not yet hit their community, there would be little interest in devoting considerable air time to the subject. There were also concerns about how such an effort, which was sure to be costly, would be funded.

Group W senior management finally concluded that the project would move forward at all Group W stations, and would be packaged for national distribution as well. A national underwriter would be sought to help defray expenses. But even if none was found, the project would be done. It was simply a matter, as one executive put it, "of doing the right thing—at the right time."

On October 19, 1987, Group W Television, in consultation with the World Health Organization's Global Programme on AIDS, announced AIDS LIFELINE, television's first ongoing national AIDS education and prevention campaign, the first such campaign in the media's history. AIDS LIFELINE was to be programmed and coordinated from KPIX in San Francisco, and marketed to television stations by Group W Television Sales, which had successfully marketed "For Kid's Sake" to more than 100 stations that year.

The announcement was made by Tom Goodgame, president of the Group W Television Stations and Dr. Jonathan Mann, director of the World Health Organization's Global Programme On AIDS (GPA), at a national tele-conference at the studios of WNET-TV, Channel 13 in New York City. U.S. Surgeon General C. Everett Koop, a leader in the drive for public under-standing of the issue, joined the teleconference from Washington, D.C. to express his support.

The World Health Organization, established in 1948 as a specialized agency of the United Nations, is the directing and coordinating authority on international health. Its 166 member countries cooperate toward a common goal of global health protection and promotion. On February 1,

1987, the Global Programme on AIDS was formally established to direct and coordinate the global strategy for AIDS prevention and control.

"This type of project is essential in the fight against AIDS," said Dr. Jonathan Mann, director of the Global Programme on AIDS at that time. "It is only through this type of massive effort that we can ensure that people are educated and informed about AIDS. Education is the key to AIDS prevention, and it is the position of the World Health Organization that the only way to stop AIDS is through a world–wide effort. What's exciting about this is that it's the private sector. That's important. And it's using a medium that speaks to people."

"There is no more serious public issue now confronting our world community than AIDS," said Tom Goodgame in announcing the national campaign.

"We have all come to see that the best defense against AIDS is information—current, frank, dispassionate and ongoing data to all segments of the population. We are gratified to be associated with the World Health Organization in this effort to get the AIDS message out worldwide. We think we can make a contribution through our medium, and we mean to do so, both on a national and international basis."

"AIDS is not simply a medical challenge, it is also a challenge to our social, legal and moral institutions," said U.S. Surgeon General C. Everett Koop.

"No other recent medical or social issue has generated a more acute and dramatic need for public information and education. We applaud Group W and the World Health Organization for their efforts to provide accurate information to both national and international audiences. We especially commend them for their intention to conduct a long–term, ongoing education campaign. The battle against AIDS will not be won overnight. Those who want to provide a lasting service to society in the fight against this deadly disease must be committed, as are Group W and the World Health Organization, to continuing their efforts for as long as is necessary."

Following the news conference, Group W conducted a live, seven–city symposium, distributed via satellite, addressing the issues surrounding the subject of AIDS. Experts in each of the five Group W cities—San Francisco, Philadelphia, Boston, Baltimore and Pittsburgh—were on hand to contribute to the discussion, which was moderated by KPIX news anchor Dave McEI-hatton, in New York. Members of the media and the community were also present in the five locations to question participants.

Production and distribution costs of the AIDS LIFELINE campaign were initially borne solely by Group W. License fees generated by the project were waived by the company. Instead, Group W requested that participating stations make a charitable donation to a local AIDS care–giving organization, the size of such donation to be based on the size of the market involved. Eventually, funds raised for either local AIDS care–giving organizations or for the National AIDS Network exceeded one million dollars. (The National AIDS Network is an organization representing more than 300 community–based service organizations. It was started by the five pioneering AIDS organizations in this country: the AIDS Project Los Angeles, the Gay Men's Health Crisis in New York City, the San Francisco AIDS Foundation, the AIDS Action Committee in Boston, and the Health Education Resource Organization in Baltimore.)

The national AIDS LIFELINE campaign eventually was syndicated to such cities as New York, Los Angeles, Chicago, Detroit, Cleveland, Atlanta, Seattle, Minneapolis, Chicago, Washington, D.C., Tampa, Denver, Salt Lake City, Green Bay, Portland, Maine, Colorado Springs and Springfield, Massachusetts, as well as the five Group W markets—in all, some 55 television stations covering 55.64% of the American public.

In 1988, the Metropolitan Life Insurance Company became the sole and exclusive national underwriter of Group W's AIDS LIFELINE public service and programming campaign. Met Life pledged one million dollars in funds to support production and programming for AIDS LIFELINE, enabling the company to concentrate its funding on providing participating stations with the most comprehensive campaign possible.

BEYOND AIDS LIFELINE

The AIDS LIFELINE campaign continued nationwide, and Group W journalists investigated and informed the public on virtually every aspect of the evolving story. Medical reporter Jeanne Blake in Boston, for instance, filed more than 100 stories between 1985 and 1989. In the past several years, it became increasingly clear that the group perhaps most at risk, at least in respect to its lack of education and sophistication on the subject of AIDS, was no longer the gay community, but IV drug users. The challenges of reaching that group were, and remain, significant.

As time passed, the company's dedication to providing information was joined by another motivation—to keep the issue before the public and to engender compassion in the audience, the sense that it could happen here. The techniques of reporting on these tragic and delicate stories had evolved from those days when medical facts were the primary burden of the story to be told. In 1989, Blake reported about the spread of AIDS to the suburbs. She chose Dick and Cheryl to convey the story. Dick, a recovering drug addict, became infected by sharing needles. He infected his wife, Cheryl, through sexual intercourse. Blake remembers the day she videotaped the story:

"My camerawoman, Terri, and I pulled our news–van up to the country antique house in Beverly, Massachusetts. We followed the stone and grass path to the back door where we were greeted by the director of a local AIDS service organization. We were led through the kitchen into a cozy living room. It was filled with huge overstuffed chairs and a big, soft orange and green plaid sofa. Too many places to sit for such a small room. Terri and I studied a portrait hanging over the sofa. We were told 'That's Dick and Cheryl.' Cheryl looked plump and proper in the picture. Her fingernails were manicured and painted. Her hair is poofed like a cheerleader in the 1960s. Dick is a big man with a salt and pepper mustache and a full beard. He was wearing a black leather vest and a black baseball cap with a Harley Davidson emblem stitched on the front. 'Hello. Isn't that a beautiful picture? I made Dick sit for it. He hates to pose. I love it so much.' We turned to see Cheryl. She was obese by medical standards. Her face was made up. Her exhaustion was apparent, the circles deep and dark under her eyes. Cheryl took my arm with her soft, pudgy hand and led me to a chair. She snuggled into a putty–colored recliner and pulled her legs up under her. 'I am going to sit here, this is Dickie's chair.' She pointed to a ham radio next to the chair. 'When he could still get up and around, Dickie would sit here and listen to this thing. That's how he would keep up with what was going on in town.' The camerawoman scoped the room checking for electrical outlets and mentally rearranging furniture to accommodate camera and lights.

"'How is Dick?' I asked. 'We had a rough night. He's very restless.' Cheryl told me he had become progressively weaker and depressed since losing his vision a few months earlier. Pointing to family photos hanging on the wall behind me, she described their life together before AIDS. His love for motorcycles, his Hell's Angels friends, his drinking and drugs and their chance meeting. I did not signal the camerawoman to start rolling videotape. 'Not yet.' I told myself. As she described the day she learned of Dick's AIDS diagnosis, she wept. I reached for her hand. I wondered, 'How can Terri NOT turn on the camera?' I was glad she resisted. We talked more. Cheryl told that she, too, was infected. 'I don't resent him. He didn't know. I tell him when I die, I know he will be at heaven's gate to pick me up on his big, red Harley.' I realized I wasn't talking only to the wife of a recovering drug addict or a person with a disease. I knew they didn't see themselves as victims of AIDS but two people, best friends, battling together through living hell. Cheryl was telling me their love story.

"I thought of the image of the drug addict we and so many other television stations have reinforced by the pictures we have repeatedly aired on the nightly news. To our viewer, a drug addict was the shooting gallery junkie, barely able to talk. Cheryl and Dick did not fit the stereotype. The story showed that a recovering drug addict is a person who may well have made contributions to his world and was capable of loving and being loved.

"Later, it was clear to me that we were only able to hear their story, and record it, because we didn't rush. Terri and I sat with Cheryl and listened before turning on a camera and shoving a microphone in her face. Fortunately, the assignment editor is a sensitive, insightful man. He knew we weren't going to cover a three–alarm fire. This story would take time. He didn't pull us out of

Dick and Cheryl's for a press conference at the State House or a drug bust in Dorchester. As a result, we gained Cheryl's trust. She allowed us to interview Dick and photograph his tortured daily walk to the backyard to breathe fresh air and feel the sunlight on his face. It was important to get those pictures. That is what makes television different from radio.

"And that, I think, is what makes covering AIDS different than many other stories a journalist will cover."

Has Group W's effort made a difference? Larry Kessler is Executive Director of the AIDS Action Committee, Boston. He has seen WBZ–TV's coverage of the crisis from its beginnings back in 1984. Perhaps his can be the final voice on the subject.

Larry Kessler, Executive Director, AIDS Action Committee Boston:

"There is a big difference in the climate in the greater Boston area than other cities, how they approach education, treat people with AIDS, how they respond to appeals for money from AIDS groups, how they deal with the politics around it. We have been able to accomplish a lot because you at WBZ–TV and *The Boston Globe* did the right thing—thoughtful, sensitive, thorough stories and on the mark. In some cities I talk to directors of AIDS organizations who never talk to the media. They have no relationship with the media. That is key to me. The media helps form/mold public opinion by presenting the options objectively. Through its coverage, WBZ made it easier to do the right thing, to educate people.

"WBZ gave people with AIDS a forum. Every research study around shows the best teachers were people with AIDS. Through you, people with AIDS got out there. You helped care–givers and doctors understand what people with AIDS were about. A lot of doctors had an image of what AIDS was like which was shattered when they saw people interviewed by you. It for many was the first time they saw people with AIDS.

"By putting articulate, clearly bright people on T.V. who talked sensibly about what their risk was, how they got AIDS and what they were doing to help educate others helped turn that around... it helped people understand there is no one model of the person with AIDS.

"People follow the lead of the T.V. station they watch. When they see over and over again the same reassuring messages, they get less anxious. We know anxiety makes it difficult for people to hear the facts. Through your coverage, people were able to hear the facts. They picked up human elements of the disease and learned prevention.

"No doubt, Westinghouse has saved lives by slowing and in some cases stopping the spread of AIDS."

Until a cure for AIDS is discovered, Westinghouse Broadcasting Company will provide its audiences with information that allays fears, gains understanding and, hopefully, encourages compassion.

APPENDIX 15–A: THE NATIONAL AIDS LIFELINE CAMPAIGN

The national AIDS LIFELINE campaign consisted of the following elements:

DOCUMENTARIES

- "AIDS 101": A one–hour, studio format show with pre–produced inserts designed to bring viewers basic information about AIDS transmission and prevention. Produced by KPIX so each station could address local issues. Aired nationally in first quarter of 1988.
- "Sexual Roulette": A one–hour pre–produced special produced by KPIX addressing heterosexual risk of AIDS. Aired nationally second quarter of 1988.
- "Critical Condition": A one–hour, pre–produced special also produced at KPIX addressing how the AIDS epidemic is exposing weaknesses within the U.S. health care system. Aired nationally third quarter of 1988. This special was nominated for a 1988 National Emmy in the area of Outstanding News and Documentary.
- "Talking With Teens": This special tackled the tough subject of how parents can discuss AIDS with teenagers. Produced as a home video for distribution through local video stores, this special also aired locally on KPIX July 23, 1988. Produced by KPIX in cooperation with the San Francisco AIDS Foundation. A collateral piece, "Talking With Your Teen About AIDS," was developed in conjunction with the special and make available through local video stores.
- "Remember My Name": A one–hour pre–produced documentary focusing on the first national tour of the Names Project Quilt, a national memorial to the thousands of people who have died of AIDS. This special was honored with a Northern California Emmy Award for Best Documentary of 1988. This special aired fourth quarter nationally. Produced by KPIX.

INFORMATION PAMPHLETS

- AIDS LIFELINE information pamphlet: Re–printed for national distribution in conjunction with the campaign. Over one million copies currently in circulation. Produced by KPIX and the San Francisco AIDS Foundation, and reprinted nationally with local information in each market. The pamphlet was made available in four languages, including Braille. Copies were produced print–ready for each market, along with suggested methods of distribution.

- AIDS LIFELINE volunteer directory: Developed by KPIX for Northern California, in conjunction with KPIX's first sponsorship of the display of the Names Project Quilt. KPIX developed this brochure to give viewers information about the many AIDS service organizations throughout the Bay Area, and how they might volunteer.
- *Talking With Your Teen About AIDS*: Developed in conjunction with the home video "Talking With Teens" and reprinted for national distribution. Produced by KPIX and the San Francisco AIDS Foundation.

PUBLIC SERVICE ANNOUNCEMENTS

The national AIDS LIFELINE campaign included two sets of nationally distributed public service announcements:

- Celebrity Public Service Announcements: January, 1988. A series of 28 public service announcements featuring nine celebrities distributed to all member AIDS LIFELINE stations. These direct and non–sensational messages talked about safe sex and AIDS awareness, and included a tag with information on how to get help locally. Produced by KPIX in San Francisco, and distributed beginning January 21, 1988. Featured Ted Danson, Quincy Jones, Ali McGraw, Marlee Matlin, Ally Sheedy, Jimmy Smits, Justine Bateman, Alyssa Milano and David Steinberg.
- Faces Of AIDS Public Service Announcements: May, 1988. A series of 16 public service announcements highlighting the faces and stories of sixteen national unsung heroes of the AIDS epidemic. Produced by KPIX in San Francisco, and distributed beginning May 23 to all member AIDS LIFELINE stations. Nominated for a 1988 National Emmy Award.

NEWS REPORTS

- A weekly AIDS update news report, produced by KPIX–San Francisco, was fed on Group W's NEWSFEED NETWORK, offering the latest stories on developments in the AIDS epidemic. These stories were satellite fed weekly to member AIDS LIFELINE stations throughout the country. Anchored by KPIX news reporter Hank Plante, and other AIDS reporters throughout the country.

V. REFLECTIONS ON EDUCATION TO PREVENT AIDS

The Impact of AIDS, and AIDS Education, in the Context of Health Problems of the Developing World

David J. Hunter
Lincoln C. Chen

Most of the five to ten million people estimated to be currently infected with the HIV[1] reside in countries of the developing world. These nations have limited financial and human resources to cope with yet another cause of morbidity and mortality. The AIDS epidemic is similar to most of the challenges to the global goal of "health for all" in that it takes a greater toll on economically disadvantaged nations. Therefore we must consider not only the unique characteristics of the AIDS epidemic that give it a high profile, but also attempt to evaluate its impact in comparison with other causes of (often preventable) morbidity and mortality in the developing world. In this chapter we first endeavor to assess the AIDS epidemic in the context of other health problems of the developing world. Then we discuss some aspects of AIDS education efforts of particular importance to developing countries. Finally, we stress the need to consider AIDS education, not just as a response to a major public health challenge of our time, but as another weapon in the fight for a general improvement in health.

AIDS: A UNIQUE DISEASE

AIDS was first clinically described in 1981, and in a short time we have learned an immense amount about the molecular biology of the causative

[1] World Health Organization, *Weekly Epidemiology Record* 63 (1988): 357–60.

virus, the epidemiology of the infection and the clinical course of the disease. The novelty of the AIDS epidemic is not due merely to the short time we have been able to observe it, but to several unique epidemiological features.

The virus

As a retrovirus, HIV integrates its genome into the cells of its host, making complete elimination of established infection difficult for the host immune response, or by conventional chemotherapeutic strategies. Although other viruses can establish lifelong infection, and can often become resurgent many years after first infection, none is known to have the pathogenic potential of HIV. In addition, HIV appears to undergo a high rate of genomic change, which alters its appearance to the immune system, thus contributing to the apparent ineffectiveness of the immune response.[2]

The host

Evidence is emerging that the infectious potential of persons infected with HIV changes over time, being higher in the first few weeks after infection, rapidly lessening, and then gradually increasing as immune function declines.[3] Unexplained individual differences also appear to exist in infectiousness (and perhaps susceptibility to infection).[4] However, an HIV–infected person is potentially infectious lifelong. The fairly long median latency between infection and the development of clinical symptoms of AIDS (at least eight years and probably longer),[5] means that many people infected with HIV are unaware of this infection. Therefore, they may be less likely to modify their behavior to prevent infecting others. This characteristic may be the single most important contributor to the spread of HIV infection.

AIDS: ANOTHER DISEASE IN THE SPECTRUM

Despite its unique features, AIDS is just one among many causes of mortality in developing countries. A study of causes of death at all ages in the developing world estimated that diarrhea caused about 4 300 000 deaths a year, measles 2 000 000, malaria 1 500 000, tetanus 1 200 000, tuberculosis 900 000, hepatitis B 800 000, whooping cough 600 000, typhoid 600 000, meningitis

---

[2] T. J. Matthews and D. P. Bolognesi, "AIDS vaccines," *Scientific American* 259 (1988): 120–27.

[3] R. R. Redfield and D. S. Burke, "HIV infection: The clinical picture," *Scientific American* (1988): 90-8.

[4] W. L. Heyward and J. W. Curran, "The epidemiology of AIDS in the U.S.," *Scientific American* (1988): 72–81.

[5] P. Bacchetti and A. R. Moss, "Incubation period of AIDS in San Francisco," *Nature* 338 (1989): 251–3.

350000, schistosomiasis 250–500000, and syphilis 200000 (table 16–1).[6] Approximately 400–500000 women die each year from pregnancy, childbirth or abortion.[7] Most of these deaths are potentially preventable. The cumulative total of cases of AIDS reported to the World Health Organization's Global Programme on AIDS (GPA) as of August 3rd, 1990, was 273425, and most of these were from developed countries.[8] After allowing for the major underreporting of the disease from countries without comprehensive disease surveillance systems, the WHO estimated that by mid–1989 a cumulative total of about 500000 cases had occurred worldwide, and that approximately 700000 new cases would occur in the three–year period 1989–91, of which more than 300000 would occur in Africa alone.[9] It can be estimated from these statistics that in 1988, of approximately 150000 cases estimated to have occurred, 80–90000 occurred in developing countries. In 1992, of approximately 320000 projected new cases, as many as 200000 may occur in developing countries. Compared with other causes of death in developing countries (table 16–1), AIDS currently accounts for a very small proportion of preventable premature mortality worldwide (although it should be noted that this proportion is relatively greater in severely affected areas, e.g. some African countries). Why then should AIDS occupy such a prominent place on the international and national public health agendas?

The fundamental reason for the priority given to the AIDS epidemic is its potential impact. The impact on public consciousness has been large in many countries; it is more difficult to assess the potential impact of the epidemic on demographic, economic, social and institutional structures. Much of this uncertainty is due to the limited information we have on the natural history of HIV infection. Information is also limited on the true extent of infection with HIV in most countries, due to inadequate health infrastructures, and to ethical considerations in population screening. Background information needed to assess impact, such as routine health and demographic statistics, or information on the population distribution of sexual behaviors, may also be scarce. These information deficits are usually more acute in developing countries, making the business of forecasting more difficult. What then do we really know about the potential impact of AIDS on developing countries?

[6] J. A. Walsh, *Establishing health priorities in the Developing World* (New York: United Nations Development Programme, 1988).

[7] M. Potts, "The most presumptuous pox." *The AIDS Reader* (Brookline, Massachusetts: Branden, 1988).

[8] World Health Organization, *Weekly Epidemiology Record* 65 (1990): 237-44.

[9] J. Mann, "Global AIDS into the 1990s," Address presented 4 June 1989 at the V International Conference in AIDS, Montreal, Canada; and J. Chin and J. Mann, "Global surveillance and forecasting of AIDS," *Bulletin of the World Health Organization* 67 (1989): 1–7.

Table 16–1. *Selected causes of death for individuals of all ages in the developing world.*

Condition	Deaths
Respiratory Disease	10 000 000
Circulatory System	8 000 000
Diarrhea	4 300 000
Measles[†]	2 000 000
Injuries	2 000 000
Neoplasms (excluding hepatoma)	2 000 000
Malaria	1 500 000
Tetanus[†]	1 200 000
Tuberculosis[†]	900 000
Hepatitis B (including hepatoma)[†]	800 000
Whooping Cough[†]	600 000
Typhoid[†]	600 000
Maternal mortality	500 000
Menigitis[†]	350 000
Schistosomiasis	250–500 000
Syphilis	200 000
AIDS (new cases 1992)[*]	200 000
AIDS (new cases 1988)[*]	80–90 000
Amebiasis	70 000
Trypanosomiasis	60 000
Rheumatic Fever and Heart Disease	52 000
Rabies[†]	35 000
Diphtheria[†]	30 000
Dengue	15 000
Hepatitis A	14 000

[†] Preventable or partially preventable by vaccination.

[*] Estimated from data in J. Chin and J. Mann, "Global surveillance and forecasting of AIDS," *Bulletin of the World Health Organization* 67 (1989): 1–7.

Source: Modified from J.A. Walsh, "Establishing health priorities in the Developing World," United Nations Development Programme. New York, 1988.

INTERNATIONAL EPIDEMIOLOGY OF AIDS

We will provide only a brief overview of the salient features of the AIDS pandemic in developing countries. The predominant mode of HIV transmission in Africa, the Caribbean and some areas of South America is heterosexual intercourse. Blood transfusions account for some infections in areas where screening is not available. The reuse of contaminated needles by medical personnel and traditional healers may play a minor role. In countries in which intravenous drug abuse is prevalent, e.g. Thailand, Brazil and Argentina, sharing of unsterilized needles and syringes is an important means of HIV spread.[10]

As more detailed information becomes available on patterns of infection within countries, the extensive heterogeneity of the AIDS epidemic can be appreciated, suggesting that the impact of the epidemic will be highly focal. While generalizations may be useful in global thinking about the disease, understanding the source of the large variations in disease rates within individual countries is extremely important for national decision–makers. The rates of AIDS across the African continent, for instance, are highly variable, which is hardly surprising given that some 2 000 distinct living cultures co–exist in 51 countries with a wide diversity of political systems and degrees of development.[11] In table 16–2, estimated crude incidence rates (rates that have not been adjusted for errors in counting methods) are presented for the 30 countries with populations greater than one million with the highest reported incidence.[12] The estimates in table 16–2 are based on reported cases of AIDS to the World Health Organization, thus the ranking is only approximate as variations in underreporting, and reporting lag, mean that incidence rates are unreliable. Nevertheless, this information does give an impression of the relative severity of the epidemic in different regions of the world. Of the ten highest incidence countries, seven are in east or central Africa, and two from the Caribbean, with the United States the only developed country. A cluster of twelve countries in east, central and southern Africa (Congo, Malawi, Uganda, Burundi, Zambia, Kenya, Tanzania, Central African Republic, Rwanda, Botswana, Zimbabwe and Zaire) emerges, with a cluster of Caribbean countries (Haiti, Trinidad and Tobago, Dominican Republic, Honduras, Panama and Costa Rica) as the developing countries most severely effected by the AIDS epidemic. That this should be evident despite the probable underreporting from many of these countries is broadly consistent with seroprevalence data, and emphasizes the greater impact of the epidemic in these regions.

The AIDS epidemic shows great diversity within countries as well. In the U.S., where HIV surveillance data can be broken down to the level of postal code areas, a greater than fifteen–fold difference in the percentage of HIV–seropositive newborns has been observed between one New York City

[10] D.C. Des Jarlais and S. R. Freidman, "AIDS and IV drug abuse," *Science* 245 (1989): 578.

[11] B. O. de Zalduondo, G. I. Msamanga and L. C. Chen, "AIDS in Africa: diversity in the global pandemic," *Daedalus* 118 (1989): 165–204.

[12] R. P. Bernard, *AIDS–Feedback through 08/1989*, expanded [AF 08 89] Geneva, Switeerland.

Table 16–2. *Estimate crude incidence rates of AIDS in 1988 reported to WHO, in countries of population greater than one milliona.*

Country	Estimated crude AIDS incidence/100 000
Congo	44.13
Malawi	38.53
Uganda	25.47
Burundi	20.54
Zambia	14.31
Haiti	12.60
Kenya	12.29
U.S.	11.18
Tanzania	10.63
Trinidad and Tobago	8.35
C.A.R.	8.09
Switzerland	5.15
Burkina Faso	4.62
Dominican Republic	4.26
France	4.15
Rwanda	3.98
Spain	3.14
Canada	2.99
Italy	2.76
Australia	2.76
Botswana	2.73
Honduras	2.71
Denmark	2.40
Panama	2.33
Zimbabwe	2.28
Zaire	2.06
Netherlands	1.95
Brazil	1.93
Ghana	1.93
Costa Rica	1.87

a Data presented for the 30 countries with the highest estimated incidence. In countries in which cases are under–recognized, under–diagnosed, or under–reported these incidence rates are substantial underestimates of the true incidence (J. Chin and J. Mann, "Global surveillance and forecasting of AIDS," *Bulletin of the World Health Organization* 67 (1989): 1–7.).
Source: R.P. Bernard, *AIDS Feedback through 08/1989*, expanded [AF 08 89]. Geneva, Switzerland.

(0.09%).[13] Similar urban/rural differences exist in Africa. In the Rwandan nationwide serosurvey, the only national serosurvey so far reported from Africa, 18.6% of urban–dwellers were HIV–1 seropositive, compared with 1.3% of approximately age– and sex–matched rural dwellers.[14] Similarly in Haiti, 10% of a sample of urban adults were HIV–1 seropositive, compared with 1% of rural adults.[15] These differences may reflect differences in risk behavior, or stages of epidemic spread. Whatever underlies this diversity, it is apparent that the impact of the HIV pandemic, and thus the appropriate response, will vary substantially within and between countries of the developing world.

PROJECTIONS OF THE EPIDEMIC CURVE

Most of the cases of AIDS that will develop in the next five to ten years will occur among persons already infected with HIV.[16] An estimated five to ten million persons are currently infected. Using the lower estimate of five million for current seroprevalence, and a series of judgments from experts with extensive knowledge of HIV/AIDS epidemiology, the WHO estimates that without prevention programs, approximately 14 million new infections will occur in the 1990s, and by the year 2000 over 800000 new cases of AIDS will occur each year worldwide.[17] If the incidence of other diseases remains stable, then AIDS will rank much higher among the causes of mortality than it does now. Given the long latency between HIV infection and disease, many of these AIDS cases will occur among those already infected. This latency is among the principal reasons that immediate action to prevent infections is so important. In the absence of therapy, primary prevention of infection is the only method of slowing the epidemic. Because the effect of preventive efforts on AIDS cases will not be felt for several years, these efforts must be given immediate priority.

DEMOGRAPHIC IMPACT OF AIDS

Most of the estimates of the demographic impact of AIDS in developing

[13] L. F. Novick, D. Berns, R. Stricof, R. Stevens, K. Pass and J. Wethers, "HIV seroprevalence in newborns in New York State," *Journal of the Amercian Medical Association* 261 (1989): 1745–50.

[14] Rwandan HIV seroprevalence study group, "Nationwide community based serological survey of HIV–1 and other human retrovirus infections in a Central African country," *Lancet*, i (1989): 941–943.

[15] J. W. Pape and W. D. Johnson, "HIV–1 infection and AIDS in Haiti," in *The Epidemiology of AIDS*, eds. R. A. Kaslow and D. P. Francis (Oxford: Oxford University Press, 1989), pp. 221–230.

[16] J. Chin and J. Mann, "Global surveillance and forecasting of AIDS," *Bulletin of the World Health Organization* 67 (1989): 1–7.

[17] World Health Organization, *Weekly Epidemiology Record* 64 (1989): 229–36.

countries have been made for Africa. Early reports of very high HIV sero-prevalence in some African populations[18] led to speculation about the "devastating" effects the epidemic might have on population growth in these countries. Press accounts spoke of "entire regions being depopulated" and humanity being "wiped out."[19] The assumption that the epidemic might lead to negative population growth rates challenged the need for family planning programs. Even after the discovery that the HIV tests used in several early studies had a very high false–positive rate,[20] these concerns remained. Several groups have attempted to assess the demographic impact of the AIDS epidemic in Africa. The simplest method for projecting the incidence of AIDS is extrapolation from trends in case reports. This technique has provided reasonably accurate predictions over a period of a few years in the U.S. and the U.K.[21] In many developing countries data on case reports are inadequate for this purpose, or information on trends is unreliable due to changes in the extent of reporting, and diagnostic recognition of the disease. In any case, for long–term forecasting, complex statistical models are needed. These models must incorporate the complex dynamics of population growth and those associated with spread of the epidemic. They must attempt to do this while several key information gaps exist on important parameters in the models. Thus, projections made so far can serve only to develop possible scenarios of demographic impact.

One set of models estimates the demographic impact of AIDS in selected countries in Africa, using simulations incorporating information on current population size, age distribution and growth rate, along with plausible values of HIV seroprevalence, latency, and male–female and perinatal transmission probabilities.[22] These simulations estimate the effect of AIDS on population growth and absolute population size and the future age–specific distribution of the populations. The general conclusion of this group is that, if unchecked, the AIDS epidemic may significantly reduce population growth rates. Under their worst–case assumptions population growth may

[18] W. C. Saxinger, P. H. Levine, A. G. Dean, G. de The, G. Lange Wantzin, J. Mohhissi, F. Laurent, M. Hoh, M. G. Sarngadharan and R. C. Gallo, "Evidence for exposure to HTLV–III in Uganda before 1973," *Science* 227 (1985):1036–8.

[19] R. Klingholz, "The march of AIDS." reprinted from *World Press Review*, in *The AIDS Reader*, eds. L. K. Clarke and M. Potts (Brookline, Massachusetts: Branden, 1988).

[20] R. J. Biggar, "The AIDS problem in Africa," *Lancet*, i (1986): 79–82.

[21] M. McEvoy and H. Tillet, "Some problems in the prediction of future numbers of cases of the acquired immunodeficiency syndrome in the U.K.," *Lancet*, ii (1985):541–2; and W. N. Morgan and J. W. Curran, "Acquired immunodeficiency syndrome: Current and future trends," *Public Health Reports* 101 (5) (1986): 459–65.

[22] R. M. Anderson, R. M. May and A. R. McLean, "Possible demographic consequences of AIDS in developing countries," *Nature* 332 (1988): 228–234; and R. M. May, R. M. Anderson and S. M. Blower, "The epidemiology and transmission dynamics of HIV–AIDS," *Daedalus* 118 (2) (1989): 163–201; and R. M. Anderson, "Mathematical and statistical studies of the epidemiology of HIV," *AIDS* 3 (1989): 333–46.

become negative, although the predicted time to onset of a decline in population is long, on the order of several decades. These models do not predict that the age structure of these populations will change dramatically, as the direct effects of mortality among adults is approximately cancelled out by the direct effect of increased infant mortality due to HIV infection, with a decline in birth rate due to adult deaths. However, this loss of young and middle–aged adults may have substantial social and economic impact.

The authors of the study themselves describe these projections as "crude," and point to deficiencies in the model assumptions that make these estimates uncertain.[23] A major simplification is the assumption that mixing of sexual partners is homogeneous and random. More complex models that incorporate heterogeneity in sexual behavior, and pooling or networking of sexual contacts, are needed. The ultimate prevalence of infection will be lower, for instance, if there is substantial variability in rates of sexual partner change, and persons are more likely to choose sexual partners from their own sexual activity class, leading to the concentration of infection among more active groups.[24]

A model that does incorporate some basic stratification by sexual activity[25] leads to quantitatively different conclusions.[26] Growth of the epidemic is slower under these assumptions, with the population growth rates in a hypothetical African country remaining substantially positive after 25 years of projection. Interestingly, this model also predicts little impact on the age structure of the population.

While the general conclusions of these models may seem reassuring (at least to proponents of the "depopulation" and "apocalypse" scenarios), the fact remains that population growth is only preserved by the very high prevailing birth rates in these countries. These models still predict a doubling of the mortality rate in severely affected countries. This is equivalent to 1.3% of the entire population dying of AIDS each year, over and above the 1.3% dying of all other causes (this figure is a projection for the year 2000, overall mortality in most African countries is currently between 1.5% and 2.3%[27]). Thus, for a country of 20 million, the second model predicts 260 000 deaths due to AIDS annually. This, then, is the most powerful rationale for treating AIDS as an urgent health priority. Unless we slow the growth of the

[23] R. M. Anderson, R. M. May and A. R. McLean, "Possible demographic consequences of AIDS in developing countries," *Nature* 332 (1988): 228–34.

[24] R. M. Anderson, "Mathematical and statistical studies of the epidemiology of HIV," *AIDS*, 3 (1989): 333–46.

[25] J. Bongaarts, "A model of the spread of HIV infection and the demographic impact of AIDS," *Stats Med* 8 (1989): 103–20.

[26] J. Bongaarts and P. Way, *Geographic variation in the HIV epidemic and the mortality impact of AIDS in Africa* (New York: Population Council, 1989).

[27] *World Health Statistics Annual* (Geneva: World Health Organization, 1988).

epidemic in high prevalence areas, the impact on population will be devastating in these areas. Unless we slow the growth of the epidemic worldwide, AIDS will take its place among the leading causes of death worldwide. The high cumulative incidence of AIDS among infected persons, and the long latency of the disease, means that to prevent these future deaths, we must prevent infections now. The models cited assume no change in high–risk sexual behavior, and demonstrate what could happen without behavior change. The possibility exists that further deterioration in the economies of the developing world, rapid urbanization and improved transport, may combine to further foster social conditions in which HIV is encouraged to spread. The challenge is to resist this tendency, and to promote sexual behavior change, and the aim should be to prevent even the most optimistic projections of these models from becoming reality.

ECONOMIC IMPACT

The economic impact of AIDS in developing countries is likely to be directly proportional to the magnitude of the epidemic. With this magnitude only crudely estimated, estimates of economic impact are even more uncertain. The focal nature of the epidemic further complicates economic forecasting, difficult enough at the national level. There are few studies of the costs of HIV infection in specific developing countries, although guidelines for the rapid estimation of these costs have been proposed.[28] Again, some qualitative statements can be made.

The direct costs of AIDS are the costs of health care, social care and public sector costs such as surveillance, blood screening, health education and research. Indirect costs are principally those of lost economic production. For the United States, the cost of AIDS in 1991 was estimated to be $66.5 billion, of which $10.8 billion were direct costs and $55.6 billion, indirect costs.[29] Although estimates of costs in developing countries are at least an order of magnitude lower, a similar preponderance of indirect over direct costs is predicted.

Scarce technology and treatment resources limit the direct costs of AIDS in developing countries. Indeed, in a transnational comparative study of estimated direct costs of AIDS, a strong correlation was observed between annual cost per patient–year of AIDS treatment and per capita gross national

[28] M. Over, S. Bertozzi and J. Chin, "Guidelines for rapid estimation of the direct and indirect costs of HIV infection in a developing country," *Health Policy* 11 (1989): 169–86.

[29] A. A. Scitovsky and D. P. Rice, "Estimates of the direct and indirect costs of acquired immunodeficiency syndrome in the United States 1985, 1986, and 1991," *Public Health Report* 102 (1987): 5–17.

product.[30] In a study of costs in Zaire and Tanzania, for instance, annual direct costs for AIDS cases were estimated at $132 U.S. dollars to $1582 in Zaire, and $104 to $631 in Tanzania. Compare this to the annual gross national product per capita of $290 and $170, respectively. However, the lower cost structure does not imply a diminished impact on individuals. The potential impact on AIDS patients and their families is overwhelming. In a study of families of children with symptomatic AIDS, the cost of a single hospitalization was four times the average monthly income, and funeral expenses were 11 times this average.[31] Few developing countries have insurance or welfare systems to help with these expenses, thus the burden of direct costs will be borne by families and their communities, already struggling for subsistence.

Lifetime indirect costs have been estimated to be at least four times greater than direct costs in Zaire and Tanzania,[32] and in Puerto Rico.[33] Data on projected case loads are still too scanty to make firm estimates of the impact of total costs on overall economic performance. Secondary costs such as a possible decline in tourism are also difficult to assess. But the concentration of the epidemic among young urban adults in their most economically productive years suggests that the economic impact will be large. A selective loss of educated and skilled workers in business and government may have profound consequences beyond what would be predicted if the distribution of disease was random.[34] In many severely affected countries in Africa, economic growth rates were slow or declining, even before the AIDS epidemic. The economic impact of AIDS is likely to exacerbate this tendency, adding another barrier to economic growth.

IMPACT ON HEALTH CARE SYSTEMS

The economic impact of AIDS in developing countries where HIV prevalence is high is felt most acutely by their health care systems. At the Mama Yemo

[30] A. A. Scitovsky and M. Over, "AIDS:costs of care in the developed and the developing world," *AIDS* 2 (Suppl.1) (1988): 571–581.

[31] F. Davachi, N. Mayemba, L. Kabongo, K. Ndoko and B. N'Galy, "The economic and social implications of AIDS in an African setting," V International Conference on AIDS, Montreal, June, 1989 (abstract W.H.P.6).

[32] M. Over, S. Bertozzi, J. Chin, B. N'Galy and Nyamuryekung'e, "The direct and indirect cost of HIV infection in developing countries: the cases of Zaire and Tanzania," in *The global impact of AIDS*, eds. A. F. Fleming, M. Carballo, D. W. Fitz Simmons, M. R. Bailey and J. Mann (New York: Alan Liss, 1988).

[33] J. I. Alameda–Lozada and A. Gonzalez–Martinez, "Economic analysis of AIDS in Puerto Rico," V International Conference on AIDS, Montreal, June 1989 (abstract W.H.P.5); and D. S. Shepard, Y. Kouri, S. Borras, J. Garib, J. Balling, "Costs of AIDS in a developing area: indirect and direct costs of AIDS in San Juan, Puerto Rico," V International Conference on AIDS, Montreal, June 1989 (abstract T.H.0.12).

[34] J. Chin and J. Mann, "Global surveillance and forecasting of AIDS," *Bulletin of the World Health Organization* 67 (1989): 1–7.

Hospital in Kinshasa, Zaire, 50% of a sample of 236 adult admissions to the Department of Internal Medicine in late 1988 were HIV seropositive.[35] In Abidjan, Ivory Coast, 49% of 1,794 hospitalized patients were HIV seropositive in 1988.[36] In Port–au–Prince, Haiti, 23% of 117 adult general admissions were HIV seropositive.[37] In Rio de Janeiro, Brazil, 19% of 496 adult medical admissions consenting to be tested at two teaching hospitals in late 1988 were HIV–1 seropositive.[38] In countries in which annual health expenditure per capita may be less than five U.S. dollars, this extra burden will seriously compromise the ability of medical facilities to respond to other types of illness. It is possible that the spread of the AIDS epidemic will also amplify the incidence of other infectious diseases. Tuberculosis, for instance, is one of the most frequent opportunistic infections among HIV–infected persons in sub–Saharan Africa,[39] and there has been a rise in the incidence of tuberculosis in some countries.[40] Tuberculosis control programs will need to be expanded to cope with this increased demand.

The recent announcement that the drug azidothymidine (AZT) not only improves survival in AIDS patients, but delays the onset of AIDS in healthy HIV–infected persons,[41] will make this drug a cornerstone of medical therapy in developed countries. The cost of this treatment, currently $2000–4000 per year, makes it effectively unavailable in developing countries. As medical therapy for AIDS improves, the disparity between treatment and survival among infected persons in developed and developing countries will increase.

SOCIAL IMPACT

While societies may share some common means of responding to an epi-

[35] S. E. Hassig, J. Perriens, E. Baende, K. Bishagara, R. W. Ryder and B. Kapita, "The economic impact of HIV infection in adult admissions to internal medicine (IM) at Mama Yemo Hospital," V International Conference on AIDS, Montreal, June 1989 (abstract T.H.O.9).

[36] K. Odehouri, K. De Cock, R. Colebunders, A. Porter, G. Adjorlolo, W. Heyward et al., "Clinical manifestations of HIV-1 and HIV–2 infections in Abidjan, Cote d'Ivoire," V International Conference on AIDS, Montreal, June 1989 (abstract T.B.O.10).

[37] M. Adrien, R. Boulos, A. Louis, F. Joseph, P. Kissinger, N. Halsey et al., "HIV–l in hospitalized Haitian pediatric and adult patients," V International Conference on AIDS, Montreal, June 1989 (abstract T.G.0.20).

[38] F. S. Sion, A. B. Serenoj, J. W. Krebs, R. S. Goncalves, E. P. Quinhoes, B. G. Weniger, M. A. Perex, E. A. Santos, C. F. Ramos Filho, P. M. Valiante, C. Ismael, and the Clinical AIDS Study Group, "Detection of HIV–2 infection and ratio to HIV–l among hospitalized patients in Rio de Janeiro, Brazil," V International Conference on AIDS, Montreal, June 1989 (abstract T.G.P.25).

[39] A. Elliot, N. Luo, G. Tembo, G. Steenbergen, P. Nunn, K. McAdam et al., "The impact of Human Immunodeficiency Virus (HIV) on Tuberculosis in Zambia: A cross–sectional study," V International Conference on AIDS, Montreal, June 1989 (abstract Th.G.0.4).

[40] World Health Organization, Weekly Epidemiology Record 64 (1989): 125–32.

[41] AIDS Newsletter 4 (1989): 1.

demic,[42] the nature of the response is powerfully determined by the nature of the society. The response to AIDS in developing countries varies with the cultures in which it appears, and evolves with the epidemic. We can analyze social response on many levels: the organized response of governments, the response of the scientific community, and the social treatment of HIV–infected persons. Only a very few generalizations can be made about the social impact of AIDS on developing countries.

While some governments in developing countries have responded with a rapidity that would shame many in developed countries, others have been slow, and some continue to be skeptical about the need for a major response. In the U.S. the failure of political response is attributed, at least in part, to the assumption that science will produce a technological solution to the problem.[43] This is unlikely to be the case in developing countries, few of which have reaped the public health benefits of technological advances for the prevention of other diseases. In many developing countries the prevailing assumption is that most disease is infectious in nature. Thus, a new infectious disease has not had the same initial impact as in countries where epidemic fatal infectious diseases were the province of historians. The large number of preventable causes of premature mortality in developing countries raises questions that have yet to be fully answered about the priority to be given to this new epidemic. The interest shown by developed countries in the AIDS problem in the developing world can easily appear to be narrow self–interest, given the poor past performance of developed countries in helping with many public health issues that are not as easily transportable.

In Haiti first, and then in Africa, the search by scientists (and journalists) from developed countries for an origin of HIV in developing countries, has led to charges of racism, and probably contributed to the reluctance of some governments to make an official response to the epidemic.[44] Alternate hypotheses about the means of HIV spread, some developed in response to the "African origin" theory, may interfere with the urgent task of education and prevention. While the effort to reconstruct the spread of the AIDS epidemic may lead to insights about prevention, the understandable perception that it is an exercise in the allocation of "blame" for the epidemic means that it should only be pursued with the collaboration of, and sensitivity for the feelings of, colleagues in Africa.

Much of what is known about the impact of AIDS on social relations of individuals in developing countries is similar to the experience of persons

[42] C. E. Rosenberg, "What is an epidemic?" *Daedalus* 102 (1989): 1–17.

[43] J. E. Osborn, "Public Health and the politics of AIDS prevention," *Daedalus* 118 (1989): 123–144.

[44] R. Chirimuuta and R. Chirimuuta, *AIDS, Africa and racism* (London: Free Association Books, 1989).

with AIDS in developed countries. But most of this information is anecdotal and research into the impact of AIDS on individuals and their families is needed to define their needs more accurately. In the U.S., grass roots organizations dedicated to the needs of people with AIDS have served as advocates, attempting to obtain access to health and social services for AIDS patients, and as care–providers, picking up where organized societal response leaves off.[45] But many of these non–profit, community–based organizations originate in a shared minority identity, specifically among homosexual men, and it is not obvious how successfully these groups can organize when the principal risk group is in the majority, i.e., heterosexuals in developing countries. Stigmatization against AIDS is still a powerful force suppressing the formation of such groups in many countries, and the absence of this source of advocacy may be one reason that AIDS is not a matter for public debate in some countries.[46] Methods to catalyze the formation of these groups in developing countries need to be explored. Preliminary data from Kinshasa, for instance, suggest that community acceptance of, and family support for, AIDS patients is high.[47] This suggests that the formation of these groups would be possible. As persons currently infected with HIV become symptomatic, the need for community support will intensify.

OPTIONS FOR AIDS PREVENTION

The above emphasizes the importance of slowing the epidemic of HIV infection, but the critical question remains: what are the most cost–effective approaches? Elimination of transfusion–associated HIV infection is possible, for instance, through increased availability of testing technology and training. However, given the high costs of screening relative to average per capita health expenditure in many developing countries, sustained external assistance is likely to be necessary. Currently, blood screening is one of the few demonstrably effective AIDS prevention options,[48] and it is important to recognize that there are additional potential benefits to screening: a means of monitoring seroprevalence, increased public confidence in hospital treatment and safety, the potential to boost morale in National AIDS Control Programs, the secondary prevention of transmission from transfusion–infected

[45] H.V. Fineberg, "The social dimensions of AIDS," *Scientific American* 259 (1988): 128–34.

[46] A.J. Fortin, "The politics of AIDS in Kenya," From *The Third World Quarterly*, reprinted in *The AIDS Reader* (Brookline, Massachusetts: Branden, 1988).

[47] A. A. Scitovsky and M. Over, "AIDS: costs of care in the developed and the developing world," *AIDS*, 2(Suppl.1) (1988): 571–81; and P. Onyango and P. Walji, "The family as a resource," in eds. A. F. Fleming, M. Carballo, D. W. Fitz Simmons, M. R. Bailey and J. Mann, *The global impact of AIDS* (New York: Alan Liss, 1988).

[48] D. Shepard and J. Eichner, "Cost–effectiveness of screening to reduce transfusion–related AIDS in developing areas," IV International Conference on AIDS, Stockholm, June 1988 (abstract 5127).

persons. In response to these considerations, approximately 10% of the WHO GPA budget is dedicated to preventing this means of transmission, compared with only 15% devoted to the prevention of sexual transmission.[49] The attributable risk due to infection via blood transfusion is low in most countries, however, thus the relative priority given to this route of infection will need to be re–examined as information improves on the cost–effectiveness of other approaches.

Few studies of the cost–effectiveness of specified interventions in developing countries exist however, and fewer still have compared the relative cost–effectiveness of different interventions. A framework for these analyses[50] offers some important insights. Preventing HIV infection in an individual also prevents infection among those the individual may subsequently infect. Reproductive rates (the average number of secondary infections generated by one primary infection in a susceptible population) have been estimated to range from 4.0 to 11.3 for several populations in East Africa, implying that these numbers of new cases would be prevented by prevention of the single primary case.[51] This amplification substantially increases the cost–effectiveness of many AIDS interventions, in relation to the use of similar interventions to prevent diseases that are not transmissible. Another important principle is that the cost–effectiveness of an intervention depends on the prevalence of HIV at the time of intervention. Once prevalence is high, the increased probability of future infection reduces the gain from preventing an episode of transmission.[52] Both principles tend to suggest that in countries where the prevalence of HIV infection is detectable, interventions may be more cost–effective early in the epidemic than later.

The few studies of the cost–effectiveness of AIDS interventions in developing countries that exist are consistent with this result. Modeling interventions in sub–Saharan Africa stress that early introduction of control measures decreases the long–term severity and costs of the epidemic.[53] For each dollar spent on AIDS prevention in Puerto Rico, as many as ten might be saved in direct and indirect costs of AIDS cases prevented.[54] Where possi-

[49] Anonymous, "Editorial," *Lancet*, i (1989): 1111–3.

[50] M. C. Weinstein, J. D. Graham, J. E. Seigel and H.V. Fineberg, "Cost–effectiveness analysis of AIDS prevention programs: concepts, complications, and illustrations," in *aids Sexual behaviour and intravenous drug abuse*, eds. C. F. Turner, H. G. Miller and L. E. Moses (Washington, D.C.: National Academy Press, 1989).

[51] R. M. Anderson, "Mathematical and statistical studies of the epidemiology of HIV," *AIDS* 3 (1989): 333–46.

[52] J. Rowley, T. W. Ng and R. M. Anderson, "Some economic implications of introducing control measures to reduce the spread of HIV infection in sub–Saharan Africa," V International Conference on AIDS, Montreal, June 1989 (abstract T.H.O.16).

[53] *Ibid.*

[54] D.S. Shepard, "Costs of AIDS in a developing area: Indirect and direct costs of AIDS in Puerto Rico," in *Economic Aspects of AIDS and HIV Infection*, eds. D. Schwefel, R. Leidl, J. Revira and M. F. Drummond (New York: Springer-Verlas, 1990).

ble, studies of the effectiveness of prevention programs should be incorporated into their design. But introduction of prevention programs can not await definitive demonstration of cost–effectiveness. As all indications suggest that early intervention is important, programs modeled on other countries' experience, or campaigns demonstrated to be effective in modifying other behaviors, should be used in all developing countries where HIV is present.

PROBLEMS FOR AIDS EDUCATION PROGRAMS IN DEVELOPING COUNTRIES

In addition to these uncertainties about AIDS prevention options, developing countries have additional problems in mounting effective AIDS education programs. In many developing countries, great heterogeneity exists in ethnicity, language and culture. Since education efforts should "reflect the particular needs and characteristics of target audiences,"[55] diversity in the targets increases the work required to develop, pretest, implement and assess AIDS prevention strategies.

Our knowledge base on the determinants of human sexuality and mechanisms for influencing behavior is poor. The developed world is hardly better off than developing countries in this respect. In culturally heterogeneous societies improving this knowledge base is likely to take more effort than in more homogeneous populations.

A major barrier to both research and action is the diminished infrastructure in many developing countries. Even if funding is available, a lack of trained personnel with experience in health education, social marketing and program implementation is a major barrier to progress.

Just as AIDS education efforts have been "crippled" in the U.S. by forces such as right–wing moralism and homophobia,[56] many developing countries face powerful institutional pressures against high–profile AIDS campaigns. AIDS education messages about safer sex and condom use may come into conflict with religious proscriptions. The centralization of power in many developing countries often means that policies on AIDS education are totally dependent on the personal beliefs and priorities of national leaders. In this regard again, many developed countries are similar, e.g. the Presidential inaction in the U.S., and the recent cancellation of a nationwide survey on sexuality by the Prime Minister of the U.K. In countries where the leadership has encouraged or demanded action on AIDS education, large campaigns and innovative programs have been possible.

We must overcome these difficulties to limit the spread of AIDS. The het-

---

[55] World Health Organization, *Weekly Epidemiology Record* 64 (1989): 13–20.
[56] H. V. Fineberg, "The social dimensions of AIDS," *Scientific American* 259 (1988): 128–34.

erogeneity of the AIDS epidemic calls for heterogeneity in research, and part of this diversity must derive from the instincts of local researchers adapting to their own situations. The paucity of these researchers, and the urgent need for cost–effective AIDS interventions and their use in all settings in which they are effective, makes international collaboration more necessary than usual.

PRIORITIES FOR RESEARCH IN AIDS EDUCATION

It has become almost banal to assert that in the absence of an effective vaccine or treatment, education is our only weapon against the AIDS epidemic. Yet most AIDS funding worldwide still goes to clinical or laboratory research. In the U.S. in 1987, for instance, only two percent of Public Health Service AIDS research funds were allocated to social and behavioral research,[57] and the situation seems little different in most other countries. To our knowledge no in depth analysis of the reasons for this disparity has been done. Possible causes include lack of communication between the competing scientific cultures of the biomedical and social sciences, the influence in AIDS funding decisions of representatives of developed countries trained to look for technological solutions, and the frequent dominance of medically trained scientists with the same technological orientation in national AIDS committees in all countries.

An idealized paradigm for research in AIDS education might go as follows: improved information on human sexuality and the determinants of sexual behaviors; selection of target groups for cost–effective intervention; design of pilot education programs; testing and evaluation of these programs; larger–scale implementation combined with evaluation and refinement. Given the urgency of the situation in countries where prevalence is high, AIDS education cannot await full completion of this research and design process. To improve education programs over the long term while responding to immediate needs, in–depth research must go hand in hand with action based on incomplete knowledge, and evaluation of this action. AIDS educators face the challenge of simultaneously building a knowledge base while implementing and evaluating programs. The heterogeneity of the AIDS epidemic implies that these activities need to be locally focussed, increasing demands on funding and personnel. How can we respond effectively to this overwhelming need?

---

[57] J. E. Seigal, J. D. Graham and M. A. Stoto, "Allocating resources among AIDS research strategies," *Policy Sciences* 1989 (In press).

INTERNATIONAL COOPERATION FOR AIDS EDUCATION

Few countries in the developing world have formal systems in place adequate to respond to this challenge. International cooperation is thus vital. Developed countries have considerable self–interest in assisting developing countries in AIDS control, as isolationism is a poor defense against pandemic infectious disease,[58] particularly one as adapted to different cultures and environments as AIDS. But the nature of the pandemic requires that this cooperation be sensitive to local priorities and needs.

The major formal mechanism for international cooperation in promoting AIDS education has been the Global Programme on AIDS (GPA) of the World Health Organization. Perhaps the most important achievement of the GPA has been its success in placing AIDS on the international health agenda, drawing initially skeptical or unwilling nations into the international response to the pandemic. The GPA has also used its moral authority to temper authoritarian public health responses to persons with AIDS is some countries.

The GPA has also played the major role in coordinating the global response to the pandemic. Through the mechanisms of national medium—term plans, countries have formulated the goals and objectives of their governmental response. On the research front, a GPA–coordinated set of surveys of sexual behavior in 20 countries across the world promises to provide useful comparative data, as well as locally needed information to design intelligent interventions. Through its staff and consultants, GPA offers technical assistance to national AIDS committees who request it.

Multilateral organizations such as the World Bank and the United Nations Development Programme, and many non–governmental organizations, are playing a major role in funding and technical assistance for AIDS education. Still more cooperative work is needed to expand the scope of intervention efforts. Many problems in conducting AIDS research in developing countries and dilemmas about the appropriate role of the international community have their origin in the scarcity of trained public health professionals. Research, program design and implementation, and policy making all require skills that are in short supply in many developing countries, with training in behavioral sciences and health education particularly scarce. It is unfortunate that the urgent need for action frequently argues against taking key personnel from their posts for training at institutions in developed countries. To effectively deal with all their health problems, not just AIDS, developing countries need public health professionals trained in–country, as well as overseas. Strengthening public health capacity is an area in which developed country institutions could play a much–needed

---

[58] L. C. Chen, "The AIDS pandemic: An internationalist approach to disease control," *Daedalus* 116 (2) (1989): 181–95.

role; current models for short–term training need to be extended. Fostering of this capacity for local research independence is crucial if developing countries are to assess and begin to deal with their own public health problems.

AIDS EDUCATION FOR THE FUTURE

Just as the AIDS epidemic has demonstrated the essential interdependence of the health of populations around the world, so AIDS itself reminds us of the connections between our environment, behavior and health that underlie the preventable diseases which account for most of the premature morbidity and mortality in the world. AIDS education is specifically designed to prevent the transmission of HIV, but also offers opportunities for broad—based health improvement. The fact that syphilis causes more deaths annually in developing countries than AIDS (table 16–1) is a reminder that other, older, diseases can be addressed in the context of AIDS prevention. A broad–based STD control program may help prevent HIV infection and the morbidity associated with other STDs and their long–term sequelae such as infertility, ectopic pregnancy, opthalmia neonatorum and congenital syphilis. Indeed, in areas in which genital ulcer diseases (chancroid, syphilis and herpes simplex II) are widely prevalent, HIV may not be controlled until these diseases are.[59]

Much of the world's preventable disease depends upon human behaviors such as smoking, eating patterns, exercise, hygiene and sanitation. In the developing world, choice of behaviors may be limited by economic circumstance. However, personal and community decisions about allocation of scarce resources often determine behaviors such as nutrition and hygiene. Lack of health education may expose whole populations to avoidable risks. Beyond the immediate goals of AIDS prevention, two challenges exist for AIDS education personnel: First, to use knowledge of the determinants of behavior and behavior change gained from AIDS–related research to explore strategies of inducing behavior change beneficial against other preventable diseases; second, to integrate these strategies into AIDS prevention programs, whenever this can be done without compromising the AIDS prevention goals.

In the specific context of AIDS prevention, numerous needs exist. We must rapidly add to our stock of knowledge on human sexual behavior and its determinants. We need to enhance our experience in behavioral interventions, and evaluate these whenever possible. Information systems

[59] W. Cates and G. S. Bowen, "Education for AIDS prevention: Not our only voluntary weapon," *American Journal of Public Health* 79 (1989): 871–4.

are needed that can cope with the explosion of new data and research and operational findings, and distribute these efficiently around the world so that all applicable experiences can be shared. Above all, we must build up local expertise and strengthen local resources, in order to create relevant, sustainable AIDS education systems.

If the legacy of AIDS were the mobilization of these resources and the ultimate control of HIV infection, then much would have been achieved. But we must not forget that it is the social and economic environment, as much as the virus, which has created the conditions for its epidemic spread in developing countries. In this environment a multiplicity of other diseases produces equal or greater misery and pain. Development of channels for AIDS education offers an opportunity to affect other health–seeking behaviors. Horizontal linkages of AIDS programs into appropriate programs such primary health care and family planning can be used to strengthen these. Stronger research and implementation capability in developing countries should be of benefit to all who seek to find ways to reduce the burden of disease. One of the many important challenges of the AIDS pandemic is the challenge to direct our energy not only toward the control of a single disease, however tragic, but to use AIDS education as a weapon in the fight for broad–based social and health improvement.

This work has been partially supported by the John Merck Fund.

U.S. Response to the AIDS Epidemic: Education Prospects in a Multicultural Society

June Osborn

The earliest years of the AIDS epidemic in the United States were characterized by an illusion of relative epidemiologic homogeneity, which fostered the assumption that preventive responses could be directed at groups. Tasteless jokes grew out of the high risk identification of the "four H's": homosexuals, hemophiliacs, heroin addicts, and Haitians, and so did simplistic thinking. Only gradually did we learn how complicated the task of AIDS education was going to be. Instead of (declared) homosexuality, the real challenge would be to reach closeted gay men or bisexuals; instead of Haitians, persons of diverse Caribbean origins shared an enhanced risk relating almost surely to the timing of virus introduction into their communities. Heroin addicts concentrated risk through shared injection apparatus, but so did intravenous (IV) cocaine users and—more confounding—"crack" smokers whose barter of sex for drugs closed the loop on risk behaviors. Even the world of the hemophiliac was made complex by growing awareness of heterosexual risk to spouses.

Thus, the early efforts to streamline messages of risk to "high–risk groups" were fraught with serious hazard, and a fundamental lesson was learned: it was risk behavior, not group identification, that influenced the likelihood of HIV exposure and subsequent disease. In many countries and cultures, that lesson could spur widespread educational efforts to alert people about the hazards of multiple sexual partners, anal intercourse and drug–using behaviors.

In the United States, however, the challenge had just begun. Not only

was linguistic diversity a challenge due to the rapidly increasing representation of Hispanics and various Asians in the society, but ethnic and
cultural variety meant that the delivery of precise messages concerning risk
behaviors would require a dizzying glossary of terms relating to subcultures which varied widely in literacy and self–perception. So daunting are
the problems posed by this diversity that it is fair to say that the future
success of AIDS prevention in the U.S. hangs on the cleverness and social
organization devoted to bridging gaps of literacy, linguistics and subcultures. As an articulate Hispanic activist put it, in pleading for support from
foundations for her organization's AIDS educational activities at the community level, "it will take you a lot less time to teach us what we need to know
about AIDS than it would for us to teach you how to be Hispanic."

CULTURAL DIVERSITY

The strict dependence of the human immunodeficiency virus on specific
human behaviors for its transmission has great significance in the context of
cultural diversity. To take a specific example, anal intercourse is clearly the
most efficient variation of sexual intercourse in spreading the virus from
infected to uninfected partners. This fact has been well–documented in
prospective studies of homosexual male couples and serves as a fundamental tenet of "safer sex" education. However, if that lesson is directed solely
to "homosexual males," many bisexual men who think of themselves as
heterosexual but who have intermittent same–sex intercourse will miss the
message and remain at risk. Similarly, while the frequency of heterosexual
anal intercourse is poorly documented, it appears to play a frequent role as
a "poor man's contraceptive" and/or a strategem to maintain the anatomic
"proof" of female virginity in cultures where that holds high value.

Thus, discussions of anal intercourse must vary greatly depending on
the cultural setting and the intended audience. But the complexity does not
stop there, for bisexuality has a far greater and somewhat less controversial
presence in some minority cultures than does avowed homosexuality (in
either minority or majority cultures). While homosexuality is met with
deep hostility, same–sex intercourse may sometimes be relatively common,
and the language used to describe such interaction can be quite distinctive.
For instance, in 1987 there was an effort by the U.S. Centers for Disease
Control to broaden the self–exclusionary warning to blood donors by changing the phrase "homosexual men" to "men who have had sex with other
men." That well–intended effort may have fallen short, however, for in some
American black communities that activity, while fairly frequent, is not
referred to as "sex."

LINGUISTIC DIVERSITY

The example just cited could be viewed equally as a matter of cultural or of linguistic diversity. In the more usual sense of linguistic variation, other kinds of problems arise. While these may be generally obvious, one example might serve to demonstrate how intractable they may be to resolution. In an effort to adapt a proposed (English language) questionnaire about variations in sexual practices, highly trained, Spanish–speaking translators were employed to try to assure that answers to the same intended question could be melded meaningfully between English– and Spanish–speaking respondents. So profound were the etymologic divisions, however, that the Spanish version of "vaginal intercourse" was invariably misunderstood to mean "lesbianism."

It is to be hoped that sufficient effort can be mustered to overcome such obvious linguistic gaps and ethnic/cultural variations. However, it is likely that much indigenous talent will be needed to do so.

SOCIOECONOMIC EFFECTS

The challenges posed by linguistic and cultural variations pale next to the difficulties posed when AIDS–preventive education is directed to hopeless and/or deeply impoverished people. An alienated, homeless adolescent may be almost completely impervious to the warning that HIV acquired now might cause awful illness five or ten years later. A sobering statistic recently appeared that, of U.S. black men aged 16, only one in four could expect to reach the age of 25 without being involved with drugs, in prison or dead. The awesome statistic that 80% of HIV–infected people will be sick or dead of AIDS 10 years after infection tends to fade into the background when compared with those more immediately dismal odds.

This socioeconomic gradient presents a direct impasse to AIDS education in America's disadvantaged communities, and it is no coincidence that both illicit drug use and HIV infection are now focussed disproportionately on those groups of young people (and their children). It is very likely that significant inroads can be made into the drug and AIDS (and STD and teenage pregnancy) epidemics only by recognizing and attacking the debilitating hopelessness and poverty that serves as a common fuel for those several conflagrations.

COMMUNICATION ACROSS BARRIERS

A final set of considerations adds to the challenge of multicultural education in the United States, and that is the perceived threat of unaccepted behavior. Many of the populations at unduly high risk of HIV (because of characteristics discussed above) perceive themselves to be at risk from majority legal and social forces. Clearly "illegal aliens" are one such group, but so are many families whose status is somewhat more secure but nonetheless tenuous. The most extreme examples occur in the context of illicit drug use and/or homosexuality in states where the latter is illegal. If AIDS education must be visible and actively sought under the aegis of authority, it may not reach its mark when to participate is to condemn oneself in the eye of the law. A more subtle but equally compelling example is the education (in the majority community) aimed at "homosexual men." While openly gay advocates of "safer sex" have had great impact in reducing HIV transmission in declared gay communities in the United States, deeply "closeted" homosexual men—who may barely admit their risk behavior to themselves—are likely to be the last, not the first, to benefit from such straightforward messages and entirely different strategies may be needed to alert them effectively to their risk.

CONCLUSION

These several paragraphs barely scratch the surface of the barrier presented by cultural diversity to efforts at universal HIV preventive education. Were the stakes less high, the impediments might seem overwhelming. But those stakes are the very future of our children's children, so much talent and energy will be needed to be sure of long–term success.

These generalizations seem clear at the outset. First, since very new issues are posed in the challenge (to convey information about intimate behavior to diverse populations), there is much yet to be learned. Furthermore, as a fringe benefit of success in such efforts, many areas of public and human health can be improved significantly with the fresh insights and techniques likely to be needed.

Second, the complex tasks of spreading information across barriers of language, culture and socioeconomic status are likely to prove impossible without the complicity and primary participation of members of targeted communities. A central role from community–based organizations is sure to be essential for the success of such efforts. As a corollary, those groups must be given a major say in determining the specific wording and mode of communication of pertinent HIV education, for there is no way to be understood if one does not speak in language comprehensible to one's intended listener.

Finally, this will all be somewhat easier if attention is paid quickly to school education at the earliest possible stage. Given the structure of American society, the early (required) school years provide the major—if not the sole—opportunity for a universal audience. HIV and AIDS will not go away; they will be a fact of life for generations to come. Just as traffic signals were unnecessary in the 19th century but indispensable in the 20th, so will knowledge of AIDS avoidance be a crucial element for survival as the 21st century dawns. The earlier and more pertinently we attack the problems limiting effective education, the more profoundly can we contribute to the richness inherent in humanity and its cultural diversity.

AIDS Education and Politics

Mervyn F. Silverman

In the best of all possible worlds, a public health crisis would be met swiftly and surely, with adequate resources directed toward the appropriate entities, with experts in the field and an educated community working together to make the best use of funds and personnel in an efficient, effective and compassionate manner. Sadly, in the world we live in, solutions to even the least complex public health problems are often elusive, with political interests interfering with and, at times, obstructing proper planning and implementation of the needed programs.

With AIDS, the most glaring example in modern medical history of an epidemic that has been complicated by issues scientific and religious, ethical and legal, financial and social, the response has been political in the extreme. At least six elements present in relation to this disease have given rise to anxiety and confusion in the United States which have in turn placed enormous pressure on the political system.

First, AIDS is a sexually transmitted disease. We have never responded sensibly to sexually transmitted diseases and today we still see many examples of our historic tendency to resort to irrationality, blame and victimization. Frank and informative discussion of these illnesses is still not in our repertoire. Secondly, in the United States, AIDS initially struck predominantly homosexual and bisexual men, a population separate in many American minds from the general community. Anyone uncomfortable with this lifestyle might experience greater anxiety concerning this disease, and this discomfort has extended far beyond the lay community to some leaders and health workers. Furthermore, politicians could easily dismiss the severity of the problem because it seemed to be an isolated situation affecting only a small and relatively disenfranchised segment of the overall society. However, since it is the nature of epidemics to ignore social, sexual, political and geographic boundaries, many public health professionals considered AIDS not only a problem for a certain group of people, but a serious threat to the health of the general population.

The third element, the long incubation period between infection and the appearance of signs and symptoms suggestive of AIDS, creates not only a great sense of insecurity, but an artificially low indication of the prevalence of infection. Fourth, to date we have no cure. In the developed world, we have come to expect an answer to almost every medical problem, especially infection. Added to this is the fifth element, which is the lack of a vaccine to protect the public from the spread of the epidemic, fueling demands for containment of the individuals who have already been infected. Finally, because AIDS is almost universally fatal, anxiety has understandably reached very high proportions.

All of the above factors have caused a fearful public to urge its politicians to "do something." Often this pressure results in reactions which are meant to be visible, but which are at best ineffective in the long run and are at worst harmful. For example, some of the repressive legislation that has been proposed, lacking any basis in science, requiring precious resources to defeat, and creating distrust among those most at risk and in need of government information.

THE RESPONSE OF THE U.S. FEDERAL GOVERNMENT TO AIDS

Throughout the industrialized world, there has been a wide variation in responses by national governments. A good example of a bad response —one based almost exclusively on politics— has been that of the United States presidential office. During the first six years of the epidemic, the most media–wise president in the history of the United States, Ronald Reagan, stood by silently while tens of thousands of his countrymen and women were becoming infected, developing ARC and AIDS, or were dying as a result of this disease. Because the problem seemed initially to reside almost exclusively in the gay community, President Reagan apparently did not feel it important enough to address the issue in any of his State of the Union Addresses or make mention of AIDS in any public utterance whatsoever. Finally, in May, 1987, during his first speech on the subject, he used a major portion of his presentation to urge mandatory testing of individuals, in contradiction to his own head of public health, the Surgeon General.

Pressure from the conservative elements of American society was effective in preventing the federal government from assuming the leading role in educating the public. Fear of appearing to condone the homosexual lifestyle and of encouraging sexual behavior among adolescents and the unmarried literally paralyzed the response of the government. Unlike Switzerland, where brochures were mailed to every household early in the epidemic, it was not until the epidemic was fairly advanced that such a mailing, *Understanding AIDS*, was made in the United States. Although mailed to 107 million homes, its promotion was so ineffectual that more than half the adults reached said they had not read it.[1] At the Centers for Disease Control, professionals labored to produce brochures, posters and educational programs only to have their efforts rebuffed by staff within the Reagan Administration attempting to "water down" the necessary messages relating to sexual behavior. No coherent national policy on AIDS was ever articulated, and no strategy for educating the public was ever developed; conflict within the Administration as to its own direction was abundantly evident.

Surgeon General C. Everett Koop, after considerable opposition from within the Reagan Administration, began to speak out forcefully on the need for clear, concise educational messages, beginning in early youth, which would explain the disease, how it is transmitted and how to prevent it. He discussed the advantages of abstinence and monogamous relationships with an uninfected person. The use of condoms as one measure to help prevent further spread among those who were not monogamous was recommended. Needless to say, this was highly offensive to some religious groups, who felt that the mere mention of non–monogamous sex would encourage sinful behavior in those who had never thought of it themselves. At the same time, the Secretary of Education, William Bennett, urged discussion of sexual matters within the context of marriage only—a message that, for many at highest risk, would fall on deaf ears. No attempt was made to place the Surgeon General, or any other expert, in charge of the fight against AIDS; instead the battles raged within and outside the White House.

While the Executive branch of government (except for the Surgeon General) remained essentially paralyzed in its response to the AIDS epidemic, the Legislative branch also had significant difficulty dealing with it. Although increased funding was approved for research, care and education, some legislators proposed their own solutions to the problem. Jesse Helms, a conservative southern senator, was attempting to prohibit funding for any educational programs which discussed homosexual sexual activities. Given the heavy concentration of AIDS cases within the gay

[1] *The Gallup Poll*. July 20, 1988. Los Angeles Times Syndicate.

community, this was analogous to establishing an educational program to reduce drunken driving while being prohibited from discussing alcohol and cars. While Senator Helms' proposals were prevented from being completely successful, valuable time and energy were expended in opposing him. The damaging effect he had on educational programs is still being felt. One might say that these contradictions, inconsistencies and confusions at the federal level created a distrust of government and official information such that a lack of confidence in the leadership became itself yet a seventh element adding to irrationality and fear in regards to AIDS.

Finally the lack of federal leadership in the educational campaign is best symbolized by a particularly clear case of administrative bumbling. October, 1988, had been designated by the government as AIDS Awareness Month in the United States. President Reagan announced this important month–long event, encouraging the public to "commemorate it with appropriate ceremonies and activities." Unfortunately, his statement was not made until November first!

THE SAN FRANCISCO MODEL

Those closely involved with AIDS quickly realized that unless local governments and community–based groups became involved, there would be little education available, either for those at greatest risk or for the general public. Relative to the federal response and that of many state and local governments across the nation, San Francisco's official reaction was timely and constructive. There was financial support for educational programs as early as December, 1981.

Yet, in spite of these advantages, educating about AIDS in San Francisco was difficult, due to the close association of the epidemic to sexual behaviors and because relevant information needed to be conveyed both to the community most directly affected and to the public in general. Because of a history of tolerance toward differences in lifestyles and sexual attitudes, San Francisco was the recipient of a major influx of lesbians and gay men in the late 1970's. Gay men in San Francisco were experiencing at the time a significant phase of "Gay Liberation," of which sexual expression was an important aspect. Bath houses catering to the wish for more sexual openness flourished, providing a safe haven and meeting place for a number of gay men. Early in the AIDS epidemic it was hoped that these locations could serve as places to provide targeted education and information, especially to those engaging in the highest–risk sexual behaviors. The intention was to engage these men in the battle without alienating them from the process of government oversight and regulation. The bath houses later proved to be relatively ineffective sites for education, because their owners were still encouraging multiple anonymous sexual contacts with little or no reinforcement of safer sex guidelines.

Since the United States government, at local, state and national levels, has historically been a poor educator in the area of sexuality, it was felt the best way to reach the gay community in San Francisco was to work through that community, encouraging organizational and grass roots participation. The best role for local government would be as convener, funder and evaluator of educational and community service programs rather than their implementer. Representatives from the gay community, people with AIDS, the medical profession and the Department of Public Health were brought together in the spirit of cooperation: the medical experts would assure the scientific validity of the information; the Department of Public Health would assist in the planning and evaluation of educational programs; the gay community and people with AIDS would provide advice on the appropriateness of the messages and gay agencies would provide the actual educational services.

Although many measure the impact of an educational program in terms of its output, clearly judgment concerning the effectiveness of any educational message is in the determination of its ability to be "heard," internalized and acted upon. Thus, over time, in–depth studies of the community and focus groups made up of volunteers from the gay (and later straight) communities would review both old and new approaches and provide important input as to the receptiveness to the messages and the levels of knowledge obtained.

In anticipation of the large influx of gay men to San Francisco for the 1983 Gay Freedom Day Parade, the Department prepared the first poster dealing with AIDS. It said simply:

- Enjoy more time with fewer partners.
- Avoid any exchange of body fluids.
- Use condoms.
- Limit your use of recreational drugs.

This first effort was criticized from both ends of the political spectrum. Some felt that the message should have been, "Stop using drugs!" "Don't have sex with more than one person!" "Don't share semen, vaginal fluids, etc!" At the same time, the National Lesbian/Gay Task Force at their annual meeting "booed" the poster as being inappropriate because the exact means of spread of this disease had not been proven. Locally, one group of lesbians and gay men objected to the open discussion of gay sexual practices while another group believed it was wrong not to state the facts as clearly as possible because of the seriousness of the problem. This disagreement was manifested in vitriolic diatribes made against one another during meetings and in the gay press. The Department of Public Health believed that more explicit language on publicly displayed posters would have been inappropriate and would have raised opposition to its publicly funded educational programs. It also felt that individuals have so often been told by their parents to stop doing what is harmful or sexual or both, that a Health Department admonishment would probably have as poor results as parental warnings have often had. In encouraging at least a gradual change in what is, after all, a most intimate and personal part of life, the Department hoped to foster safer practices.

As the epidemic grew, the disagreements among various factions within the gay community disappeared and future educational efforts were based on the premise that the only audience we should worry about offending was the audience we wished to reach. All of the materials planned for distribution which had been created by community groups were reviewed by the Director of Health for appropriateness, and if they contained explicit language or visuals, they did not carry the Health Department's name on them in order to avoid criticism by politicians or objections by members of the general community regarding the use of public funds for this purpose. Departments of health in some other cities were not as careful, with the unfortunate result that certain very effective but explicit materials were prohibited from being disseminated. Regretfully, in the case of San Francisco, the education has been reinforced by the sad fact that virtually everyone in the city has known at least one person who is infected, is ill, has died or has lost someone to AIDS. Many are faced with friends newly diagnosed every day as these tragic statistics continue to rise. Obviously, we must figure out how to motivate individuals to change unsafe behaviors without a "body count."

Fortunately in San Francisco and other major cities in the United States, there were a number of gay publications which were widely used to convey important information regarding AIDS and were as explicit as necessary. But these publications could not be carried home by those homosexual and bisexual men who had not "come out" to their families and friends, or by other groups such as those blacks, Hispanics and Asians who were either unaware of the publications or who did not identify with the gay community. It was important, therefore, to attempt to educate as effectively as possible through the medium of the general lay press so that at least the basic preventive message could be seen by everyone regardless of their ethnicity or sexual preference. Gradually terms used to inform the public became more precise: "body fluids" was replaced with "semen and vaginal fluids" and "unsafe sex" became "anal or vaginal intercourse without the use of condoms and spermicide."

Utilizing press releases, public service announcements, public appearances, pamphlets, focus groups, support groups, bus signs, telephone hot lines and conferences, and with minimal political interference, San Francisco was able to educate and inform those at highest risk for infection, as well as the community at large. One result was a dramatic decline in rectal gonorrhea cases by over 75% in three years, indicating a significant reduction of the highest–risk behavior, unprotected anal intercourse. This could not have been accomplished without the cooperation of the executive and legislative branches of local government, an active and involved lesbian and gay community, a committed community of health workers, a supportive media environment (both gay and mainstream), and the general support of the citizenry.

THE NATIONAL RESPONSE

Sadly, other locales have not been as successful. This has been due in part to the inability or unwillingness of their health departments to serve in a coordinating, central capacity. In a number of locations there has been a demonstrated lack of leadership and integrity on the part of executive or legislative leaders. Some places have been burdened with little or no state support, lack of media involvement and a less visible gay presence. Furthermore, in those places characterized by a social and political conservatism, motivation has been high to avoid subjects and materials likely to be shocking or controversial.

The net effect of governmental inaction at all levels has been a tremendous response from non–governmental organizations. Many of these organizations deserve much credit for their efforts to meet the educational and informational needs of those at greatest risk. Others have found themselves ill–equipped to do a job which requires official attention, oversight and resources. Many associations, such as Gay Men's Health Crisis in New York City, AIDS Project/Los Angeles and the San Francisco AIDS Foundation, have produced relevant, timely and effective educational materials. In recent years, as the epidemic has grown in minority populations, non––governmental agencies from these communities have also been attempting to meet their own special cultural and linguistic needs. This has proven difficult because of the sensitivities toward homosexuality, cultural attitudes toward sexuality and, in some cases, the prevalence of drug use within these groups. The intentions and results of these local, grass roots efforts are often laudable; the fact that they are necessary in the absence of a well–planned and carefully implemented national education program leads to a situation in which there is both an inconsistency in substance and quality of education and a great inequality of coverage across age, socio–cultural and geographical boundaries.

Furthermore, the patchwork variability of the information that is publicized leads to confusion and inconsistency in the thinking of many. For example, while only 11% of Americans said that working near someone poses a risk for AIDS, 25% would refuse to work alongside a person with AIDS, and an equal number believed employers should be able to fire a person with AIDS solely because of the disease.[2] Only one in ten believed that a child could contract AIDS by sitting in the same classroom with an HIV–infected child, but one in three would keep their child home under these circumstances.[3] While one opinion poll reported that only six percent of Americans were "very worried" about their own risk, other polls have revealed that 30% support quarantine, 29% would vote for a politician who endorsed it, and 17% would support a landlord's right to evict people with AIDS from their home.[4]

A Gallup Poll reported that over 90% understand the risks of needle sharing and unprotected sexual relations. But 29% still believe that donating blood can cause infection, 22% still believe they can become infected from a drinking fountain, 20% from a toilet seat, and 25% from a cough or sneeze.[5] The findings remain essentially unchanged as reported in the January–March, 1989, National Health Interview Survey.[6]

These beliefs have given tacit approval to increased discriminatory practices on the part of employers, insurance companies, landlords and schools. Such irrational fears also underlie the obsession of some of our politicians with mandatory testing and the maintenance of registries of seropositives. Needless to say, it is extremely difficult to educate those at high risk in such an atmosphere of danger and distrust. Because of their fear of breaches of confidentiality and consequent exclusion from obtaining life's necessities (jobs, homes, health care, the company of others), many refuse to take part in programs associated with testing and may not attend to

---

[2] *The Gallup Poll.* November 26, 1987. (Storrs, CON.: Roper Center for Public Opinion Research).

[3] G. Gallup Jr. ed., *The Gallup Poll: public opinion 1985* (Wilmington, DE.: Scholarly Resources. 1986); and Louis Harris and Associates, *Harris survey*, (Storrs, CON.: Roper Center for Public Opinion Research, September 23, 1985).

[4] H. Quinley, "The new facts of life: heterosexuals and AIDS," *Public Opinion* (May/June 1988): 53–5; and *Gallup Poll*, (Storrs, CON.: Roper Center for Public Opinion Research, November 22, 1987); and ABC News (Storrs, CON.: Roper Center for Public Opinion Research, June, 1987); and "Human immunodeficiency virus infection in the United States: a review of current knowledge," *Morbidity and Mortalitay Weekly Report* 36 (Suppl. 6) (1987): 1–48; and D.F. Musto, "Quarantine and the problem of AIDS," *Milbank Memorial Fund* 64 (Suppl. 1) (1986): 97–117.

[5] Louis Harris and Associates, *AIDS survey* (Storrs, CON.: Roper Center for Public Opinion Research, August 1987); and Gallup Poll, (Storrs, CON.: Roper Center for Public Opinion Research, November 26, 1987)

[6] D.A. Dawson, *AIDS Knowledge and Attitudes for January–March, 1989, Provisional Data From the National Health Interview Survey.* Advance Data. August 15, 1989, p. 176.

messages from governmental institutions which they see as inimical to their best interests. Admiral James T. Watkins, Chairman of the President's Commission on HIV, stated in his press conference of June 2, 1988, that discrimination is the most significant obstacle to progress in our fight against AIDS. "If the nation does not address this issue squarely," he said, "it will be very difficult to solve most other HIV–related problems."[7] Like the other findings of this commission appointed by President Reagan, this warning was ignored by him. President Bush has supported and signed the Americans with Disabilities Act in 1990 which will have a positive impact on this issue.

SUGGESTIONS FOR THE FUTURE

What, therefore, must be done so that a country can reach all the communities within its borders? First and foremost, we must learn from the past and recognize that the presence of strong public health and medical leadership is an absolute necessity to control this epidemic. Ongoing evaluations of the various interventions and strategies need to be made so that ineffective programs can be eliminated and promising ones can be expanded and duplicated by others. Part of a national approach should be the funding of local communities to help plan for and implement prevention programs targeted to specific at–risk populations.

Any reliance on compulsory or restrictive public health measures designed out of irrational fear or political motivation will not only be counterproductive, but actively destructive of our efforts. Expanded research into the epidemiology of HIV infection must take place in order to fully understand the impact of this disease and refine our projections for the future. We need the cooperation of people with HIV infection and we need the trusting ear of the public so that we can convey to them the facts as they are uncovered. We also need dedicated and sensitive health care workers; they themselves need opportunities for continuing education and they need emotional support.

No disease in the history of mankind has ever been eliminated through treatment. Only through prevention can we hope to conquer AIDS. Since an effective vaccine is not expected for general distribution in the near future, the only vaccination we have available now is education. If today we could educate everyone and if they comprehended and followed our direction, we could stop the spread of the virus without any drugs or vaccines. The reality is we can not and they will not. Each nation must find its own way

[7] K.A. Fackelmann, ed., "An AIDS battleplan," *Medicine and Health Perspectives*, June 13, 1988: 1–4.

to address this need. In order for effective educational programs to be planned, careful studies of the target audiences must be made in order to better understand the determinants of behavior change relative to HIV infection. For example, intensive outreach to street youth and prostitutes, many of whom are on drugs and who sell themselves for money and/or drugs, must be made in the cities. (We must not lose sight of the fact that even "socially" acceptable drugs such as alcohol and other mind—altering substances lead to risk—taking behavior normally avoided when not under their influence.)

In the United States an important weapon in our educational "arsenal" is the media, a subject covered very well by others in this book. Given the U.S. government's abdication to date of a leadership role in preventing the spread of AIDS, we have had to rely more heavily on the print and electronic media to inform, to educate, and to help reduce discrimination by exposing it where it exists. Through sensitive human interest stories, the media have the power to motivate people to be more compassionate. In essence, the media can bring to the far corners of the country the human side of the tragic statistics. The federal government still needs to establish an effective national media campaign and pay for prime time airing of public service messages. (I believe this also applies to other countries in which the media play an important role and which have not yet utilized this valuable resource.) The President himself needs to participate in some of the messages, stressing the need for compassion, and encouraging reasonable precautions while quieting the irrational anxieties rampant in our nation. He might even consider having "Fireside Chats" like those of President Roosevelt during Word War II. This would be most appropriate because, as in the early 1940s, we too are at war. The enemy is not only a virus, but bigotry, ignorance and apathy. And it is winning. The vanquished are the more than 500 000 with AIDS, the over five million who are infected with HIV, and the untold numbers who have died worldwide. We owe it to them to wage a full—scale attack on this epidemic.

CONCLUSION

The story of AIDS must not end; it must continue to be told. If we are going to be effective in slowing the spread of the virus and providing the best care possible for those infected, we must "secularize" this disease. The Names Project, with its quilt of over 12 000 panels memorializing some of those who have died of AIDS, is the most eloquent testimony I know to the fact that, regardless of age, sex, sexual preference, color of skin or ethnic background, everyone who is infected, has AIDS or has died, is someone's child. The quilt represents, among other things, a creative and loving way to bring a very powerful educational message to people. As long as individuals can separate themselves from others based on differences in sexual preference, culture or lifestyle, there will never be the necessary public support for an appropriate and compassionate approach to the AIDS crisis. We need compassion not only in our hearts, but in the form of national anti–discrimination laws. In our zeal to "secularize," however, we should never "normalize" this disease, as we have with so many others which have been accepted as part of the fabric of society and to some extent forgotten. We must never lose sight of the fact that AIDS will outlive us all. This does not diminish the urgency, but recognizes the long–term aspects of this epidemic and highlights the futility of denial and apathy. In recognizing the persistence of AIDS we must help those in the front lines with support and appreciation; theirs is often an exhausting and sad, if otherwise rewarding, job.

The educational ideal would be to have everyone, from the world's leaders to the individual members of each community, understand that AIDS is a global problem that affects each one of us, and threatens to rob us of an individual and collective future. When communities and nations are willing to dedicate the necessary resources to prevent its spread, when individuals are willing to take personal responsibility for preventing infection, and when we can have a loving attitude toward those who are already affected by this disease, we will be united in purpose such that together we can be victorious over AIDS.

Conclusion: Reflections on Education to Prevent AIDS

Jaime Sepulveda
Harvey Fineberg
Jonathan Mann

It is certainly a lot easier to write about AIDS education, or to read about it, than to do it—and do it well. Conscious and concerned about the gap between theory and practice, the editors and authors of this book have tried to maintain a positive, helpful and pragmatic tone. We believe this is important because it can be very discouraging when the reader turns from a book on a complicated subject like AIDS education to the real world of health departments, health educators and target populations. Accordingly, this book has sought to stimulate the reader, to present and illustrate several key concepts and to reinforce the idea that AIDS education is highly complex. Yet the book should also have encouraged the reader, particularly through the descriptions of practical experience and media strategies, to realize that a combination of sound reasoning, attention to key issues, and commitment to preventing HIV infection is enough to get started.

Despite the urgency of the epidemic, it is important to consider carefully the different options for planning, implementing, monitoring and evaluating AIDS education programs. The single largest error would be to design such a program in a vacuum; the planning process, implementation of the program and its review (monitoring and evaluation) must involve diverse disciplines and, most critically, must involve those to whom the program will be directed. If this principle were enshrined, much wasted energy and resources could be saved; nevertheless, participation of the target population alone, without technical and professional guidance, is never enough.

The many contributions made from various disciplines in the fight against AIDS should be recognized. In the early phases of the AIDS pandemic, the largest contribution to prevention efforts came from epidemiological studies. Even before the etiologic agent was recognized, epidemiologists had identified the magnitude of the epidemic, the modes of transmission and associated risk-factors, and proposed preventive measures. Later on, basic scientists discovered HIV, the causative agent of AIDS, which in turn led to the development of laboratory reagents that permitted the screening of blood and blood products and the testing of individuals.

Clinical trials with drugs effective *in vitro* promoted the discovery of the therapeutic benefits (and limitations) of AZT and other pharmaceuticals in AIDS patients. The social sciences then joined with medicine in developing initial studies to assess knowledge, attitudes, practices and beliefs about AIDS, and in designing of studies of sexual behavior and drug use, key elements in the transmission of AIDS. Finally, the communication sciences have proposed strategies to reach audiences through diverse channels and with appropriate messages.

The obstacles to a good prevention campaign against AIDS are great, both in number and in complexity. They can be divided into two groups, intrinsic and imposed: the first refers to inherent difficulties due to our own ignorance and to the complexity of human sexuality; the second is related to societal reaction to a new and frightening disease.

Human sexual impulse has a clear biological base, and its various expressions should be regarded as natural. However, many of these expressions are often stigmatized. Sexually transmitted diseases (STDs) may be treated secretly; sex and death are difficult to discuss openly. Therefore, although clearly present and growing, AIDS is ignored or minimized by some sectors of society.

We must admit our own ignorance and limitations about the best way to combat AIDS. It is now a commonplace to say that in the absence of drugs or vaccines our only alternative is education. It is still valid and true, yet easier said than done. A universally valid or accepted educational model does not exist. Messages and channels of communication must vary depending on the audience. The epidemic is not static but quite dynamic, affecting increasingly larger geographical areas and populations. Finally, information alone is not enough to change sexual and drug using habits.

External or imposed obstacles include moral, political and financial issues. Some think that advocating modification of behavior to prevent HIV transmission without condemning the underlying behavior (e.g. needle exchange, condom distribution) is equivalent to condoning or even promoting the activities through which AIDS transmission occurs. The challenge is to find educational strategies which maintain a delicate balance between effectiveness and acceptability.

AIDS prevention is a world-wide political and financial problem. AIDS is the only disease that has merited a declaration from the United Nations General Assembly, which demonstrated its concern about the epidemic's global threat. AIDS also led to the largest gathering in history of health ministers for a coordinated action. However, globally, interest in AIDS appears to be declining. AIDS, a chronic problem rather than an immediate crisis, has lost its novelty. Worse, AIDS is a very expensive disease, individually and collectively; for the person who has the disease and for the governments of poor countries, the expenses are extraordinary. Neither the treatment of AIDS nor preventive campaigns are cheap, especially in a world in which the per capita health budgets of some African countries are less than ten dollars annually.

Managerial difficulties also impede AIDS prevention efforts. Throughout the world we are rapidly losing international, national and local AIDS leaders. Two circumstances explain this loss. First, since AIDS became a global problem, emerging leaders have received intense political pressure and media attention, often to the irritation of supervisors and politicians, reluctant to share the limelight. Second, the lack of quick and tangible results from AIDS prevention activities caused frustration and fatigue among program managers. The constant criticism both from the outside and from other health programs competing for attention and resources frequently results in the departure of the original creative leaders and in a shift towards more conservative, even "business as usual" style programs.

From the standpoint of the health authorities, there are two antagonistic conceptions about strategies to confront the AIDS pandemic. The first assumes that because of the ways AIDS is transmitted it will affect some groups before others, and therefore society as a whole will be best protected by taking measures against those affected groups or individuals. The second considers AIDS itself to be the real enemy, and that protecting society implies protecting all of its members.

Three reasons have been proposed to explain (but not justify) the lack of compassion for people with AIDS.[1] The first has to do with the fear of contagion. The second is associated with the low social value assigned to those who belong to "high risk groups." A third reason is the rejection of any reminder of our vulnerability, our susceptibility to the images of the plague.[2]

[1] G. Friedland, "AIDS and Compassion," *Journal of the American Medical Association* 259(19) (1988): 2898–9.

[2] *Ibid.*

AIDS has provoked an intense social response. This response has been diverse throughout different societies, but has evolved in general from violence and discrimination toward increasing tolerance. Further progress is needed to ensure that the human rights of people with AIDS or HIV infection are not violated, particularly in places where no "ombudsman" or equivalent agency for the defense of human rights exists.

We would like to offer some specific recommendations for program managers:

A. Elements of Planning[3]
  1. Establish clear goals in a national AIDS plan, using all epidemiological and social research data available.
  2. Develop strategies to reach targeted audiences with appropriate messages through all available channels of communication.
  3. Make information and support services available to the general public and to those affected by AIDS.
  4. Establish a sound plan for monitoring and evaluation.
  5. Involve all segments of society in the fight against AIDS.
B. Elements of human rights[4]
  1. AIDS is an infectious disease and should not be considered in a separate category.
  2. Discrimination against HIV–infected people and people with AIDS is both scientifically and ethically unjustified.
  3. Health care providers have a duty to serve all patients to the best of their abilities.
  4. Governments and institutions have a duty to provide information and health care to all.
  5. Existing laws and legislation should be revised and adapted to ensure their effectiveness, ethical acceptability and capacity to protect human rights.

We close this book in a spirit of cautious optimism. Key concepts have been articulated, many tools are well–tried and ready to be used, and the dangers of the AIDS pandemic are pressing. The success of AIDS education will depend, as always, on informed leadership, vision and personal commitment. In AIDS education, mistakes will of course be made, as experience is gained and lessons are learned; the only tragedy would be never to start the process, or to allow the extraordinary complexity of human behavior and AIDS education to lead to intellectual paralysis or programmatic passivity.

---

[3] WHO, "Guide to Planning Health Promotion for AIDS Prevention and Control," WHO AIDS Series 5 (Geneva: World Health Organization, 1989).
[4] WHO–Norway, MOH 1988.

Profiles on Contributors

JEANNE BLAKE

Jeanne Blake is the medical reporter for WBZ-TV. In that capacity, Ms. Blake has broken dozens of stories about advances in medicine. Her coverage of the AIDS epidemic has earned her local and national recognition. In 1987 and 1988, Jeanne Blake received Associated Press awards for continuing coverage of AIDS. Governor Michael Dukakis presented Ms. Blake with the Governor's Recognition Award for her "outstanding contributions to AIDS education in Massachusetts." In 1988, the Massachusetts Human Rights Campaign honored Ms. Blake for her sensitive coverage of AIDS issues. Also, the Massachusetts Chapter of Americans for Democratic Action presented Blake with an Achievement Award in recognition of "outstanding leadership in the field of health care." In 1989, the Massachusetts Public Health Association presented Blake with its Public Service Award in recognition of her "significant contributions of public service in behalf of public health." In addition, the Massachusetts Visiting Nurses Association has presented its annual award to Ms. Blake for her contributions in educating the people of Massachusetts about health care issues. In the spring of 1989, Jeanne Blake hosted a Public Broadcasting System (PBS) program about AIDS.

CLAIRE MONOD CASSIDY, PH.D.

Claire Cassidy is presently a writer, a consultant to AIDSCOM, and a lecturer in anthropology at the University of Maryland–College Park. Dr. Cassidy was formerly the Associate Coordinator for International Programs at the University of Maryland, and has also taught at the University of Minnesota. She received her Ph.D in human biology with a specialty in applied medical anthropology. Her career interest in communications is expressed in numerous publications in the fields of AIDS prevention, mother and child nutrition, and food habits research. Besides work in several of the United States, she has completed research in Belize, Sri Lanka and Mauritania.

LINCOLN C. CHEN, M.D., M.P.H.

Lincoln C. Chen is presently the Taro Takemi Professor of International Health, the Director of International Health Programs, Chairman of the Harvard Committee for the Takemi Program, Chairman of the Department of Population Sciences, Director of the Harvard Center for Population Studies and a Faculty Fellow at the Harvard Institute for International Development, all at the Harvard School of Public Health. He received his bachelor's degrees from Princeton, his medical degree from Harvard and his master's in public health from the Johns Hopkins School of Hygiene and Public Health. Dr. Chen worked in Bangladesh with the International Center for Diarrheal Disease Research, and also held the post of Program Officer for Population and the Social Sciences, for the Ford Foundation. Before joining the Harvard faculty, Dr. Chen was the Ford Foundation representative for India, Nepal and Sri Lanka from 1981–1986. Dr. Chen is the director of the AIDS and Reproductive Health Network Facilitation Group and a member of the ARHN Steering Group.

Dr. Chen has published, among other articles, "The AIDS Pandemic: An Internationalist Approach to Disease Control," "Summary, AIDS and Reproductive Health: Research Priorities for an International Scientific Network," and co–authored "AIDS in Africa: Diversity in the Global Pandemic," published in the journal *Daedalus*. He also presented "Looking to the Future: A Revolution in Health Communications through AIDS Control," at the Symposium on Communication and Education on AIDS, Ixtapa, Mexico.

MARCIE L. CYNAMON, M.A.

Marcie L. Cynamon received her master's in demography with a specialty in fertility patterns from Georgetown University in 1977. Since that time, she has worked as a survey statistician and more recently as the Special Assistant to the Director of the Division of Health Interview Statistics, at the National Center for Health Statistics. Ms. Cynamon's work in survey research includes the design, development and management of large national surveys on a wide range of health issues including AIDS knowledge and attitudes, sexual behavior, disabilities and adolescent health risk behaviors. She has published several articles on the level of knowledge about AIDS in the U.S. and has presented papers on AIDS–related issues at numerous professional meetings. In her current position, she has coordinated HIV–related research and served on several advisory panels on matters pertaining to AIDS survey research.

MARY DEBUS

Mary Debus is Senior Vice President and Director of the International Division for Porter/Novelli—a public relations company known for its work in health communications and social marketing. Ms. Debus is responsible for managing Porter/Novelli's work in developing countries on AIDS prevention, child survival, nutrition communications and family planning.

Previously, Ms. Debus was President and CEO of Business Decisions Inc., an international market research company specializing in the development of cross–cultural marketing and communication research tools. She was also Senior Vice President at ASI Market Research, where she developed a variety of innovative techniques for evaluating the effectiveness of print and broadcast advertising materials.

Since beginning a second career in international development, Ms. Debus has designed research to support social marketing and health communications projects in Mexico, Ghana, Egypt, Indonesia, Nepal, the Dominican Republic, Panama, Barbados, Trinidad and Tobago, and the Philippines. She has developed training programs for health professionals on marketing communications and marketing research, and written articles on qualitative research and focus group techniques. As an advisor to the World Health Organization's Global Programme on AIDS, she has also helped to plan educational and promotional strategies for AIDS prevention.

WILLIAM DEJONG, PH.D.

William DeJong has a Ph. D. in psychology from Stanford University. He presently holds the position of Director of Research for the Center for Health Communication at Harvard School of Public Health, and is Deputy Director for the Harvard Alcohol Project. His publications include "Recommendations for Future Mass Media Campaigns to Prevent Preteen and Adolescent Substance abuse,"in *Health Affairs*, "Condom Promotion: The Need for a

Social Marketing Program in America's Inner Cities," in the *American Journal of Health Promotion*, "Preventing AIDS and Other STDS through Condom Promotion: A Patient Education Intervention," in the *American Journal of Public Health*, and "Recent STD Prevention Efforts and Their Implication for AIDS Health Education," from the *Health Education Quarterly*.

HARVEY V. FINEBERG, M.D., M.P.P., PH.D.

Dean of the Harvard School of Public Health (HSPH), Harvey V. Fineberg is a graduate of Harvard College, Harvard Medical School, and Harvard's John F. Kennedy School of Government. Prior to his appointment as dean in 1984, he was professor in health policy and management at the School of Public Health.

Since 1970's , Dean Fineberg has been a leading figure in the health policy field. As a member of the Public Health Council of Massachusetts from 1976-1979, he participated in decision-making matters of hospital investment and health policy. from 1982- to 1985 he served as chairman of the Health Care Technology Study Section of the National Center for Health Services Research.

His past research focused on several areas of health policy, including the process of policy developmentand implementation, assessment of medical technology, and dissemination of medical innovations. He helped found and has served as president of the Society of Medical Decision Making and has also served as consultant to the World Health Organization. As a member of the Institute of Medicine, he has served on numerous panels dealing with topics of health policy, ranging from AIDS to vaccines to new medical technology.

Dean Fineberg is co-author of the books *Clinical Decision Analysis and The Epidemic that Never Was*, an analysis of the controversial federal immunization program against swine flu in 1976. He recently chaired the Institute of Medicine Committee that produced the report, *Adverse Effects of Pertussis and Rubella Vaccines*. He has also authored numerous journal articles, including the recent pieces "Education to Prevent AIDS: Prospects and Obstacles" in *Science* and "The Social Dimensions of AIDS" in *Scientific American*. In 1988 he received the Joseph W Mountin Prize from the Centers for Disease Control and the Wade Hampton Frost Prize from the Epidemiology Section of the American Public Health Association

LAURIE GARRETT

Laurie Garrett is the medical reporter for *Newsday*, a metropolitan New York newspaper that is the sixth largest daily in the United States. A U.S.

citizen, she studied biochemistry at the University of California at Santa Cruz. As a graduate student, she studied immunology at the University of California at Berkeley.

Laurie Garret joined *Newsday* in 1988 after more than seven years at National Public Radio where as science correspondent she reported on AIDS from San Francisco, Los Angeles, Washington, East Africa, London, Geneva and Paris. She has earned numerous journalism awards including the Peabody, Armstrong, National Press Club and World Hunger Awards for her work.

THOMAS GOODGAME

Thomas Goodgame has served as president of Westinghouse Broadcasting Company's Group W Television Stations since April of 1986. He is responsible for the operation of Group W's five owned and operated television stations; Group W Television Sales; and NEWSFEED, Group W's television satellite news gathering cooperative.

Mr. Goodgame has held posts in Group W including vice president and general manager of KDKA-TV in Pittsburgh and vice president and general manager of WBZ-TV in Boston. While he was at KDKA and WBZ, those stations won the coveted Gabriel Award as the finest television stations in the nation. Before joining the Westinghouse Broadcasting Company, he served as vice president and general manager of KTUL-TV in Tulsa, Oklahoma and held the same post at KATV in Little Rock, Arkansas. Mr. Goodgame was President of the New England Chapter of the National Association of Television Arts and Sciences (NATAS). He serves on the Television Board of the National Association of Broadcasters (NAB), and is a member of the NBC affiliates' Board of Directors. He is also past chairman of the ABC affiliates' Board.

STEVEN LAWRENCE GORTMAKER, M.S., PH.D.

Dr. Steven Gortmaker is the Director of the Harvard Institute for Social Research in the Department of Sociology and also a senior lecturer in the Department of Health and Social Behavior, at the Harvard School of Public Health (HSPH). Dr. Gortmaker studied math statistics and sociology at the University of Michigan and received his master of science degree and his doctorate from the University of Wisconsin, also in sociology. Dr. Gortmaker has taught as an assistant professor in the Department of Health Services at HSPH, as a research and teaching assistant at the University of Wisconsin and as a research assistant at the University of Michigan.

Dr. Gortmaker has received numerous grants to research topics related to child health, especially rural infant care, chronic illness and obesity in children and poverty and child health, as well as research on worksite-based health promotion programs and the AIDS epidemic in Mexico. His numerous publications focus on prenatal care, infant health, poverty and child health, Medicaid in the U.S., sex education for children, child obesity, children with chronic illnesses, seropositivity and behavioral and sociological risks among homosexual and bisexual men in Mexico, poverty and AIDS in relation to infant mortality in the U.S., applications of logistical models, and measures of fatness. Dr. Gortmaker is a member of the American Statistical Association, the American Sociological Association and the American Public Health Association.

MILTON GOSSETT

Milton Gossett joined Compton Advertising in 1949, became a copywriter in 1951, Vice President and Associate Creative Director in 1961, President in 1968, Chief Executive Officer in 1975 and Chairman in 1977. As a result of a merger with Saatchi & Saatchi, a European advertising agency, Mr. Gossett became Chairman and CEO of the combined organization. He was a leading force in building Saatchi & Saatchi Advertising Worldwide into one of the world's largest advertising networks, with associate agencies in 44 countries around the world.

Milton Gossett is a member of the Board of the Eye–Bank for Sight Restoration, a member of the Business Council of New York State and director of the Advertising Council. He serves on the Board of Directors of the National Center for Health Education and is a member of the Board of the Terri Gotthelf Lupus Research Institute. He is on the Advisory Board of the Center for Health Communication of the Harvard School of Public Health, and also serves on the Dean's Council. In addition he is a former director of the American Foundation for AIDS Research and continues as a member of the New York City AIDS Task Force.

DAVID JOHN HUNTER, M.B., B.S., M.P.H., SC. D.

David J. Hunter presently holds the posts of Assistant Professor of Epidemiology at the Harvard School of Public Health, Research Associate in Medicine at Channing Laboratory, also at Harvard, and Associate Epidemiologist at Brigham and Women's Hospital, Boston. Dr. Hunter received his medical degree from the University of Sydney, and went on to study a master's in public health and a doctorate in epidemiology at Harvard University. He has presented papers at the International AIDS meetings in Atlanta, Washington, Stockholm, Montreal and San Francisco. His research activities include responsibility for advising on the design of research projects conducted by AIDS and Reproductive Health Network members around the world. For this work, the unique features of AIDS have required combining principles of both infectious disease and chronic disease epidemiology.

In addition to consulting, he is an active collaborator, with Professor J. Mati of the University of Nairobi, in a study of contraceptive use and HIV infection in Nairobi. During 1987–1988 he was coordinator of the Population AIDS Project for the Office of International Health Programs at Harvard. Among his publications are articles such as "Estimation of the Risk of Outcomes of HTLV-III infection," in *Lancet*, "Considerations for the Pooling of Sera to Reduce Costs of HIV Screening, presented at the International Conference on AIDS in Stockholm, and "Population–based Case–control Studies and AIDS Epidemiology", an AIDS and Reproductive Health Network background paper.

JOSE ANTONIO IZAZOLA, MD., M.Sc.

At the present time Jose Antonio Izazola is a Fogarty fellow in the doctoral program at the Harvard School of Public Health. He has a medical degree from the Autonomous Metropolitan University of Mexico at Xochimilco and a master's in demography from El Colegio de Mexico.

From 1985 to 1987 Dr. Izazola worked as an epidemiology resident in a joint program of the Mexican Directorate of Epidemiology and the U.S. Centers for Disease Control, where he initiated the Federal Program for AIDS Detection and National Committee for AIDS Prevention and Control (CONASIDA) from 1986 to 1989. From 1987 to 1989 he was head of the Department of Medical Demography, also in the General Directorate of Epidemiology. During this period, Dr. Izazola participated in several research projects as well as being in charge of the development of knowledge, attitudes and practices and AIDS surveys, the production of educational materials for AIDS prevention, marketing research on condoms, and designing ethnographic research on Mexican homosexual men. Dr. Izazola has participated as principal investigator on a variety of research projects which have focused on topics such as the evaluation of mass media campaigns for AIDS prevention, and the design, distribution and evaluation of condom promotion campaigns for female sex workers and for gay and bisexual men.

His publications include articles on cognitive and epidemiological characteristics of HIV transmission in Mexico, on epidemiological patterns of AIDS in Mexico, on risk factors for HIV infection in gay and bisexual men in Mexico City, and a chapter of the book *AIDS, Science and Society in Mexico* entitled "Knowledge, Attitudes and Practices about AIDS: Basis for the Design of Educational Programs."

MUKESH KAPILA, M.A., M.Sc., B.M,. B.Ch., M.R.C.G.P., M.F.C.M.

Mukesh Kapila is former Deputy Director of the AIDS Programme of the Health Education Authority in the U.K. He is also a consultant in public health medicine and works as the Director of Action Health 2000, an international, non–governmental organization. From time to time, he is also an advisor to the WHO Global Programme on AIDS. Dr. Kapila has a degree in medicine from Oxford University. He has a master's in public health from the University of London, School of Hygiene and Tropical Medicine.

Mukesh Kapila has experience in community and public health work in Africa and Asia, including recent AIDS planning and training done with national governments on WHO assignments. He is a member of the Royal College of General Practitioners and of the Faculty of Community Medicine and is a Fellow of the Royal Society of Tropical Medicine. He has given numerous lectures and presentations at international conferences, in London, Stockholm, Cologne, Madrid, Bangkok, Ixtapa and Montreal. He has written many papers on AIDS education, evaluation of programs and on other communicable disease and public health issues. Dr. Kapila is the editor of the periodicals *AIDS U.K.* and *AIDS DIALOGUE* and of forthcoming monographs on local AIDS programs in the U.K. He is senior adviser for the Overseas Development Administration. His research interests include monitoring and evaluation, policy analysis and operational research.

LLOYD J. KOLBE, PH.D.

Lloyd J. Kolbe is Director of the Division of Adolescent and School Health at the U.S. Centers for Disease Control (CDC). The division implements a national program that helps schools, and other agencies that serve youth, provide effective HIV education. The division also conducts research to assess, and consequently improve, HIV education for school–age youth. Dr. Kolbe also presently serves on the editorial board for *AIDS Education and Prevention: An Interdisciplinary Journal*; and chairs the AIDS Task Force for the International Union for Health Education.

Before joining the CDC, Dr. Kolbe served as assistant professor of health sciences at the University of Northern Colorado and also worked as an associate professor at the University of Texas School of Public Health. He held the posts of director of evaluation and director of school health education programs at the National Center for Health Education, chief of evaluation for the U.S. Office of Disease Prevention and Health Promotion, and associate director of the University of Texas Center for Health Promotion Research and Development.

Dr. Kolbe has written several journal articles and book chapters on HIV education for school–age youth. He was the chairman of the Symposium on Applying Behavioral Science to Control the AIDS Epidemic for the American Association for the Advancement of Science and also of the U.S. Public Health Service Liaison Panel to the National Academy of Sciences Committee on AIDS Research and the Behavioral, Social, and Statistical Sciences. Dr. Kolbe served on the steering committee for the Second International Symposium on AIDS Information and Education (in Yaounde, Cameroon).

FREDERICK KROGER

Fred Kroger is Director of the National AIDS Information and Education Program at the U.S. Centers for Disease Control (CDC) in Atlanta, Georgia. This program includes the National AIDS Hotlines, the national AIDS Information Clearinghouse, the "America Responds to AIDS" public service advertising campaign, and several grant programs for national and regional organizations.

Mr. Kroger joined the CDC in 1968, following four years of classroom teaching, and served in several state and local health departments as a sexually transmitted disease (STD) educator. In 1977, Mr. Kroger became the head of CDC's national STD education program. Prior to joining the AIDS program, Mr. Kroger served for three years as Deputy Director of CDC's Division of Health Education.

Mr. Kroger has spoken at numerous national, regional and state conferences in the United States and been published in medical and education journals on subjects associated with health communications.

PETER LAMPTEY, M.D., DR.P.H.

Peter Lamptey is presently the Director of the AIDSTECH Project at Family Health International (FHI), which is a project designed to provide technical assistance and funding to prevent the spread of HIV infection in developing countries.

Dr. Lamptey studied at the University of Ghana Medical School. He has a master's in public health from the University of California, Los Angeles, and studied at the Massachusetts Institute of Technology in the international nutrition policy program. Dr. Lamptey received his doctorate in public health, focusing on population and nutrition, from the Harvard School of Public Health in 1980.

Dr. Lamptey has been a lecturer and Maternal and child health and family planning (MCH/FP) specialist in the Department of Community Health at the University of Ghana Medical School. He was also a Senior Program Development Associate for Africa FHI in Accra, Ghana, where his responsibilities included managing the Regional Office for Africa, identifying and recruiting African researchers in the field of reproductive health, and organizing workshops and training researchers in research methodology. He was the Associate Medical Director for Clinical Trials at FHI. In this post his responsibilities included assisting with the development of FHI research policy, goals and objectives and developing and reviewing research designs for clinical and social science research. Dr. Lamptey also served as the chairman for FHI's Task Force on AIDS and was responsible for the development of projects in AIDS research, prevention and control in developing countries; the review of proposals on AIDS from investigators and program managers; and supervision of FHI's activities on AIDS. Dr. Lamptey has attended the III, IV, V, VI International Conference on AIDS as well as the I International Conference on AIDS Education and the Pan American Tele–Conference on AIDS.

JONATHAN M. MANN, M.D., M.P.H.

Jonathan M. Mann is at present Professor of Epidemiology and International Health at the Harvard School of Public Health and Director of the International AIDS Center of the Harvard AIDS Institute. From 1986-90, he was director of the World Health Organization's Global Program on AIDS, based in Geneva, Switzerland. From 1984-86, Dr. Mann directed the Project SIDA, a collaborative AIDS research Project involving the Centers for Disease Control, the National Institute of Allergy and Infectious Diseases, the Institute of Tropical Medicine (Antwerp, Belgium) and the Ministry of Health, republic of Zaire. Prior to working in Zaire, Dr. Mann was state epidemiologist and assistant director of the health department in New Mexico.

Dr. Mann received his bachelor's degree from Harvard College, his M.D. from Washington University in St. Louis (1974)and M.P.H. from the Harvard School of Public Health (1980).

Dr Mann interests involve public health at the national and international levels. He is focusing on specific issues, involving both AIDS and broader public health concerns, including: human rights; AIDS and public health; global learning and exchange of experience and strategies; the role of community-based organizations in health; global equity in accessibility of diagnostic, therapeutic and preventive technologies; research in human behavior as a fundamental need for progress in public health; Women AIDS and health; pandemic recognition and response; and the development of new concepts of globalism in international health.

THOMAS W. NETTER

Thomas W. Netter was the Public Information Officer for the World Health Organization's Global Programme on AIDS. until 1990. Mr. Netter worked as a staff correspondent for the Associated Press in Omaha and Lincoln, Nebraska, New York City and Geneva, Switzerland and was the chief correspondent for the Associated Press in their Warsaw bureau. Mr. Netter has also worked as a free–lance correspondent, writing articles for *The New York Times*, *The International Herald Tribune*, *The Daily Telegraph of London*, and broadcasting for the National Broadcasting Company. Therefore, he has extensive publications on AIDS, general science, politics, arms control and financial matters in these periodicals, as well as in the *Chicago Tribune*. In addition, he has edited of magazine articles for a variety of publications in the U.S. and Europe. He was also the editor and responsible officer for the publication of AIDS *Prevention and Control: Invited Presentations and Papers from the World Summit of Ministers of Health on Programmes for AIDS Prevention*, published by WHO/Pergamon Press in 1988.

Dr. Netter delivered presentations at the Joint Media Workshop of the WHO, the International Development Research Council of Canada for Developing Country Journalists and at the First Regional Workshop on AIDS and Broadcast Journalists held in Japan. He also attended the World Summit of Ministers of Health on Programmes for AIDS Prevention, the Global Impact of AIDS Conference, the International Conferences on AIDS in Stockholm and Montreal, the I International Symposium on Information and Education on AIDS, the I International Conference on AIDS in Asia and the II Regional Conference on AIDS in Europe. Dr. Netter is currently working at Harvard University.

JUNE E. OSBORN, M.D.

Dr. June Osborn is the Dean of the School of Public Health at the University of Michigan. She is also a professor of epidemiology at the School of Public Health and a professor of pediatrics and communicable diseases at the Medical School of the University of Michigan. She has recently been appointed the post of Chairperson for the U.S. National Commission on AIDS.

Dr. Osborn received her bachelor's degree from Oberlin College and her M.D. from the Case Western Reserve University. She did pediatric residency at the Harvard hospitals and postdoctoral training in virology and infectious disease at Johns Hopkins and the University of Pittsburgh.

Dr. Osborn has worked as a professor of medical microbiology and pediatrics at the University of Wisconsin Medical School and held the post of Associate Dean of the Graduate School for Biological Science for the University of Wisconsin. She has numerous publications about the AIDS epidemic.

RICHARD G. PARKER, PH.D.

Richard G. Parker received his doctorate in social and cultural anthropology from the University of California, Berkeley. Although he is originally from the United States, he currently lives in Rio de Janeiro, where he is a professor of anthropology at the Institute of Social Medicine at the State University of Rio de Janeiro. He has published extensively on gender and sexuality in Brazil, and is currently completing a book on Brazilian sexual culture. He has been involved in research on the social dimensions of AIDS in Brazil since 1985, and his recent publications include "Acquired Immunodeficiency Syndrome in Urban Brazil," *Medical Anthropology Quarterly*, "Sexual Culture and AIDS Education," *AIDS 1988: AAAS Symposia Papers*, and "Responding to AIDS in Brazil,"in *Action on AIDS: National Policies in Comparative Perspective*, in press.

MARYAN PYE, M.B.B.S., M.F.C.M.

Maryan Pye is the Special Advisor to the AIDS Programme for the Health Authority in the U.K.. She graduated in medicine from the University of London, Charing Cross Hospital Medical School. Dr. Pye has also worked as a specialist in community medicine for the Cambridge Health Authority, where he was responsible for health promotion and health education. Maryan Pye has done work in the area of women's health as well, including contraception and cervical screening.

Maryan Pye is a member of the Faculty of Community Medicine. He is an editor of *AIDS UK* and of a forthcoming monograph on local AIDS programs in the United Kingdom. Dr. Pye has co–authored, with Mukesh Kapila, papers on AIDS presented at conferences in London and Montreal. His major research interest is operational research in AIDS programs.

MICHAEL L.E. RAMAH

Michael Ramah, joined Porter/Novelli, Washington, D.C. in 1987, bringing 10 years of marketing experience in over 45 countries to the International Division. Applying a range of marketing, advertising, promotion and research tools from the private sector to social marketing in the developing world, Mr. Ramah has contributed to child survival, family planning, AIDS/HIV, and substance abuse prevention. He is the former Latin America/Caribbean regional director for the USAID funded AIDSCOM Project.
Mr. Ramah, who began his work in AIDS/HIV prevention in New York in the early 1980's, has presented papers at the International Conferences in Montreeal and San Francisco, as well as at numerous regional conferences throughout Latin America, the Caribbean, Africa and Asia.

A graduate of Williams College, Mr. Ramah has completed coursework at the University of Madrid as well as Georgetown University.

MARK L. ROSENBERG, M.D., M.P.P.

Mark Rosenberg is currently the Director of the Division of Injury, Control at the Center for Environmental Health and Injury Control which is part of the U.S. Centers for Disease Control (CDC) of Atlanta, Georgia. Dr. Rosenberg previously worked as the Special Assistant for Behavioral Science in the Office of the Deputy Director, HIV, at the CDC.

Dr. Rosenberg received his B.A. from Harvard University, his M.D. from the Harvard Medical School and a master's in public policy from Harvard's Kennedy School of Government. He trained in internal medicine and infectious diseases at Massachusetts General Hospital and completed a residency in psychiatry at the Beth Israel Hospital in Boston. He has also served in the Epidemic Intelligence Service and completed a residency in preventive medicine at the CDC.

Mark Rosenberg is a clinical assistant professor in the Emory University School of Public Health and an associate clinical professor in the Department of Psychiatry at Emory University School of Medicine. He is a clinical associate professor in community medicine at Morehouse Medical School and a lecturer in the Department of Health Policy and Management at the Harvard School of Public Health. Dr. Rosenberg has directed a number of projects at the CDC focusing on the role of the behavioral sciences, communication and evaluation in HIV research and interventions. He is also the author of the book, *Patients: The Experience of Illness*, a series of photographic essays and interviews portraying the effects of serious illness on patients, families and caregivers.

GIL SCHWARTZ

Gil Schwartz is the Vice President of Communications at Group W Television of Westinghouse Broadcasting Company, Inc. Mr. Schwartz has a bachelor's degree in English from Brandeis University. In his role as vice president of communications for Group W Television, Mr. Schwartz managed the national media communications surrounding the company's "AIDS LIFELINE" campaign. In that effort, he maintained contact with all participating "AIDS LIFELINE" stations, monitoring their programs and progress in what was a unique information and education campaign in media history. In addition to his role at Westinghouse Broadcasting, Mr. Schwartz is a playwright and journalist whose articles have appeared in a wide variety of trade and consumer publications.

JAIME SEPULVEDA, M.D., M.P.H., DR.SC.

Jaime Sepulveda is presently Vice-Minister of Health in the Mexican Secretariat of Health and was previously General Director of Epidemiology. He was appointed coordinator of Mexico's National Committee for the Prevention and Control of AIDS (CONASIDA) in 1988, a position he continues to hold. From 1983 to 1985, he served as Deputy Director of the National Institutes of Health.

Born in Mexico City, Jaime Sepulveda received his medical degree from the National Autonomous University of Mexico (UNAM) School of Medicine. He continued his education at the Harvard School of Public Health (HSPH), where he received his master's in public health specializing in tropical medicine, and his doctorate in population sciences. He has had teaching appointments at UNAM and HSPH in subjects primarily dealing with epidemiology of infectious diseases. Dr. Sepulveda has participated and directed various research projects in Mexico, primarily related to AIDS and HIV transmission. He is the president of the Mexican Association of Epidemiologists, the chairman of the AIDS and Reproductive Health Network (ARHN) at Harvard, and is currently a member of the National

Academy of Medicine, Mexico's highest award for a physician. He has been the organizer for the I through the VII International Course on Applied Epidemiology given by Harvard and UNAM in Mexico from 1983 to 1989. He was also a fellow of the Takemi program at Harvard from 1984–1985.

Dr. Sepulveda has recently published three books: *AIDS in Mexico*; *AIDS, Science and Society*; and *Malnutrition and Infectious Diseases*. He has also contributed chapters to several other books and published articles in various international medical journals. Dr. Sepulveda is also the editor of several epidemiological bulletins.

Mervyn F. Silverman, M.D., M.P.H.

Mervyn Silverman is the president and the national spokesperson for the American Foundation for AIDS Research (AmFAR). He is also the director of the AIDS Health Services Program at the Robert Wood Johnson Foundation.

Dr. Silverman graduated with a B.S. from Washington and Lee University and received his M.D. from Tulane University. He received his M.P.H. from Harvard University. Mervyn Silverman worked as a Peace Corps physician in Thailand, and then held the position of Regional Medical Director for Southeast Asia and the Pacific. He also worked for the Food and Drug Administration in Washington, D.C. as the Special Assistant to the Commissioner and later as the Director of the Office of Consumer Affairs. Dr. Silverman has worked as the Medical Director for Planned Parenthood of Kansas and the Director of Health of the Wichita–Sedgewick County Department of Community Health, also in Kansas. From 1977 to 1985 Dr. Mervyn Silverman directed the Department of Health for the City of San Francisco.

Among Dr. Silverman's publications are journal articles on AIDS, especially AIDS care, the San Francisco experience of AIDS care and public policy concerning AIDS. He has also contributed chapters on various topics such as AIDS care, public policy and the community response, to a variety of books, including *Charting the Future of Health Care*; *AIDS: Public Policy Dimensions*; *What To Do About AIDS*; *AIDS and Patient Management: Legal, Ethical and Social Issues* and *AIDS: Facts and Issues*.

William A. Smith, Ed.D.

William Smith currently serves as Executive Vice President and Director of Social Development Programs at the Academy for Educational Development.

In this position, he manages and coordinates a division serving 35 countries through communication programs in health, population, nutrition and agriculture. During his twenty years of work in development, he has specialized in the application of communication to behavior change. As senior technical advisor to the Academy's AIDSCOM Project (Public Health Communication for AIDS Prevention), he supervises the integration of social marketing and behavioral analysis as tools for promoting the prevention of AIDS.

Dr. Smith helped organize both the International Symposium on Education and Information on AIDS and the World Summit on AIDS. He served as advisor on communication and health promotion to the WHO's Global Programme on AIDS. Dr. Smith was also chairperson of the National Council on International Health Conference in Washington, D.C. in 1987.

In addition to his work in AIDS prevention, Dr. Smith has a background in non–formal education, communication, marketing and child survival. Dr. Smith earned his Ed.D. degree in Non–formal Adult Education and Curriculum Design from the University of Massachusetts, Amherst, and his B.A. degree in Education from the University of South Florida, Tampa.

Dr. Smith has authored or co–authored over forty publications on health and development with topics including education for prevention, innovative approaches to the use of media and education, condom promotion and use assessment, social marketing in West Africa and the use of mass media for health education in less developed countries. Among these publications are three books which he co–authored: AIDS: *Reducing HIV Transmission through Education and Communication*; AIDS *Education: Lessons from International Health*, and *Drug Abuse Prevention: Voices from the Front Line*.

DENNIS D. TOLSMA, M.P.H.

Dennis Tolsma is Senior Advisor for Preventive Health Services at the Centers for Disease Control (CDC). He also has a faculty appointments at the School of Public Health and at the Department of Community Health of the Emory University School of Medicine. He has a B.A. from Calvin College, Michigan and a master's in public health from Columbia University.

Mr. Dennis Tolsma's entire career has been devoted to education and public health. His 25 years of service at the CDC cover such activities as infectious and chronic disease control, evaluation, policy studies, strategic planning in international health and prevention. He also directed the CDC's Center for Health Promotion and Education, which included responsibility for the Office on Smoking and Health as well as the Divisions of Nutrition, Reproductive Health, and Health Education, and the school health education component of the AIDS information and education program. His current position includes responsibility for strategies to foster workplace health promotion, prevention as an element of health services research, and linkage of worker health objetives to the growing corporate interest in Total Quality Management. He is one of the principal architects of two major prevention policy documents issued by the Public Health Service, entitled *Healthy People and Disease Prevention* and *Health Promotion: Objectives for the Nation*, as well as the *Model Standards for Community Preventive Health Services*. Mr. Tolsma holds an appointment in the Federal Senior Executive Service, and in 1988 was one of six charter members selected government–wide for the Senior Executive Service Fellows Program.

Mr. Tolsma has received several awards and honors, including the Public Health Service Superior Service Award; the Distinguished Service Award of Eta Sigma Gamma, the professional society of the health sciences; and the Recognition Award of the Asia Pacific Academic Consortium for Public Health. He has authored a number of scientific articles and many presentations, including a chapter on health behavior and health promotion in the 1992 edition of Maxcy–Rosenau–Last *Public Health and Preventive Medicine.*. From 1988 to 1991, Mr. Tolsma was President of the International Union for Health Education, a private voluntary organization that addresses health promotion and education issues globally.

JEREMY S. WARSHAW

Jeremy Warshaw is the senior vice president and management supervisor of Saatchi & Saatchi Advertising. Mr. Warshaw received his undergraduate degree from the University of London.

Jeremy Warshaw has a well–rounded, 11–year experience in the communications industry on both sides of the Atlantic. He has worked on a full range of advertising accounts including Schweppes, Black & Decker, Volvo, Evian mineral water, Paine Webber, U.K. Department of Health Blood Donor campaign, LIVE AID pro–bono campaign, and anti–AIDS advertising for New York City.

SHARON WEIR

Ms. Sharon Weir is a research associate with the AIDSTECH program at Family Health International. She is a member of the operations research team and is responsible for developing and monitoring AIDSTECH's operations research programs to answer critical questions on the most effective, culturally appropriate, and sustainable strategies to prevent the sexual transmission of HIV infection in the developing world. She has worked with AIDS control programs in developing countries to design and implement strategies for targeted education, condom distribution, and STD control programs.

Sharon Weir is currently enrolled as a doctoral student in epidemiology at the University of North Carolina. She holds a master's degree in policy sciences and public affairs from Duke University and a master of public health in maternal and child health from the University of North Carolina. Prior to joining the AIDSTECH team in March, 1988 she was a senior research analyst in the Program Evaluation Department of Family Health International where she evaluated components of family planning programs in Zimbabwe, Nigeria and Sri Lanka.

Her most recent presentations include two oral presentations on lessons learned in evaluating educational interventions at the Assessing AIDS Prevention Conference in Montreux, Switzerland, 1990; an oral presentation on a method for program evaluation at the International Conference on AIDS in Africa, Kinshasa, Zaire, 1990; and a poster presentation on an AIDS in San Francisco, California, 1990.

JAY A. WINSTEN, PH.D.

Dr. Jay A. Winsten presently occupies the post of Associate Dean for Public and Community Affairs at the Harvard School of Public Health. He is also Director of the Harvard Alcohol Project and Director of the Center for Health Communication, also at Harvard. Dr. Winsten has a Ph. D. in biology from Johns Hopkins University. Among other publications, he has been featured in *The New York Times* writing on AIDS, and is the author of "Science and the Media: The Boundaries of Truth," which was published in *Health Affairs*. In addition, he co–wrote, with William DeJong, "Recommendations for Future Mass Media Campaigns to Prevent Preteen and Adolescent Substance Abuse," also published in *Health Affairs*. He has also published on the origins of human cancer.

Printed in Mexico
EDICIONES COPILCO, S. A. de C. V.